MEASUREMENT BY THE PHYSICAL EDUCATOR: WHY AND HOW

David K. Miller, Ph.D.

University of North Carolina at Wilmington

Benchmark Press, Inc.
Indianapolis, Indiana

Library of Congress Cataloging in Publication Data:

Miller, David K. 1942-

Measurement by the Physical Educator: Why and How

Cover Design: Gary Schmitt and Kathryn Miller
Copy Editor: Lynn Hendershot

Library of Congress Catalog Card number: 86-71384

ISBN: 0-936157-05-4

Printed in the United States of America
10 9 8 7 6 5 4 3 2 1

DEDICATED TO

My wife Roselyn and our daughter Kathryn
for their love, encouragement, and patience

IN APPRECIATION OF

Dr. Harold M. Barrow
for his professional guidance and inspiration

PREFACE

Students in measurement and evaluation classes are often bombarded with an abundance of information. Regrettably, some students complete these classes with a little knowledge in many areas, but no confidence and skills to perform the responsibilities expected of a physical educator. As a physical educator, these students often do not measure knowledge, physical performance and affective behavior in the proper way. If in a teaching position, these individuals construct poor knowledge tests, fail to correctly select, administer and use physical performance tests, and grade students with methods that require little effort.

Upon successful completion of a measurement and evaluation class, the physical education major should be able to:
1. use and interpret fundamental statistical techniques;
2. select appropriate knowledge and physical performance tests;
3. construct good physical performance tests;
4. construct good objective and subjective knowledge tests;
5. objectively measure and grade students who participate in a physical education class;
6. administer physical performance and sports skills tests, interpret the results and prescribe activities for development of physical performance skills and sports skills;
7. administer body structure and composition tests, interpret the results and prescribe scientifically sound methods for attainment of a healthy percent body fat;
8. administer posture and body mechanics tests, interpret the results, and prescribe activities for development of proper posture and body mechanics;
9. administer physical performance tests to special populations, interpret the results and prescribe activities for development of physical performance skills; and
10. administer affective behavior tests and interpret the results.

The purpose of *Measurement by the Physical Educator: Why and How* is to assist the physical education major in the development of these abilities.

Performance objectives are presented at the beginning of each chapter, and throughout the chapters there are inserts to remind the students of these objectives. The statistical concepts are simplified and examples related to physical education are provided. Review problems are presented at the conclusion of sections in Chapter 2; the student is encouraged to complete these problems before continuing to another section. Review problems are provided at the conclusion of other chapters. The chapters on written test construction and grading are inclusive, emphasizing the important responsibilities of the physical education teacher in these areas. Many practical and easy to administer tests for the measurement of agility, balance, cardiorespiratory fitness, flexibility, muscular strength and endurance, body composition, posture and physical fitness are described. At the conclusion of the chapters with these tests, activities for development of the components are provided. Additionally, tests for the measurement of affective behavior and special populations are presented, with emphasis on how these tests should be used.

I am indebted to the individuals who reviewed this manuscript and offered suggestions for improvements — P. Graham Hatcher, University of North Carolina at Wilmington; Robert L. Johnson, Appalachian State University; and Arthur W. Miller, University of Montana. I also would like to express my gratitude to The Graphic Spectrum of Wilmington, North Carolina for the artwork, Paul E. Hosier for the photography, and Andrea Williams and Donna Cheatham for their technical assistance. Finally, sincere thanks are extended to the staff of Benchmark Press for all the time and effort they put into the preparation of this book.

CONTENTS

1

Measurement, Evaluation and Statistics

Upon completion of this chapter, you should be able to:
1. Define measurement and evaluation;
2. List and describe the reasons for measurement and evaluation by the physical educator; and
3. State why the ability to use statistics is important for the physical educator.

"Why statistics? I don't need statistics to be a good teacher." "I don't need statistics. I plan to work in a health fitness center."

Perhaps you have made comments similar to these, or have heard some of your classmates make them. If you do not plan to perform your responsibilities as they should be performed, and you do not plan to continue your professional growth as a physical educator, you are correct in this belief. However, if you want to be the best physical educator you can possibly be, the study of statistics should be included in your professional preparation.

Statistics involves the collection, organization and analysis of numerical data. Statistical methods require the use of symbols, terminology and techniques that may be new to you, but you should not fear these methods. The idea that statistics is a form of higher mathematics is incorrect. To successfully perform the statistics presented in this book, you need only a basic knowledge of arithmetic and some simple algebra. Actually, the most complex formula in statistics can be reduced to series of logical steps involving adding, subtracting, multiplying and dividing. If you are willing to study the statistical concepts and perform the provided exercises, you will master the statistics presented to you.

Before finding an answer to "Why statistics?" you should understand the meaning of measurement and evaluation, and the reasons for measurement by the physical educator. Measurement is not a new concept to you. You measured your height and weight throughout your growing years. You have read how fast athletes have run, how high some have jumped, and how far a baseball or golf ball has been hit. All of these are examples of measurement. When you assume a position as a physical educator, you will perform measurement tasks. On many occasions this measurement will be administered in the form of a test, resulting in a score. Examples of these tests are cardiovascular fitness tests, flexibility tests and sports skills tests. On other occasions measurement may not involve a performance by a person, but will consist of the measurement of a particular attribute. Anthropometric and body fat measurements are such examples. You should recognize that in all of the above examples, a number, or numbers, is obtained. So we can say that **measurement** is usually thought of as quantitative; it is the process of assigning a number to a performance or an attribute of a person. There may be instances when you measure and the score is a term or phrase, but usually measurement will involve the use of numbers. Of course, measurement of objects is done, but as a physical educator you will be concerned primarily with people.

Once you have completed the measurement of a particular attribute of an individual, you must give meaning to it. For instance, if you administer a cardiovascular fitness test to participants of an adult fitness group, they will immediately want to know the status of their cardiovascular fitness. Without an interpretation of the quality of the test scores, the test has no meaning to the group. If you perform skinfold measurements on a 10th-grade physical education class, the students will want to know what the sum of the measurements means in relation to body fat; otherwise, the measurements will have no meaning. The same can be said for written tests. There must be an interpretation of the tests scores if they are to have meaning. This interpretation of measurement is **evaluation**: You will make a judgement about the measurement. For measurement to be effective, it must be followed by evaluation.

> Are you able to:
> define measurement and evaluation and give examples of each?

REASONS FOR MEASUREMENT AND EVALUATION BY THE PHYSICAL EDUCATOR

Now that you know what measurement and evaluation are, consider how you will use them in your profession. It is assumed that you will always follow measurement with evaluation.

Motivation: If used correctly, measurement can highly motivate most individuals. In anticipation of a test, students usually study the material or practice the physical tasks that are to be measured. This study or practice should improve performance. Skinfold measures might encourage overfat individuals in health fitness programs to lose body fat. A sports skills test administered to inform individuals of their ability in the sport might motivate them to improve their skills. This motivation is more likely to occur, however, if you as the instructor provide positive feedback. Always try to keep your evaluation in the positive frame rather than in the negative.

Finally, most everyone enjoys comparing past performances with current ones. Knowing that a second measurement will take place, students and adults often work to improve on the original score.

Diagnosis: Through measurement you can diagnose the weaknesses (needs) and strengths of a group or individuals. Measurement prior to the teaching of a sports skill, physical fitness session, or other events you teach as a physical educator, may cause you to alter your initial approach to what you are teaching. For example, you may discover, before you do anything else in a softball class, you need to teach the students how to throw properly. You also may find that some individuals need more or less attention than others in the group. Identifying those students who have the ability to throw with accuracy and good form will enable you to devote more time to the students who cannot perform the skill. If you serve as an adult fitness leader, the identification of individuals with a higher level of fitness than the rest of the group will enable you to begin their program at a different level.

In certain settings it may be possible that you are able to prescribe personal exercises or programs to correct the diagnosed weaknesses. Exercise prescription is a popular term in fitness programs, but appropriate activities may be prescribed in other programs as well. Diagnostic measurement is valuable also after a group has participated in a class for several weeks. If some students are not progressing as you feel they should, testing may enable you to determine why they are not.

Classification: There may be occasions when you would like to classify students into similar groups for ease of instruction. In addition, individuals usually feel more comfortable when performing with others of similar skill. Sometimes, even in so-called noncontact sports, homogeneous grouping should be done for safety reasons. Also, homogeneous grouping is occasionally necessary in aerobic and fitness classes so individuals with a low level of fitness will not attempt to perform at the same intensity as individuals with a high level of fitness.

Achievement: The most common reason for measurement is to determine the degree of achievement of program objectives and personal goals. Students certainly like to know how far they have progressed in a given period of time, and you need to know their achievement in order to better evaluate the effectiveness of your instruction. Individuals in wellness programs like to know the progress toward their health goals, and measurement can often best provide this information.

Achievement is often used to determine grades in physical education. If administered properly, performance tests and written tests certainly are appropriate for grading, and they serve to decrease the need of subjective grading of the students. Many physical education teachers, however, mistakenly use tests only for determining grades. The assigning of grades will be discussed at length in Chapter 6.

Evaluation of instruction and programs: With any responsibilities you assume as a physical educator, there will be occasions that you will have to justify the effectiveness of your instruction and/or program to your employer. For instance, when budget cuts are anticipated in the public schools, physical education and the arts are often the first programs considered. It is also necessary to justify a program when budget increases are requested. It will be difficult for you to provide data that supports a program without testing to determine if unit objectives have been met.

Measurement of each student's skill at the beginning of an activity unit will enable you to determine the effectiveness of previous instruction and programs and at what point you should begin your instruction. If the students are not knowledgeable of basic rules and cannot demonstrate the elementary playing skills of an activity, it will be necessary that you begin your instruction at that level. In addition, there may be occasions that you wish to compare different methods of teaching sports skills or fitness. If you can be confident that the different groups are of equal initial ability, it is possible to compare the results of test scores at the conclusion of instruction and determine if one method of teaching is better than another. This procedure will be discussed in greater detail in Chapter 2.

Prediction: Measurement to predict future performance in sport has increased in popularity, but this type of testing usually requires expertise in exercise physiology and psychology. Maximum oxygen uptake, muscle biopsies, and anxiety level are examples of tests that are used to predict future performance in sport.

Research: Research is used to find meaningful solutions to problems and as a means to expand a body of knowledge. It is of value for program evaluation, instructor evaluation, and improvement in performance, as well as other areas related to physical education. There are many opportunities for physical educators who wish to perform research.

Now that you are aware of the primary reasons for measurement in physical education, you are ready to know "Why Statistics?"

Are you able to:
list and describe the reasons for measurement and evaluation by the physical educator?

WHY STATISTICS?

Whether you are a teacher, an instructor in a fitness center, an administrator, or have responsibilities in a corporate setting, the ability to use statistics will be of value to you. While no attempt will be made in this book to provide an extensive coverage of statistics, after you have completed Chapter 2 you should have the skill to:

Analyze and interpret data: The data gathered for any of the measurement reasons described above should be statistically analyzed and interpreted. It is a mistake to gather data and make important decisions about individuals without this analysis. Decisions regarding improvement in group performance and differences in teaching methodology should not be made without statistical analysis. Also, if you are willing to statistically analyze and interpret test scores, you can better inform all participants of the test results than you can with a routine analysis of the scores. So, using statistical analysis and interpretation, you are able to provide a more meaningful evaluation of your measurement.

Interpret research: As a physical educator you should read research published in professional journals. After completion of this book you will not understand all statistical concepts, but you will have enough of an understanding to accurately interpret the results and conclusions of many studies. This ability will enable you to put into practice the conclusions of research. Too many physical educators fail to use research findings because they do not understand them. If you are to continue your professional growth, it is essential that you are able to interpret research related to physical education.

Standardize test scores: Many measurements performed by the physical educator will be in different units, for example, feet, seconds and numbers. To compare such measurements it is best to convert the scores to standardized scores. A popular form of standardized scores is percentile scores (as reported SAT scores).

Determine the worth (validity and reliability) of a test: Validity and reliability of a test may not mean much to you now, but by knowing how to interpret statements about these characteristics, you are more likely to select the appropriate test to administer to your students, clients or customers. In addition, you will be able to estimate the validity and reliability of tests that you construct.

> Are you able to:
> describe why the ability to use statistics is important to the physical educator?

You have read the reasons for measurement and evaluation and the uses of statistics by the physical educator. Now you need to develop the ability and confidence to use statistics in the performance of your responsibilities as a physical educator.

2

Statistical Tools For The Physical Educator

Upon completion of this chapter, you should be able to:
1. Define all statistical terms that are presented;
2. Describe the four scales of measurement and provide examples of each;
3. Describe a normal distribution;
4. Define the three measures of central tendency, identify the symbols used to represent them, describe their characteristics, calculate them with ungrouped and grouped data and state how they can be used to interpret data;
5. Define the four measures of variability, identify the symbols used to represent them, describe their characteristics, calculate them with ungrouped and grouped data and state how they can be used to interpret data;
6. Define percentile and percentile rank, identify the symbols used to represent them, calculate them with ungrouped and grouped data and state how they can be used to interpret data;
7. Describe a histogram and a frequency polygon;
8. Define standard scores, calculate z-scores and T-scores and interpret their meanings;
9. Define correlation, interpret the correlation coefficient and use the rank-difference and product-moment methods to determine the relationship between two variables;
10. Define the null hypothesis;
11. Use and interpret the t test for independent groups and the t test for dependent groups; and
12. Use and interpret analysis of variance for independent groups and analysis of variance for repeated measures.

Before you begin to develop the skill to use statistics, you should be able to define the following terms.

Data: The result of measurement is called data. Data usually means the numerical result of measurement, but it can also mean verbal information.

Variable: A variable is a trait or characteristic of something which can assume more than one value. Examples of variables are cardiovascular endurance, percent body fat, flexibility, and muscular strength. Their values will vary from one person to another, and they may not always be the same for one individual.

Population: A population includes all subjects (members) within a defined group. All subjects of the group have some measurable or observable characteristic. For example, if you wanted to determine the physical fitness of 12th-grade students in a particular high school, the population would be all students in the 12th grade.

Sample: A sample is a part or subgroup of the population from which the measurements are actually obtained. Rather than collect physical fitness data on all students in the 12th grade, a smaller number could be chosen to represent the population.

Random sample: A random sample is one in which every subject in the population has an equal chance of being included in the sample. A sample could be formed by randomly selecting a group to represent all 12th graders. The selection could be done by placing the names of all 12th-grade students in a container and randomly drawing the names out of it, or with a table of random numbers.

Parameter: A parameter is a value, a measurable characteristic, that refers to a population. The population mean (the average) is a parameter.

Statistic: A statistic is a value, a measurable characteristic, that refers to a sample. The sample mean is a statistic. Statistics are used to estimate the parameters of a defined population. (NOTE: When used in this manner the word "statistics" is plural. If used to denote a subject or body of knowledge, the word "statistics" is singular.

Descriptive statistics: When every member of a group is measured and no attempt is made to generalize to a larger group, the methods used to describe the group are called descriptive statistics. Conclusions are reached only about the group being studied.

Inferential statistics: When a random sample is measured and projections or generalizations are made about a larger group, inferential statistics are used. The correct use of inferential statistics permits you to use the data generated from a sample to make inferences about the entire population. Suppose you were in charge of a physical fitness program at a wellness center and wished to estimate the physical fitness of all 300 female adults in the program. You could randomly select 30 of the females, test them, and through the use of inferential statistics, estimate the physical fitness of the 300 females.

Discrete data: Discrete data are measures that can have only separate values. The values are limited to certain numbers, usually whole numbers, and cannot be reported as fractions. Examples of discrete data are the sex of the individual, the number of team members, the number of shots made, and the number of hits in a softball game.

Continuous data: Continuous data are measures that can have any value within a certain range. The values can be reported as fractions. Running and swimming events (time) and throwing events (distance) are examples of continuous data.

Ungrouped data: Ungrouped data are measures not arranged in any meaningful manner. The raw scores are used for calculations as recorded.

Grouped data: Grouped data are measures arranged in some meaningful manner to facilitate calculations.

Are you able to:
define these statistical terms?

SCALES OF MEASUREMENT

Variables may be grouped into four categories of scales depending on the amount of information given by the data. Different rules apply at each scale of measurement, and each scale dictates certain types of statistical procedures. As measurement moves from the lowest to the highest scale, the result of measurement is closer to a pure measure of a count of quantity or amount.

Nominal Scale

The nominal scale is the most elementary scale and is used to identify objects or persons. Names are given to the variables; the categories are exclusive of each other; and each category is assumed to be as valuable as the other. Some nominal scales have only two categories, but others may have more. Classification of positions on a baseball team, and individuals as college graduate/noncollege graduate are examples of the nominal scale.

Ordinal Scale

The ordinal scale provides some information about the order or rank of the variables, but it does not indicate how much better one score is than another. No determination can be made of the relative differences from rank to rank. For example, the order of finish in a 10-kilometer race provides information about who is fastest, but it does not indicate how much faster the number one finisher is than the number two finisher, or any of the other runners.

Interval Scale

An interval scale provides information about the order of the variables, using equal units of measurement. The same distance exists between each division of the scale, so it is possible to say how much better one number is than another. However, the interval scale has no true zero point. A good example of an interval scale is temperature. It is possible to say that 90° F is 10° warmer than 80° F and that 55° F is 10° warmer than 45° F, but it cannot be said that 90° is twice as hot as 45°. Since 0° F does not mean the complete absence of heat, there is no true zero point. Many measurements in physical education are in the interval scale.

Ratio Scale

A ratio scale possesses all the characteristics of the interval scale and has a true zero point. Examples of ratio scales are height, weight, time, and distance. Ten feet is twice as long as 5 feet; 9 minutes is 3 times longer than 3 minutes; and 20 pounds is 4 times heavier than 5 pounds. (Table 2-1 summarizes the major differences among these four scales of measurement.)

> Are you able to:
> define the four scales of measurement and give examples of each?

Table 2-1. *Scales of Measurement*

Scale	Characteristics	Examples
Nominal	Numbers represent categories. Numbers do not distinguish groups and do not reflect differences in magnitude.	Divisions by sex or race, eye color
Ordinal	Numbers indicate rank order of measurements, but they do not indicate the magnitude of the interval between the measures.	Order of finish in races, grades for achievement
Interval	Numbers represent equal units between measurements. It is possible to say how much better one measure is than another, but there is no true zero point.	Temperature, year, IQ
Ratio	Numbers represent equal units between measurements, and there is an absolute zero point.	Height, weight, distance, time

NORMAL DISTRIBUTION

Most of the statistical methods used in descriptive and inferential statistics are based on the assumption that a distribution of scores is normal, and that the distribution can be graphically represented by the normal curve (bell-shaped), as shown in Figure 2-1. For example, the distribution of the college entrance test scores of all test takers would be normal. However, the distribution of test takers who are primarily in advanced classes would not be normal. It would be positively skewed. This concept will be discussed later in the chapter. As with all graphic representations of frequency distributions, the score values are placed on the horizontal axis, and the frequency of

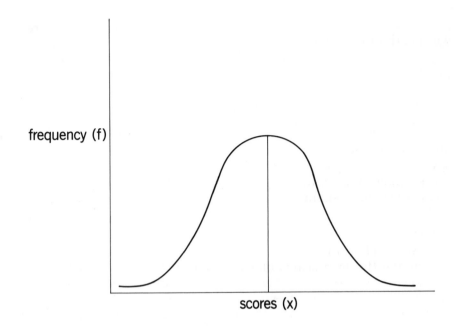

Figure 2-1. *Normal curve.*

each score is plotted with reference to the vertical axis. The two ends of the curve are symmetrical, and represent the scores at the extremes of the distribution.

The normal distribution is theoretical and is based upon the assumption that the distribution contains an infinite number of scores. Since you will not measure groups of infinite size, you should not be surprised when you have distributions that do not conform to the normal curve. If the distribution is based on a large number of scores, however, it will be close to normal distribution. You can have a large number of scores if you administer the same test to several groups, or if you combine your test scores from several years of testing into one distribution. A normal distribution has the following characteristics:

1. A bell-shaped curve.
2. Symmetrical distribution about the vertical axis of the curve; whatever happens on one side of the curve is mirrored on the other.
3. Greatest number of scores found in the middle of the curve, with fewer and fewer found toward the ends of the curve.
4. All measures of central tendency (mean, median, mode) at the vertical axis.

NOTE: Distributions that are not close to normal will have different curves. The curve may be pointed (scores are similar, group is very homogeneous); flat (scores are not similar, group is very heterogeneous); skewed (scores are clustered at one end of curve); u-shaped (scores are clustered at two ends of curve); or have two or more high points (scores have more than one mode). Skewed curves will be described later.

Are you able to:
describe a normal distribution?

ANALYSIS OF UNGROUPED DATA

Imagine that you have given a volleyball knowledge test to a group of 30 seventh-grade students, and you wish to have a better understanding of the test results as well as interpret the scores to the students. With the aid of an inexpensive calculator, you can fulfill both of these objectives. This portion of the chapter will show you how to use descriptive statistics to analyze and interpret the volleyball knowledge test scores as well as other ungrouped test scores. A test with high scores has intentionally been selected as an example to demonstrate that the procedures are not difficult. Tables 2-2, 2-3 and 2-4 report the results of the volleyball knowledge test analysis.

Score Rank

Although you will be able to perform statistical analysis without putting the scores in rank order, you may first want to carry out this procedure. This will provide you with information about each person's rank in the score distribution. Be careful how you use the rank of scores. Sometimes, all the scores will be above what you consider a satisfactory score. Since someone has to be at the bottom when scores are ranked, you may not want to share this information with the group. Do not create alarm or embarrassment when there is no need. Table 2-2 has the ranking of the 30 volleyball knowledge test scores. The steps for ranking the scores are:
1. List the scores in descending order.
2. Number the scores. The highest score is number 1 and the last score is the number of the total number of scores. (Table 2-2 has 30 scores, so the last score is number 30.)
3. Since identical scores should have the same rank, average the rank, or determine the midpoint, and assign them the same rank.

Measures of Central Tendency

Measures of central tendency are descriptive statistics that describe the middle characteristics of a distribution of scores. The most widely used statistics, they represent scores in a distribution around which other scores seem to center. Measures of central tendency are the mean, median and mode.

The Mean: With any test, the first question usually asked by the students upon knowing their individual scores is, "What is the class

Table 2-2. *Rank of Volleyball Knowledge Test Scores*

Rank		Score
1		96
2		95
3		93
4	] 4.5	92
5		92
6	] 6.5	91
7		91
8		90
9	9	90
10		90
11		89
12	12	89
13		89
14		88
15		88
16	16	88
17		88
18		88
19		87
20	20	87
21		87
22	] 22.5	86
23		86
24	] 24.5	85
25		85
26	] 26.5	84
27		84
28		83
29		82
30		81

average?" The **mean**, the most generally used measure of central tendency, is the arithmetic average of a distribution of scores. It is calculated by summing all the scores and dividing by the total number of scores. Some important characteristics of the mean are:

1. It is the most sensitive of all the measures of central tendency. It will always reflect any change within a distribution of scores.
2. It is the most appropriate measure of central tendency to use for ratio data, and may be used on interval data.
3. It considers all information about the data, and is used to perform other important statistical calculations.
4. It is influenced by extreme scores, especially if the distribution is small. For example, when one or more scores are high in relation to the other scores, the mean is pulled in that direction. This characteristic is the chief disadvantage of the mean.

The symbols used to calculate the mean and other statistics are:

$\overline{X}$ = the mean (called X-bar)

Σ (Greek letter sigma) = "the sum of"

Table 2-3. *Measures of Central Tendency and Variability and Percentiles (deciles) Computed from Ungrouped Volleyball Knowledge Test Scores (N=30)*

Score	X^2	cf	Percentile
96	9216	30	
95	9025	29	
93	8649	28	
92	8464	27	90
92	8464	26	
91	8281	25	
91	8281	24	80
90	8100	23	
90	8100	22	
90	8100	21	70
89	7921	20	
89	7921	19	
89	7921	18	60
88	7744	17	
88	7744	16	
88	7744	15	50
88	7744	14	
88	7744	13	
87	7569	12	40
87	7569	11	
87	7569	10	
86	7396	9	30
86	7396	8	
85	7225	7	
85	7225	6	20
84	7056	5	
84	7056	4	
83	6889	3	10
82	6724	2	
81	6561	1	
$\Sigma X = 2644$	$\Sigma X^2 = 233,398$		

R = 96 − 81 = 15

$$\bar{X} = \frac{\Sigma X}{N} = \frac{2644}{30} = 88.1 \qquad Q = \frac{Q_3 - Q_1}{2} = \frac{90 - 85.5}{2} = 2.25$$

$P_{50} = 88$

$$s = \sqrt{\frac{N\Sigma X^2 - (\Sigma X)^2}{N(N-1)}} = \sqrt{\frac{30(233,398) - (2644)^2}{30(30-1)}}$$

Mo = 88

$$s = 3.6$$

X = individual score
N = the total number of scores in a distribution
The formula for calculating the mean is:

$$\bar{X} = \frac{\Sigma X}{N}$$

Simply, to calculate the mean, you add all the scores in a distribution and divide by the number of scores you have. The calculation of $\overline{X}$ from the distribution in Table 2-3 is:

$$\overline{X} = \frac{2644}{30} = 88.1$$

Since you probably would report the scores to the students in whole numbers, you should round the mean to 88.

Are you able to:
identify the symbol for the mean?
define the mean?
describe the characteristics of the mean?
calculate the mean with ungrouped data and use it to interpret the data?

The Median: The **median** is the score that represents the exact middle in the distribution. It is the 50th percentile, the score which 50% of the scores are above and 50% of the scores are below. Some important characteristics of the median are:
1. It is not affected by extreme scores; it is a more representative measure of central tendency than the mean, when extreme scores are in the distribution. As an example of this fact, consider the height of five individuals. If the heights are 71", 72", 73", 74" and 75", the mean height of the five people is 73", and the median height is 73". Now imagine that we exchange the individual that is 75" in height for an individual that is 85" in height. The mean is now 75", but the median remains at 73".
2. It is a measure of position; it is determined by the number of scores and their rank order. It is appropriately used on ordinal or interval data.
3. It is not used for additional statistical calculations.

The median may be represented by Mdn or P_{50}. The steps for calculation of P_{50} are:
1. Arrange the scores in ascending order.
2. Multiple N by .50 to find 50% of the distribution.
3. Count up from the bottom score until you reach the number determined in step 2. This score is P_{50}.

The calculation of P_{50} from the distribution in Table 2-3 is:
1. .50(30) = 15
2. The 15th score from the bottom is 88. $P_{50} = 88$

Since you will be using this same procedure to calculate any percentile, you may want to place a cumulative frequency (cf) column with the ascending listing of scores. The cumulative frequency is an accumulation of frequencies beginning with the bottom score. In the cf column the highest score will have the same number as N.

The Mode: The **mode** is the score that occurs most frequently. In a normal distribution the mode is representative of the middle scores. If a distribution has two modes, it is bimodal, and it is possible for a distribution to be multi-modal, or have no mode at all. Since no symbol is used to represent the mode, Mo is sometimes used. Some characteristics of the mode are:

1. It is the least used measure of central tendency. It might be useful when estimating what sizes to order in equipment, such as helmets, caps, pants or shirts. If you did not know how many of each size to order, you could order more of the most popular size.
2. It is not used for additional statistical calculations.
3. It is not affected by extreme scores, the total number of scores or their distance from the center of the distribution.

The mode of the distribution in Table 2-3 is 88.

Which Measure of Central Tendency is Best for Interpretation of Test Results?

You have studied the definitions of the three measures of central tendency, calculation procedures and some characteristics of each. Do you know which of the three is best for interpreting test results to any group that you might be testing? In making your decision, you should consider the following:

1. The mean, median and mode are the same for a normal distribution (symmetrical curve), but you often will not have a normal curve.
2. The farther away from the mean and median the mode is, the less normal the distribution (i.e., the curve is skewed). Figure 2-2 shows the relationship of these measures to a symmetrical curve, a positively skewed curve, and a negatively skewed curve. In a positively skewed curve the scores are clustered at the lower end of the scale; the tail of the curve is to the right and the mean is higher than the median. In a negatively skewed curve the scores are clustered at the upper end of the scale; the

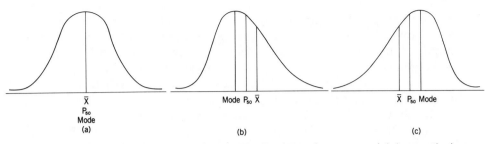

Figure 2-2. (a) Normal curve, (b) positively skewed curve, and (c) negatively skewed curve.

tail of the curve is to the left and the mean is lower than the median. An extremely difficult test where most of the scores are low but a few high scores increase the mean often results in positively skewed curve. An easy test where most of the scores are high but a few low scores decrease the mean usually results in a negatively skewed curve.

3. The mean and median are both useful measures. If the curve is badly skewed with extreme scores, you may wish to use only the median. You must decide how important the extreme scores are. If the curve is approximately normal, use the mean and median.

4. In most testing the mean is the most reliable and useful measure of central tendency. It also is used in many other statistical procedures.

Are you able to:
use the three measures of central tendency to interpret test results to a group?

Measures of Variability

You now are prepared to use the mean, median and mode to interpret data in relation to a central grouping of scores. However, to provide a more meaningful interpretation you also need to know how the scores spread, or scatter. For example, it is possible for two classes to have the same mean on a skills test, but the spread of the scores be entirely different. To illustrate this point, consider the following two sets of scores:

Group A : 80, 82, 83, 84, 86 $\overline{X} = 83$
Group B : 65, 75, 90, 90, 95 $\overline{X} = 83$

Both groups have a mean of 83, but the spreads of the scores are very different. The spread, or scatter, of scores is referred to as **variability**. When groups of scores are compared, measures of variability should be considered as well as measures of central tendency. By knowing the measures of variability you can determine the amount that the scores spread, or deviate, from the measures of central tendency. The measures of variability are: the range, quartile deviation, mean deviation and standard deviation.

STATISTICAL TOOLS 17

The Range: The **range** is determined by subtracting the lowest score from the highest score. It is the easiest measure of variability to compute, but since it represents only the extreme scores and provides no distribution information, it is also the least useful. Two groups of data may have the same range, but have very different distributions. Consider the following example of scores:

Group A: 97, 95, 89, 87, 86, 85, 83, 80, 75, 72

Group B: 81, 77, 75, 73, 70, 68, 64, 61, 58, 56

Both groups have a range of 25, but the distributions are not similar. It is possible for you to have completely different distributions when you administer the same knowledge or physical performance test to different groups.

Some characteristics of the range are:

1. It is dependent on the two extreme scores.
2. Since it indicates nothing about the variability of the scores between the two extreme scores, it is the least useful measure of variability.

The formula for determining the range is:

R = High score - Low score

You may see this formula also:

$R = H_x - L_x$

The range for the distribution in Table 2-3 is: R = 96 - 81 = 15

Are you able to:
identify the letter used to represent the range?
define the range?
describe the characteristics of the range?
calculate the range with ungrouped data and use it to interpret the data?

The Quartile Deviation: Sometimes called the semi-quartile range, the **quartile deviation** is the spread of the middle 50% of the scores around the median. The quartile deviation is not reported often, but is of value if the distribution is on the ordinal scale. The extreme scores will not affect the quartile deviation; thus, it is more stable than the range. Much like the other measures of variability, the quartile deviation is useful when comparing groups.

Some characteristics of the quartile deviation are:

1. It uses the 75th percentile and 25th percentile to determine the deviation. The difference between these two percentiles is referred to as the interquartile range.
2. It indicates the amount that needs to be added to, and subtracted from, the median to include the middle 50% of the scores.
3. It usually is not used in additional statistical calculations.
   The symbols used to calculate the quartile deviation are:
   Q = quartile deviation

Q_1 = 25th percentile or 1st quartile (P_{25} may be used also) = score in which 25% of the scores are below and 75% of the scores are above

Q_3 = 75th percentile or 3rd quartile (P_{75} may be used also) = score in which 75% of the scores are below and 25% of the scores are above

The steps for calculation of Q_3 are:

1. Arrange the scores in ascending order.
2. Multiple N by .75 to find 75% of the distribution.
3. Count up from the bottom score to the number determined in step 2. Approximation and interpolation may be required to calculate Q_3 and Q_1 as well as other percentiles. Interpolation is necessary in the calculation of Q_1 from the distribution in Table 2-3.

The steps for calculation of Q_1 are:

1. Multiple N by .25 to find 25% of the distribution.
2. Again count up from the bottom score to the number determined in step 1.

To calculate Q, substitute the values in the formula:

$$Q = \frac{Q_3 - Q_1}{2}$$

The calculation of Q from the distribution in Table 2-3 is:

1. .75(30) = 22.5

   The 22nd score from the bottom is 90, and the 23rd score is 90. Midway between these two scores would be the same score, so the score of 90 is at the 75%.

2. .25(30) = 7.5

   The seventh score from the bottom is 85, and the eighth score is 86. Since 7.5 is midway between these two scores, the score of 85.5 is at the 25%. Calculating the average of 85 and 86 would serve the same purpose.

3. $$Q = \frac{90 - 85.5}{2} = \frac{4.5}{2} = 2.25$$

Now what does 2.25 mean? Remember we said that the quartile deviation is used with the median. So now add 2.25 to 88 (the median in Table 2-3) and subtract 2.25 from 88.

88 + 2.25 = 90.25

88 – 2.25 = 85.75

Theoretically, the middle 50% of the scores in the distribution should fall between the scores of 85.75(86) and 90.25(90). With 30 scores there should be 15 scores between the scores of 86 and 91; but you will discover that 16 scores fall between these two scores. The difference is explained in the fact that the distribution in Table 2-3 does not fulfill all requirements of normalcy. However, it is similar enough to use Q for interpretation purposes. Most of the test distributions you will use in your professional responsibilities will be similar enough to normalcy.

Are you able to:
identify the symbol for the quartile deviation?
define the quartile deviation?
describe the characteristics of the quartile deviation?
calculate the quartile deviation with ungrouped data and use it to
interpret the data?

The Mean Deviation: The **mean deviation**, sometimes called
the average deviation, is another way to determine the variability of a
distribution. To calculate the mean deviation you must consider the
deviation of each score from the mean of the distribution. A deviation
is defined as the distance any score is from the mean of the distribution. This deviation score is represented by a small "d" or a small
"x."

When determining the deviation score it is necessary to use a plus
or minus sign. If the score is above the mean, a plus sign is used, and if
the score is below the mean, a negative sign is used. In any distribution
the sum of the deviation scores from the mean is equal to zero. With a
sum of zero, no average deviation can be found unless the procedure is
changed. So, in determining the mean deviation, you ignore the plus
and minus signs and simply sum all the deviations and divide by N. In
a normal distribution, the scores between the range of the mean plus
one mean deviation, and the mean minus one mean deviation, will
include the middle 57.5% of the scores.

Some characteristics of the mean deviation are:

1. It is a more meaningful measure of variability than the range
   and the quartile deviation because it considers all scores rather
   than just the two extreme scores or the 75th and 25th percentiles.
2. It indicates the value that needs to be added to, and subtracted
   from, the mean to include the middle 57.5% of the scores. It
   includes 7.5% more scores than does the quartile deviation.
3. Although it is usually not used to analyze data, it does form the
   basis of the standard deviation.
   The symbols used to calculate the mean deviation are:
   MD = mean deviation
   Σ = sum of
   d or x = deviation score $(X - \overline{X})$
   X = individual score
   $\overline{X}$ = mean
   N = number of scores
   The formula use to calculate the mean deviation is:
   $$MD = \frac{\Sigma d}{N}$$

The steps for calculation of MD are:
1. Arrange the scores into a series.
2. Determine d for each score.

3. Determine Σd.
4. Substitute values in formula.

Table 2-4 includes the deviations of the volleyball knowledge test scores found in Table 2-3. The calculation of MD from the distribution in Table 2-4 is:

1. Σd = 82.4
2. $MD = \dfrac{82.4}{30}$

   = 2.74

   MD = 2.7

To determine the middle 57.5% of the scores, you now add 2.7 to $\overline{X}$ and subtract 2.7 from $\overline{X}$.

$\overline{X} + 2.7 = 88.1 + 2.7 = 90.8$
$\overline{X} - 2.7 = 88.1 - 2.7 = 85.4$

If the distribution were normal, the middle 57.5% of the scores would be between the scores of 85 and 91. Again, though the distribution is not normal, it is similar enough to use MD for interpretation of the scores.

> Are you able to:
> identify the symbol for the mean deviation?
> define the mean deviation?
> describe the characteristics of the mean deviation?
> calculate the mean deviation with ungrouped data and use it to interpret data?

The Standard Deviation: The **standard deviation** is the most useful and sophisticated measure of variability. It describes the scatter of scores around the mean. The standard deviation is a more stable measure of variability than the range or quartile deviation because it depends on the weight of each score in the distribution.

The lower case Greek letter sigma (σ) is used to indicate the standard deviation of a population, and the letter "s" is used to indicate the standard deviation of a sample. Since you generally will be working with small groups, the formula for determining the standard deviation will include (N–1) rather than N. This adjustment produces a standard deviation that is closer to the population standard deviation.

Some characteristics of the standard deviation are:

1. It is the square root of the variance, which is the average of the squared deviations from the mean. The variance is used in other statistical procedures. The population variance is represented as σ^2 and the sample variance is represented as s^2.
2. It includes all scores and is the most reliable measure of variability.
3. It is used with the mean. In a normal distribution one standard deviation added to the mean and one standard deviation subtracted from the mean includes the middle 68.26% of the scores.

Table 2-4. *Mean Deviation and Standard Deviation Computed from Volleyball Knowledge Test Scores, Deviations, and Squared Deviations (N=30)*

Score	d	d²
96	7.9	62.41
95	6.9	47.61
93	4.9	24.01
92	3.9	15.21
92	3.9	15.21
91	2.9	8.41
91	2.9	8.41
90	1.9	3.61
90	1.9	3.61
90	1.9	3.61
89	0.9	0.81
89	0.9	0.81
89	0.9	0.81
88	−0.1	0.01
88	−0.1	0.01
88	−0.1	0.01
88	−0.1	0.01
88	−0.1	0.01
87	−1.1	1.21
87	−1.1	1.21
87	−1.1	1.21
86	−2.1	4.41
86	−2.1	4.41
85	−3.1	9.61
85	−3.1	9.61
84	−4.1	16.81
84	−4.1	16.81
83	−5.1	26.01
82	−6.1	37.21
81	−7.1	50.41
$\Sigma X=2644$	$\Sigma d=82.4$	$\Sigma d^2=373.50$

$\overline{X} = 88.1$

$$MD = \frac{\Sigma d}{N} = \frac{82.4}{30} = 2.7$$

$$s = \sqrt{\frac{\Sigma d^2}{N-1}} = \sqrt{\frac{373.5}{29}} = 3.6$$

4. With most of the data a relatively small standard deviation indicates that the group being tested has little variability; it has performed homogeneously. A relatively large standard deviation indicates the group has much variability; it has performed heterogeneously.
5. It is used to perform other statistical calculations. The standard deviation is especially important for comparing differences between means. Techniques for making these comparisons will be presented later in this chapter.

The symbols used to determine the standard deviation are:

s = standard deviation
$\overline{X}$ = mean
Σ = sum of
d = deviation score $(X-\overline{X})$
X = individual score
N = number of scores

Two methods for determining the standard deviation will be presented. The first method requires only the use of the individual scores and a calculator. The calculator should be able to compute the square root of a number, or you should be able to figure the square root by hand. An example of computing the square root by hand is provided in Appendix A. The second method requires the use of the squared deviations. Both methods obtain the same results.

Calculation with ΣX^2

1. Arrange the scores into a series.
2. Find ΣX.
3. Square each of the scores and add to determine the ΣX^2.
4. Insert the values in the formula:

$$s = \sqrt{\frac{N\Sigma X^2 - (\Sigma X)^2}{N(N-1)}}$$

The calculation of s from the distribution in Table 2-3 is:

1. Scores are in a series.
2. ΣX = 2644
3. ΣX^2 = 233,398
4.
$$s = \sqrt{\frac{30(233,398) - (2644)^2}{30(30-1)}}$$

$$= \sqrt{\frac{7,001,940 - 6,990,736}{30(29)}}$$

$$= \sqrt{\frac{11,204}{870}}$$

$$= \sqrt{12.8781}$$

$$= 3.59$$

$$s = 3.6$$

Calculation with Σd^2

1. Arrange the scores into a series.
2. Calculate $\overline{X}$.
3. Determine d and d^2 for each score; then calculate Σd^2.
4. Insert the values in the formula:

$$s = \sqrt{\frac{\Sigma d^2}{N-1}}$$

The calculation of s from the distribution in Table 2-4 is:

1. Scores are in a series.
2. $\overline{X}$ = 88.1
3. Σd^2 = 373.5
4.
$$s = \sqrt{\frac{373.5}{30-1}}$$

$$= \sqrt{\dfrac{373.5}{29}}$$

$= \sqrt{12.8793}$ NOTE: This value should be the same value as found in the ΣX^2 method, but due to the rounding off of $\overline{X}$, there is a slight difference.

$s = 3.6$

Since each score must be subtracted from the mean and, since the mean is often not a whole number, this method can be time-consuming. However, if you have already calculated the mean deviation, much of the necessary work has been completed.

Relationship of Standard Deviation and Normal Curve

The use of the standard deviation will have more meaning when it is related to the normal curve. Based on the probability of a normal distribution, there is an exact relationship between the standard deviation and the proportion of area and scores under the curve. The standard deviation marks off points along the base of the curve. An equal percentage of the curve will be found between the mean plus one standard deviation, and between the mean minus one standard deviation. The same is true for plus and minus 2.0 or 3.0 standard deviations.

The following observations can be made about the standard deviation and the areas under a normal curve:

1. 68.26% of the scores will fall between +1.0 and –1.0 standard deviations.
2. 95.44% of the scores will fall between +2.0 and –2.0 standard deviations.
3. 99.72% of the scores will fall between +3.0 and –3.0 standard deviations. Generally, scores will not exceed +3.0 and –3.0 standard deviations from the mean. Figure 2-3 shows these observations.

The relationship of the standard deviation and the normal curve provides you a meaningful and consistent way to compare the performance of different groups using the same test, and to compare the performance of one individual with the group. In addition, by knowing the value of the mean and standard deviation the percentile rank of the scores can be expressed. To illustrate how these procedures can be done, consider the following example.

As part of a physical fitness test, a teacher administered a 60-second sit-up test to her two ninth-grade classes. She found the mean and standard deviation for each class to be:

Class 1	Class 2
$\overline{X} = 32$	$\overline{X} = 28$
$s = 2$	$s = 4$

Figure 2-4 compares the spread of the two distributions. You can see that Class 1 is a more homogeneous group.

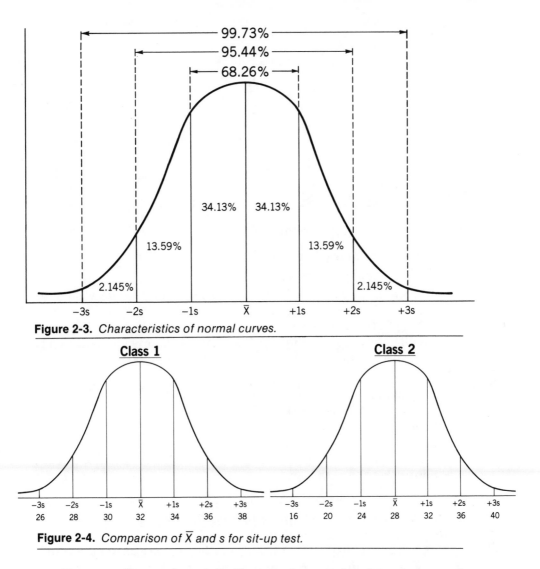

Figure 2-3. *Characteristics of normal curves.*

Figure 2-4. *Comparison of X̄ and s for sit-up test.*

Now consider student A in Class 1 who completed 34 sit-ups, and student B in Class 2 who also completed 34 sit-ups. Though both students have the same score, Figure 2-5 shows that they do not have the same relationship to their respective class mean and standard deviation. Student A is 1 standard deviation above the class 1 mean and student B is 1.5 standard deviations above the Class 2 mean. Table 2-5 shows that +1 standard deviation above the mean includes approximately 84% of the curve and that +1.5 standard deviations above the mean include approximately 93% of the curve. Though the two scores are the same, they do not have the same percentile score.

The steps for calculating the percentile rank through use of the mean and standard deviation are:

1. Calculate the deviation of the score from the mean. $d = (X - \overline{X})$
2. Calculate the number of standard deviation units the score is from the mean. Some textbooks refer to these units as z scores.

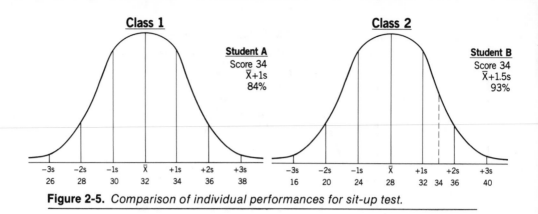

Figure 2-5. *Comparison of individual performances for sit-up test.*

The use and interpretation of z-scores are described on page 37.

No. of standard deviation units from the mean $= \dfrac{d}{s}$

3. Use Table 2-5 to determine where the percentile rank of the score is on the curve. On occasions it may be necessary to approximate the percentile rank.

NOTE: If a negative value is found in step 1, the percentile rank will always be less than 50. If a positive value is found in step 1, the percentile rank will always be more than 50.

Are you able to:
identify the symbol for the standard deviation?
define the standard deviation?
describe the characteristics of the standard deviation?
calculate the standard deviation with ungrouped data and use it to interpret the data?
describe the normal curve?

Which Measure of Variability is Best for Interpretation of Test Results?

You have studied the definitions of the four measures of variability, how to calculate them, and some characteristics of each. In deciding which of the four is best for interpreting test results of a group you might be testing, you should consider the following:

1. The range is the least reliable of the four, but it is used when a fast method is needed.
2. The quartile deviation is more meaningful than the range, but it considers only the middle 50% of the scores.
3. The mean deviation considers every score, but it is not mathematically sound (negative signs are ignored).
4. The standard deviation considers every score, is the most reliable, and is the most commonly used measure of variability.

Are you able to:
properly use the four measures of variability to interpret test results to a group?

Table 2-5. *Percentile Scores Based on the Mean and Standard Deviation Units*

$\overline{X}$ and s units	Percentile rank	T-score	$\overline{X}$ and s units	Percentile rank	T-score
$\overline{X}$ + 3.0s	99.87	80	$\overline{X}$ − 0.1s	46.02	49
$\overline{X}$ + 2.9s	99.81	79	$\overline{X}$ − 0.2s	42.07	48
$\overline{X}$ + 2.8s	99.74	78	$\overline{X}$ − 0.3s	38.21	47
$\overline{X}$ + 2.7s	99.65	77	$\overline{X}$ − 0.4s	34.46	46
$\overline{X}$ + 2.6s	99.53	76	$\overline{X}$ − 0.5s	30.85	45
$\overline{X}$ + 2.5s	99.38	75	$\overline{X}$ − 0.6s	27.43	44
$\overline{X}$ + 2.4s	99.18	74	$\overline{X}$ − 0.7s	24.20	43
$\overline{X}$ + 2.3s	98.93	73	$\overline{X}$ − 0.8s	21.19	42
$\overline{X}$ + 2.2s	98.61	72	$\overline{X}$ − 0.9s	18.41	41
$\overline{X}$ + 2.1s	98.21	71	$\overline{X}$ − 1.0s	15.87	40
$\overline{X}$ + 2.0s	97.72	70	$\overline{X}$ − 1.1s	13.57	39
$\overline{X}$ + 1.9s	97.13	69	$\overline{X}$ − 1.2s	11.51	38
$\overline{X}$ + 1.8s	96.41	68	$\overline{X}$ − 1.3s	9.68	37
$\overline{X}$ + 1.7s	95.54	67	$\overline{X}$ − 1.4s	8.08	36
$\overline{X}$ + 1.6s	94.52	66	$\overline{X}$ − 1.5s	6.68	35
$\overline{X}$ + 1.5s	93.32	65	$\overline{X}$ − 1.6s	5.48	34
$\overline{X}$ + 1.4s	91.92	64	$\overline{X}$ − 1.7s	4.46	33
$\overline{X}$ + 1.3s	90.32	63	$\overline{X}$ − 1.8s	3.59	32
$\overline{X}$ + 1.2s	88.49	62	$\overline{X}$ − 1.9s	2.87	31
$\overline{X}$ + 1.1s	86.43	61	$\overline{X}$ − 2.0s	2.28	30
$\overline{X}$ + 1.0s	84.13	60	$\overline{X}$ − 2.1s	1.79	29
$\overline{X}$ + 0.9s	81.59	59	$\overline{X}$ − 2.2s	1.39	28
$\overline{X}$ + 0.8s	78.81	58	$\overline{X}$ − 2.3s	1.07	27
$\overline{X}$ + 0.7s	75.80	57	$\overline{X}$ − 2.4s	0.82	26
$\overline{X}$ + 0.6s	72.57	56	$\overline{X}$ − 2.5s	0.62	25
$\overline{X}$ + 0.5s	69.15	55	$\overline{X}$ − 2.6s	0.47	24
$\overline{X}$ + 0.4s	65.54	54	$\overline{X}$ − 2.7s	0.35	23
$\overline{X}$ + 0.3s	61.79	53	$\overline{X}$ − 2.8s	0.26	22
$\overline{X}$ + 0.2s	57.93	52	$\overline{X}$ − 2.9s	0.19	21
$\overline{X}$ + 0.1s	53.98	51	$\overline{X}$ − 3.0s	0.13	20
$\overline{X}$ + 0.0s	50.00	50			

Percentiles and Percentile Ranks

Though you have learned to calculate percentiles and percentile rank, it will be beneficial to discuss them in greater detail. **Percentile** refers to a point in a distribution of scores below which a given percent of the scores fall. For example, the 60th percentile is the point where 60% of the scores in a distribution are below and 40% of the scores are above. To calculate a percentile, you first multiply N by the desired percentage. You then determine the score that is at that percentile in a distribution. In Table 2-3, the 60th percentile score is 89.

The **percentile rank** of a given score in a distribution is the percent of the total scores which fall below the given score. A percentile rank, then, indicates the position of a score in a distribution in percentage terms. Percentile ranks are determined by beginning with the raw scores and calculating the percentile ranks for the scores. In Table 2-3, the score of 89 has a percentile rank of 60.

Although percentiles are of value for interpretation of data, they do have weaknesses. The relative distance between percentile scores are the same, but the relative distances between the observed scores are not. Since percentiles are based on the number of scores in a distribution rather than the size of the raw score obtained, it is sometimes more difficult to increase a percentile score at the ends of the scale than in the middle. The average performers, whose raw scores are found in the middle of the scale, need only a small change in their raw scores to produce a large change in their percentile scores. However, the below average and above average performers, whose raw scores are found at the ends of the scale, need a large change in their raw scores to produce even a small change in their percentile scores. This weakness is usually found in all percentile scores.

If you do not remember how to calculate percentiles, you should refer to the sections on the median and quartile deviation. In Table 2-3 the percentile scale is divided into deciles (ten equal parts). Deciles are represented as D_1 (10th percentile), D_2 (20th percentile), D_3 (30th percentile), on up to D_9 (90th percentile).

> Are you able to:
> identify the symbol for percentiles, quartiles, and deciles?
> define percentile and percentile rank?
> calculate percentiles and use them to interpret the data?

You now should be able to statistically analyze ungrouped data. Practice using that ability by completing the review problems.

REVIEW PROBLEMS

1. Mrs. Block completed the volleyball unit with her two ninth-grade classes by administering the same volleyball skills test to both classes. One of the test items was the volleyball serve. Calculate the range, $\overline{X}$, P_{50}, mode, Q, MD, s, and deciles for the two groups of scores. Were the performances of the classes different in any way? Was one class more homogeneous?
   Class A
   42, 50, 57, 45, 56, 69, 45, 43, 46, 51, 61, 55, 40, 47, 59, 47, 46, 30, 48, 53, 40, 40, 64, 48, 41
   Class B
   51, 43, 43, 37, 33, 53, 44, 44, 38, 34, 37, 51, 20, 24, 39, 34, 38, 50, 10, 37, 39, 27, 25, 29, 23
2. Calculate the $\overline{X}$ and s for these two-minute sit-up test scores:
   42, 41, 53, 60, 84, 49, 57, 65, 61, 48, 33, 57, 55, 50, 65, 54, 55, 57, 65, 45, 58, 54, 52, 40, 55
3. Given:
   $\overline{X} = 33$
   $s = 2$
   $X_1 = 36$
   $X_2 = 29$
   $X_3 = 32$
   Use the normal curve and determine the percentile rank for the three observed scores.

ANALYSIS OF GROUPED DATA

The widespread availability of calculators and microcomputers has made the grouping of data less prevalent than it once was. However, you may have occasions when you want to analyze a large number of scores. Even with a calculator, it is difficult to work with the data unless they are arranged in a more convenient form.

A frequency distribution is one method for arranging the data in a more convenient form. Frequency distributions may be either simple or grouped. In a simple frequency distribution all scores are listed in descending order, and the number of times each individual score occurs is indicated in a frequency column. Table 2-6 shows a simple frequency distribution.

Table 2-6. *Simple Frequency Distribution of Push-Up Scores.*

X	t	f
51	1	1
50	11	2
49	111	3
48	T++1	5
47	T++1 1	6
46	T++1 1	6
45	T++1 1	6
44	T++1 11	7
43	T++1 11	7
42	T++1 111	8
41	T++1 111	8
40	T++1 T++1	10
39	T++1 1111	9
38	T++1 1	6
37	T++1 1	6
36	T++1 11	7
35	T++1	5
34	1111	4
33	1111	4
32	T++1	5
31	1111	4
30	11	2
29	11	2
28	1	1
27	1	1
		N = 125

If the scores are spread over a wide range, however, a simple frequency distribution is long and bulky. There may be gaps in the range where no scores occur or so few scores fall at each score value that the group pattern is not very clear. In such instances, it is more convenient to represent the scores in a grouped frequency distribution rather than individually.

To aid you in the understanding of the procedures for arranging data into a grouped frequency distribution, the following example will be used.

Mrs. Wren administered a tennis serve test to three 10th-grade physical education classes (N=75) and grouped the scores into a frequency distribution for analysis purposes. The scores were:

88 83 75 81 56 82 86 62 87 79 93 58 61 61 75
73 94 48 79 72 81 85 52 73 62 80 73 84 63 61
67 63 75 73 67 72 73 72 77 73 85 82 70 57 58
54 79 68 54 70 77 81 68 83 65 77 90 52 75 62
84 69 56 68 69 63 70 91 70 80 65 70 88 72 63

Table 2-7 shows the frequency distribution for scores. The steps Mrs. Wren followed to construct the frequency distribution follow:

1. Determine the range.

   NOTE: Some textbooks define the range as the highest score minus the lowest score plus one, when grouping the scores.

   R for the Table 2-7: 94 − 48 = 46

Table 2-7. *Frequency Distribution and Measures of Central Tendency and Variability for Tennis Serve Scores*

Class interval	t	f	cf	d	fd	fd²
93 – 95	11	2	75	7	14	98
90 – 92	11	2	73	6	12	72
87 – 89	111	3	71	5	15	75
84 – 86	⊺⊦⊦⊦	5	68	4	20	80
81 – 83	⊺⊦⊦⊦ 11	7	63	3	21	63
78 – 80	⊺⊦⊦⊦	5	56	2	10	20
75 – 77	⊺⊦⊦⊦ 11	7	51	1	7	7
72 – 74	⊺⊦⊦⊦ ⊺⊦⊦⊦	10	44	0	0	0
69 – 71	⊺⊦⊦⊦ 11	7	34	−1	−7	7
66 – 68	⊺⊦⊦⊦	5	27	−2	−10	20
63 – 65	⊺⊦⊦⊦ 1	6	22	−3	−18	54
60 – 62	⊺⊦⊦⊦ 1	6	16	−4	−24	96
57 – 59	111	3	10	−5	−15	75
54 – 56	1111	4	7	−6	−24	144
51 – 53	11	2	3	−7	−14	98
48 – 50	1	1	1	−8	−8	64
		N = 75			Σfd = −21	Σfd² = 973

R = 94 − 48 = 46

Mo = LL + 1/2 (i) = 71.5 + 1/2(3) = 73

$$\overline{X} = AM + i \left(\frac{\Sigma fd}{N} \right) = 73 + 3 \left(\frac{-21}{75} \right) = 72.16$$

$$P_{50} = LL + i \left(\frac{\%(N) - cf_b}{f_w} \right) = 71.5 + 3 \left(\frac{.50(75) - 34}{10} \right) = 72.55$$

$$Q = \frac{Q_3 - Q_1}{2} = \frac{80.61 - 63.87}{2} = 8.37$$

$$s = i \sqrt{ \frac{\Sigma fd^2}{N} - \left(\frac{\Sigma fd}{N} \right)^2 } = 3 \sqrt{ \frac{973}{75} - \left(\frac{-21}{75} \right)^2 } = 10.77$$

2. Determine the number of class intervals. The number of intervals depends on the number of scores, the range of the scores and the purpose of organizing the frequency table. If a frequency table has too few intervals (less than 10) the frequency of scores in each interval may be quite large, making it difficult to observe the essential characteristics of the distribution. If too many intervals are included (more than 20), several intervals may not contain any scores and too much work is required to complete the table. Generally it is best to have between 10 and 20 intervals. Fifteen intervals is usually a good number of intervals.

Once the approximate number of intervals has been decided, the size of the class interval (i) must be determined. An estimate of i can be found by dividing the range of the scores by the number of intervals wanted. If the range of a distribution happens to be 54, i could be found by:

$$\frac{54}{15} = 3.6$$

It is easier to work with whole numbers, so we have the choice of using 3 or 4 for i. When i is smaller than 10, the numbers 2, 3, 5, 7, and 9 are usually used. Even numbers other than the number 2 may be used, however. The advantage of odd numbers is that the midpoint of the intervals will be whole numbers, and it is often necessary to find the midpoint of intervals. When i is larger than 10, multiples of 5 (10, 15, 20 and so forth) are generally used.

You also may determine the number of class intervals by dividing the range by what you feel would be an appropriate i. In the above example the procedure would be:

$$\frac{54}{3} = 18 \text{ or} \frac{54}{5} = 11$$

The number of intervals may be 18 or 11, which of course means that i = 3 or 5 is acceptable.

Class intervals and i for Table 2-7:

$$\frac{46}{15} = 3.06$$

Note: With i=3, there will be 16 intervals.

3. Determine the limits of the bottom class interval. A general practice is to begin the bottom interval with a number which is a multiple of the interval size. It is acceptable, however, to begin the bottom interval with the lowest score or to make the lowest score the midpoint of the interval.

Bottom interval for Table 2-7: 48 to 50

4. Construct the table. The remaining intervals are formed by increasing each interval by the size of i until an interval is reached that includes the highest score.

NOTE: There is a difference in the "apparent limits" and "real limits" of the intervals. It can be observed in Table 2-7 that there is a one-point gap between the end of one interval and the beginning of the next interval. To avoid this gap, the real limits of the bottom interval are 47.50 to 50.4999. The real limits of the next interval are 50.50 to 53.4999, and so forth.

5. Tally the scores. The scores are counted one at a time, and a tally mark is placed to the right of the appropriate interval.
6. Record the tallies under the column headed f (which stands for frequencies). Sum the frequencies ($\Sigma f = N$).

Are you able to:
group scores into a frequency distribution?

Measures of Central Tendency

Observing Table 2-7, you notice columns other than the f column are included. These columns are used to calculate the measures of central tendency and variability. Since the definitions (with the exception of the mode), characteristics and uses for these measures are the same as when they are calculated with ungrouped data, they will not be repeated.

The Mode: The mode for grouped data is defined as the midpoint of the interval that has the largest number of frequencies. The midpoint of an interval is calculated by adding one-half of i to the real lower limit of the interval. One symbol used in the formula for this calculation is new to you.

LL = real lower limit of interval with largest number of scores

The mode in Table 2-7 is:

Mo = LL of interval + 1/2(i)
 = 71.5 + 1/2(3)
 = 71.5 + 1.5

Mo = 73

The Mean: Two symbols used in the formula for calculation of the mean of grouped data are new to you.

AM = assumed mean; midpoint of the interval you assume the mean to be

Σfd = sum of f × d

The steps for calculation of the mean are:

1. Label a column d. In the interval in which you assume (guess) the mean is located, place a 0. If the distribution is approximately normal, the mean will be close to the middle of the distribution. Do not be concerned about guessing the correct interval because the value of the mean will be the same regardless of where you assume the mean.
2. Indicate the deviation of each interval from the assumed mean by numbering consecutively above and below the interval of the assumed mean. Positive values are above the mean, and negative values are below.
3. Label a column fd. Multiple f times d for each interval.

NOTE: Be aware that you will have positive values above the interval of the assumed mean, and negative values below.

4. Calculate Σfd.

   NOTE: Be aware that you are summing positive and negative numbers. The Σfd is a correction factor. A negative value for fd indicates that you have assumed the mean to be higher than it actually is, and a positive value for fd indicates the opposite.

5. Substitute the values in the formula:

$$\overline{X} = AM + i \left(\frac{\Sigma fd}{N} \right)$$

The calculation of the mean from the distribution in Table 2-7 is:

$$\overline{X} = 73 + 3 \left(\frac{-21}{75} \right)$$
$$= 73 + 3(-.28)$$
$$= 73 - .84$$
$$\overline{X} = 72.16$$

The Median: The symbols used in the formula to calculate the median and other percentiles for grouped data are:

   LL = the real lower limit of the interval containing the percentile of interest

   % = the percentile you wish to determine

   cf_b = the cumulative frequency in the interval below the interval of interest

   f_w = frequency of scores in interval of interest

The steps for calculation of the median are:

1. Label a column cf and determine the cumulative frequency for each interval.
2. Multiple .50(N) and determine which interval P_{50} is located.
3. Identify cf_b and f_w.

   NOTE: The cf_b value will not exceed the number found in step 2.
4. Substitute the values in the formula:

$$P_{50} = LL + i \left(\frac{\%(N) - cf_b}{f_w} \right)$$

The calculation of the median from the distribution in Table 2-7 is:

$$.50(75) = 37.5$$

$$P_{50} = 71.5 + 3 \left(\frac{37.5 - 34}{10} \right)$$

$$= 71.5 + 3 \left(\frac{3.5}{10} \right)$$
$$= 71.5 + 3(.35)$$
$$= 71.5 + 1.05$$
$$P_{50} = 72.55$$

Are you able to:
calculate the measures of central tendency and percentiles with
data grouped into a frequency distribution?

Measures of Variability

Calculation of the range for grouped data was described previously. Calculation of the quartile deviation and standard deviation will be covered now.

The Quartile Deviation: The formula for the quartile deviation is the same for grouped and ungrouped data, and the technique and formula for calculating Q_3, Q_1 and other percentiles are the same as described for calculation of the median.

The calculation of Q from the distribution in Table 2-7 is:

$$Q_3$$
$$.75(75) = 56.25$$

$$Q_3 = 80.5 + 3\left(\frac{56.25 - 56}{7}\right)$$

$$= 80.5 + 3\left(\frac{.25}{7}\right)$$

$$= 80.5 + 3(.036)$$
$$= 80.5 + .11$$
$$Q_3 = 80.61$$

$$Q_1$$
$$.25(75) = 18.75$$

$$Q_1 = 62.5 + 3\left(\frac{18.75 - 16}{6}\right)$$

$$= 62.5 + 3\left(\frac{2.75}{6}\right)$$

$$= 62.5 + 3(.458)$$
$$= 62.5 + 1.37$$
$$Q_1 = 63.87$$

$$Q = \frac{Q_3 - Q_1}{2}$$

$$= \frac{80.61 - 63.87}{2}$$

$$= \frac{16.74}{2}$$

$$Q = 8.37$$

The Standard Deviation: One symbol used in the formula for calculation of the standard deviation for grouped data is new to you.

Σfd^2 = sum of d × fd

The steps for calculation of the standard deviation are:

1. Label a column fd^2 and determine fd^2 for each interval.
   NOTE: You are to multiply d × fd.
2. Calculate Σfd^2.
3. Substitute the values in the formula:

$$s = i\sqrt{\frac{\Sigma fd^2}{N} - \left(\frac{\Sigma fd}{N}\right)^2}$$

The calculation of s in the distribution in Table 2-7 is:

$$s = 3 \sqrt{\frac{973}{75} - \left(\frac{-21}{75}\right)^2}$$

$$= 3 \sqrt{12.9733 - (.28)^2}$$

$$= 3 \sqrt{12.9733 - .0784}$$

$$= 3 \sqrt{12.8949}$$

$$= 3(3.59)$$

$$s = 10.77$$

Are you able to:
calculate the quartile deviation and standard deviation with data grouped into a frequency distribution?

To test your ability to group data into a frequency distribution and to calculate the measures of central tendency and variability, complete the review problem.

REVIEW PROBLEM

1. Mr. Bird administered a badminton clear test to 60 students. Group the scores into a frequency distribution and determine the range, mode, median, mean, quartile deviation and standard deviation. The scores are:

74	75	64	86	73	74	75	70	69	67
80	78	61	81	77	78	65	65	70	69
85	84	83	62	84	74	75	81	66	74
63	73	77	64	66	72	80	77	80	70
66	69	72	83	69	67	73	72	75	75
70	67	65	73	73	72	72	73	74	73

GRAPHS

Data are often presented in a graphic form. Well-prepared graphs enable individuals to interpret data without reading the raw data or tables. Several types of graphs may be used, but only the histogram and the frequency polygon will be described here. The following guidelines should be used when constructing these graphs:

1. The length of the vertical axis (Y), called the ordinate, is about two-thirds to three-fourths the length of the horizontal axis (X), called the abscissa.
2. The vertical axis begins with zero.
3. The score values are recorded from low to high, left to right.

4. A space of one-half to one column is left between the vertical axis and the first column, and between the last column and the end of the horizontal axis.
5. The graph is given a title.

Histogram

A **histogram** is a bar graph in which the score frequencies are represented by a series of columns. The width of each column corresponds to the interval size, and the height of each column corresponds to the frequencies in each interval. The midpoint of each interval is in the middle of the column. Figure 2-6 is a histogram of the data in Table 2-7.

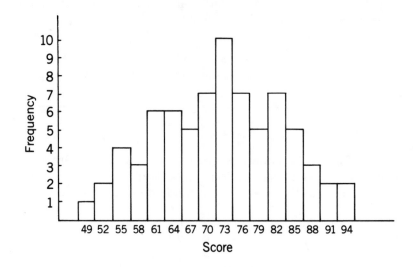

Figure 2-6. *Histogram of tennis serve scores made by 75 10th-grade students.*

Frequency Polygon

A **frequency polygon** is a line graph in which the midpoints of the intervals are plotted at a point corresponding to the frequency of the interval, and connected with straight lines. At each end of the polygon, a line is drawn back to zero. Figure 2-7 is a frequency polygon of the data in Table 2-7.

> Are you able to:
> define histogram and frequency polygon and state when they may be used appropriately?

STANDARD SCORES

After collecting scores for different performances, you may wish to combine or compare scores; but, because the scores have no similari-

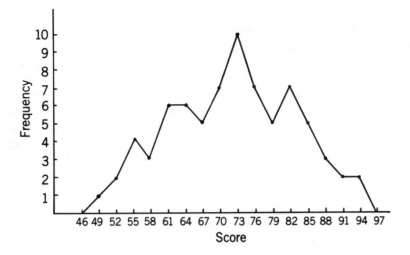

Figure 2-7. *Frequency polygon of tennis serve scores made by 75 10th-grade students.*

ties, you are unable to perform these functions. For example, suppose you are teaching a physical fitness unit to a high school class, and at the conclusion of the unit you administer a two-minute sit-up test, the sit-and-reach test, a two-mile run and a physical fitness knowledge test. How do you average the scores of the four tests? You certainly cannot add the scores and divide by four. How do you compare a student's performance on the sit-up test with her performance on the two-mile run? You cannot tell her that 55 sit-ups is a better score than a time of 15:10 — unless you have a procedure to convert the raw scores into standard scores. Procedures to make such conversions follow.

z-Scores

A **z-score** represents the number of standard deviations a raw score deviates from the mean. After calculation of the mean and standard deviation of a distribution, it is possible to determine the z-score for any raw score in the distribution through the use of this formula:

$$z = \frac{X - \overline{X}}{s}$$

Consider the example of Mrs. Wren previously described on page 30. If Mrs. Wren wanted to convert the tennis serve test scores into z-scores she would substitute each individual score in the formula. For the scores of 88 and 54 the z-scores would be:

$$z = \frac{88 - 72.2}{10.8} \qquad z = \frac{54 - 72.2}{10.8} \quad (\overline{X} \text{ and } s \text{ are rounded to}$$
$$= \frac{15.8}{10.8} \qquad = \frac{-18.2}{10.8} \qquad \text{one decimal place})$$
$$z = 1.46 \qquad z = -1.69$$

How are these z-scores interpreted? The z-scale has a mean of 0, a standard deviation of 1, and normally extends from –3 to +3 (plus and minus 3 standard deviations from the mean include 99.74% of the scores). In observing Figure 2-8, you see that a z-score of 1.46 is approximately 1.5 standard deviations above the mean, and a z-score of –1.69 is over 1.5 standard deviations below the mean. Knowing the relationship of the standard deviation and the normal curve, we can state that 1.46 is an excellent z-score and –1.69 is a poor z-score. Also, by referring to Table 2-5, we see that 1.5 standard deviations above the mean has a percentile rank of 93 and 1.7 deviations below the mean has a percentile rank of 4.

If Mrs. Wren had administered other tennis skills tests (e.g., forehand, backhand and lob tests), with similar distributions, she could convert the scores to z-scores and average them for one tennis skill score. She also could compare each student's z-scores for the four tests, and determine the strongest and weakest skills of each student.

All standard scores are based on the z-score. Since z-scores are expressed in small numbers, involve decimals and may be positive or negative, many testers do not use them.

T-Scores

The **T-scale** has a mean of 50 and a standard deviation of 10. T-scores may extend from 0 to 100, but it is unlikely that any T-score would be beyond 20 or 80, since this range includes plus and minus 3 standard deviations. Figure 2-8 shows the relationship of z-scores, T-scores and the normal curve. As the z-score is part of the formula for conversion of raw scores into T-scores, the formula is:

$$\text{T-score} = 50 + 10 \left(\frac{(X - \overline{X})}{s} \right) = 50 + 10\,z$$

Again, consider the scores of 88 and 54 for Mrs. Wren's tennis serve test. The T-scores are:

$$T_{88} = 50 + 10\,(1.46) \qquad T_{54} = 50 + 10\,(-1.69)$$
$$= 50 + 14.6 \qquad\qquad = 50 + (-16.9)$$
$$= 64.6 = 65 \qquad\qquad = 33.1 = 33$$

NOTE: T-scores are reported as whole numbers.

T-scores may be used in the same way as z-scores. However, because only positive, whole numbers are reported and the range is 0 to 100, the T-scale is easier to interpret. However, it is sometimes confusing to the individuals being tested when they are told that a T-score of 60 or above is a good score. If you use T-scores, you should be prepared to fully explain their meanings. Table 2-5 shows the relationship of the mean and standard deviation, percentile rank and T-scores.

You may prefer to convert the raw scores in a distribution to T-scores through the following procedure:
1. Number a column of T-scores from 20 to 80.
2. Place the mean of the distribution of the scores opposite the T-score of 50.

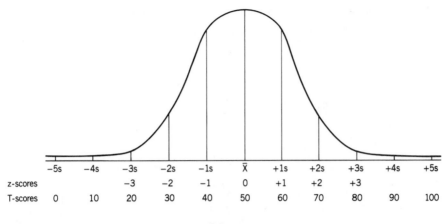

z-scores	−5s	−4s	−3s	−2s	−1s	X̄	+1s	+2s	+3s	+4s	+5s
z-scores			−3	−2	−1	0	+1	+2	+3		
T-scores	0	10	20	30	40	50	60	70	80	90	100

Figure 2-8. *z-scores and T-scores plotted on a normal curve.*

3. Divide the standard deviation of the distribution by 10. The standard deviation for the T-scale is 10, so each T-score from 0 to 100 is one-tenth of the standard deviation.
4. Add the value found in step 3 to the mean and each subsequent number until you reach the T-score of 80.
5. Subtract the value found in step 3 from the mean and each decreasing number until you reach the number 20.
6. Round off the scores to the nearest whole number.
   NOTE: For some measurements, lower scores are better (e.g., timed events and heart rate). When you are working with such scores, you should subtract the T-values toward 80 and add the values toward 20. Table 2.8 shows the conversion of Mrs. Wren's tennis serve scores to T-scores. For illustration purposes, only the T-scores 40 to 60 are included in the table. Since the value found in dividing the standard deviation by 10 is 1.08, it is rounded to 1.1.

Percentiles

Percentile scores are also standard scores, and may be used to compare scores of different measurements. Since they change at different rates (remember the comparison of low and high percentile scores with middle percentiles), they should not be averaged to determine one score for several different tests. For this reason, you may prefer to use the T-scale when converting raw scores to standard scores. Since the calculation of percentiles was previously described, it will not be described here.

Are you able to:
describe the purposes of standard scores?
convert raw scores into z-scores and T-scores and interpret them?

Table 2-8. *Conversion of Tennis Serve Scores to T-Scores*

T-score	Observed score
60	83.2
59	82.1
58	81.0
57	79.9
56	78.8
55	77.7
54	76.6
53	75.5
52	74.4
51	73.3
50	72.2
49	71.1
48	70.0
47	68.9
46	67.8
45	66.7
44	65.6
43	64.5
42	63.4
41	62.3
40	61.2

$\overline{X} = 72.2$

$s = 10.77$

$\dfrac{s}{10}\left(\begin{matrix}\text{value added to and}\\ \text{subtracted from } \overline{X}\end{matrix}\right) = \dfrac{10.77}{10} = 1.077 = 1.1$

REVIEW PROBLEM
1. To test your ability to convert raw scores to standard scores, convert the scores in the review problem on page 39 to T-scores.

CORRELATION

Correlation is a statistical technique used to express the relationship between two sets of scores (two variables). For example, is there a relationship between athletic participation and academic achievement? Do individuals with a high level of physical fitness earn higher academic grades? Is there a relationship between arm strength and golf driving distance? Is there a relationship between body fat percent and the ability to run two miles? Also, correlation techniques are used to determine validity, reliability and objectivity of tests. These techniques will be described in Chapter 3.

The number which represents the correlation is called the **correlation coefficient**. Two techniques for determining the correlation coefficient will be presented here. Regardless of the technique used, correlation coefficients have several common characteristics. (Statements 2 and 3 are general statements; size and significance of coefficient must be considered.)

1. The values of the coefficient will always range from +1.00 to

-1.00. It is rare that the coefficients of +1.00, –1.00 and 0.00 are found, however.

2. A positive coefficient indicates direct relationship; for example, an individual who scores high on one variable is likely to score high on the second variable, and an individual who scores low on one variable is likely to score low on the second variable.

3. A negative coefficient indicates inverse relationship. The individual who scores low on one variable is likely to score high on the second variable, and the individual who scores high on the first variable is likely to score low on the second.

4. A correlation coefficient near .00 indicates no relationship. An individual who scores high or low on one variable may have any score on the second variable.

5. The number indicates the degree of relationship and the sign indicates the type of relationship. The number +.88 indicates the same degree of relationship as the number –.88. The signs indicate that the directions of the relationship are different.

6. A correlation coefficient indicates relationship. After determining a correlation coefficient, you cannot infer that one variable causes something to happen to the other variable. If a high, positive correlation coefficient were found between participation in school sports and high academic grades, it could not be said participation in school sports causes a person to earn good grades. It could only be said that there is a high, positive relationship.

Scattergram

A **scattergram** is a graph used to illustrate the relationship between two variables. To prepare a scattergram:

1. Determine the range for each variable.
2. Designate one variable as the X score and the other variable as the Y score.
3. Draw and label the axes. Represent the X scores on the horizontal axis and the Y scores on the vertical axis. Begin with the lower X scores at the left portion of the X axis and the lower Y scores at the lower portion of the Y axis.
4. Plot each pair of scores on the graph by placing a point at the intersection of the two scores.

Figure 2-9 is a scattergram of the relationship between isometric and isotonic strength scores.

The scattergram can indicate a positive relationship, a negative relationship or a zero relationship. If a positive relationship exists, the points will tend to cluster along a diagonal line that runs from the lower left-hand corner of the scattergram to the upper right-hand corner. In a negative relationship, the points tend to do the opposite; they move from the upper left-hand corner to the lower right-hand corner. With a positive or negative line, the closer the points cluster

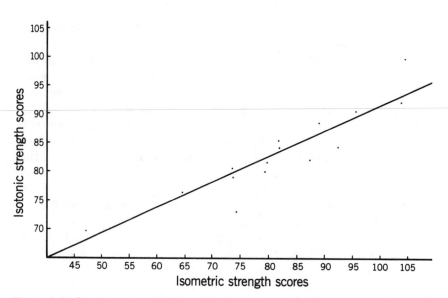

Figure 2-9. *Scattergram of relationship between isometric and isotonic strength scores.*

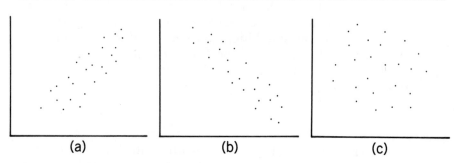

(a) (b) (c)

Figure 2-10. *Scattergrams showing (a) positive, (b) negative, and (c) zero correlation between two variables.*

along the diagonal line, the higher the correlation. In a zero relationship the points are scattered throughout the scattergram. Figure 2-10 illustrates the three types of relationships.

Spearman Rank-Difference Correlation Coefficient

The **Spearman rank-difference correlation coefficient**, also called rank-order, is used when one or both variables are ranks or ordinal scales and the number of subjects is small (30 or fewer subjects). The difference (D) between the ranks of the two sets of scores is used to determine the correlation coefficient. The following examples are relationships that could be determined through utilization of the rank-difference correlation coefficient:

- the ranking of participants in a badminton class and their order of finish in tournament play;
- the ability to serve well and the order of finish in a tennis tournament; and
- vertical jump scores and speed in the 100 meter run.

Of course, there are many other relationships that could be determined with the rank-difference correlation coefficient.

The symbol for the rank-difference coefficient is the Greek rho (ρ) or r_{rho}. To determine ρ, perform the following steps:

1. List each set of scores in a column.
2. Rank the two sets of scores.
   NOTE: This procedure was described for you earlier in the chapter.
3. Place the appropriate rank beside each score.
4. Head a column D and determine the difference in rank for each pair of scores.
   NOTE: The sum of the D column should always be 0. If it is not, check your work.
5. Square each number in the D column and sum the values (ΣD^2).
6. Calculate the correlation coefficient by substituting the values in the formula:

$$\rho = 1.00 - \frac{6(\Sigma D^2)}{N(N^2 - 1)}$$

Table 2-9 illustrates the calculation of the rank-difference correlation coefficient for sit-up and push-up scores.

Table 2-9. *Rank-Difference Correlation Coefficient for Sit-up and Push-up Scores*

Student	Sit-up Score	Rank of S-U Score	Push-up Score	Rank of P-U Score	D	D²
A	28	19.5	19	18.0	1.5	2.25
B	31	16.5	22	15.5	1.0	1.00
C	32	13.5	25	11.0	2.5	6.25
D	35	7.0	23	13.5	- 6.5	42.25
E	32	13.5	27	8.5	5.0	25.00
F	40	1.0	35	1.0	0.0	0.00
G	33	10.0	29	4.5	5.5	30.25
H	35	7.0	28	6.5	0.5	0.25
I	32	13.5	26	10.0	3.5	12.25
J	36	4.5	29	4.5	0.0	0.00
K	35	7.0	31	3.0	4.0	16.00
L	31	16.5	33	2.0	14.5	210.25
M	36	4.5	24	12.0	- 7.5	56.25
N	30	18.0	21	17.0	1.0	1.00
O	37	2.5	18	19.0	-16.5	272.25
P	37	2.5	27	8.5	- 6.0	36.00
Q	33	10.0	22	15.5	- 5.5	30.25
R	28	19.5	17	20.0	- 0.5	0.25
S	32	13.5	28	6.5	7.0	49.00
T	33	10.0	23	13.5	- 3.5	12.25

$$\Sigma D^2 = 803.00$$

N = 20

$$\rho = 1.00 - \frac{6(\Sigma D^2)}{N(N^2 - 1)}$$

$$= 1.00 - \frac{6(803)}{20(400 - 1)}$$

$$= 1.00 - \frac{4818}{7980}$$

$$= 1.00 - .60$$

$$\rho = .40$$

Pearson Product-Moment Correlation Coefficient

The **Pearson product-moment correlation coefficient**, also called Pearson r, is used when measurement results are reported in interval or ratio scale scores. (This popular correlation coefficient has many variations, but only one method will be described.) The symbol for the product-moment correlation coefficient is r.

Observed scores are used with this calculation method of the product-moment correlation coefficient. The steps for calculation are:

1. Label columns for name, X, X^2, Y, Y^2 and XY.
2. Designate one set of scores as X, the other set as Y, and place the appropriate paired scores by the individual's name.
3. Find the sums of the X and Y columns (ΣX and ΣY).
4. Square each X score, place in the X^2 column and find the sum of the column (ΣX^2).
5. Square each Y score, place in the Y^2 column and find the sum of the column (ΣY^2).
6. Multiply each X score by the Y score, place the product in the XY column and find the sum of the column (ΣXY).
7. Substitute the values in the formula.

$$r = \frac{N(\Sigma XY) - (\Sigma X)(\Sigma Y)}{\sqrt{N(\Sigma X^2) - (\Sigma X)^2} \quad \sqrt{N(\Sigma Y^2) - (\Sigma Y)^2}}$$

Table 2-10 illustrates the calculation of the Pearson product-moment correlation coefficient for isometric and isotonic strength scores.

INTERPRETATION OF THE CORRELATION COEFFICIENT

After calculating the correlation coefficient, you must interpret it. This interpretation should be done with caution. For example, a correlation coefficient of .70 may be considered quite high in one analysis, but low in another. The purpose for which the correlation coefficient is computed must be considered when making a decision about how high or low a coefficient is. Keeping the purpose of the correlation study in mind, the following ranges can be used as general guidelines for interpretation of the correlation coefficient:

r = below .20 (extremely low relationship)
r = .20 to .39 (low relationship)
r = .40 to .59 (moderate relationship)
r = .60 to .79 (high relationship)
r = .80 to 1.00 (very high relationship)

Describing a correlation coefficient as high or low is an attempt to label the magnitude of the relationship. To better determine the relationship of two variables, the **coefficient of determination** should be utilized. The coefficient of determination is the square of the correlation coefficient (r^2). It represents the common variance between two variables, or the proportion of variance in one variable that can be accounted for by the other variable. For example, suppose the correlation coefficient between standing broad jump scores and leg strength is .85. We calculate that $r^2 = .72$, which means that 72% of the variability in the standing broad jump scores is due to the individuals having different leg strength. Utilizing the coefficient of determination shows that a high correlation coefficient is needed to indicate a

Table 2-10. *Product-Moment Correlation Coefficient for Isometric and Isotonic Strength Scores*

Name	Isometric Score X	X^2	Isometric Score Y	Y^2	XY
A	63	3969	76	5776	4778
B	78	6084	80	6400	6240
C	46	2116	70	4900	3220
D	103	10609	102	10404	10506
E	74	5476	73	5329	5402
F	82	6724	87	7569	7134
G	95	9025	92	8464	8740
H	103	10609	93	8649	9579
I	87	7569	83	6889	7221
J	73	5329	79	6241	5767
K	78	6084	82	6724	6396
L	89	7921	90	8100	8010
M	82	6724	85	7225	6970
N	73	5329	81	6561	5913
O	92	8464	85	7225	7820
	1218	102032	1258	106456	103706

N = 15

$$r = \frac{N(\Sigma XY) - (\Sigma X)(\Sigma Y)}{\sqrt{N(\Sigma X^2) - (\Sigma X)^2} \ \sqrt{N(\Sigma Y^2) - (\Sigma Y)^2}}$$

$$= \frac{15(103706) - (1218)(1258)}{\sqrt{15(102032) - (1218)^2} \ \sqrt{15(106456) - (1258)^2}}$$

$$= \frac{1555590 - 1532244}{\sqrt{1530480 - 1483524} \ \sqrt{1596840 - 1582564}}$$

$$= \frac{23346}{\sqrt{46956} \ \sqrt{14276}}$$

$$= \frac{23346}{(216.69) \ (119.48)}$$

$$= \frac{23346}{25890.12}$$

r = .90

substantial to high relationship between two variables. In addition, coefficients of determination can be compared as ratios, whereas correlation coefficients cannot. For example, an r of .80 is not twice as large as an r of .40. By using the coefficient of determination, we see that when r = .80, it is four times stronger than when r = .40. (r = .80, r^2 = .64; r = .40, r^2 = .16).

Negative Correlation Coefficients

There are occasions when a negative correlation coefficient is to be expected. When a smaller score, that is considered to be a better score, is correlated with a larger score, that also is considered to be a better score, the correlation coefficient usually will be negative. The relationship between maximum oxygen consumption and the time required to run two miles is an example. Generally, individuals with high values for maximum oxygen consumption will have lower times for the two-mile run than individuals with low values for maximum oxygen consumption. In addition, a negative correlation will probably occur with performance that requires support of the body, (weight correlated with pull-ups or dips).

OTHER CORRELATION TECHNIQUES

Although the Spearman rank-difference and Pearson product-moment correlation coefficients are widely used, there are occasions when they are not the appropriate techniques to use. To keep you informed, additional techniques will be described briefly. The procedures for these techniques can be found in most statistical textbooks.

Phi Coefficient

The phi coefficient is used when both variables are true dichotomies. A dichotomous variable is one that can have only one of two possible values. Examples of studies employing the phi coefficient are:

- the relationship of the sex of an individual, and success or failure on a particular task
- the relationship of the sex of an individual, and response to the question, "Do you enjoy physical education?"

Point Biserial Coefficient

The point biserial coefficient is appropriate when one variable is continous and one variable is dichotomous. It is based on the assumption that the discrete variable is a true dichotomy. Such classifications as male-female, participant-nonparticipant, and undergraduate student-graduate student are true dichotomies. This assumption is not appropriate for artificial dichotomies such as skilled-nonskilled or enthusiastic-nonenthusiastic. Examples of studies that would employ the point biserial coefficient are:

- the relationship of the sex of an individual, and success on a standardized test

• the relationship of the graduate/nongraduate student (college) and performance on a fitness test

Biserial Correlation Coefficient

The biserial correlation coefficient is appropriate when one of the variables is continuous and the other is an artificial dichotomy. A study of the relationship between the number of miles run per week and the time for running 5,000 meters would require the use of the biserial correlation coefficient. The miles run per week is the artificial dichotomous variable and might be divided into less than 50 miles per week and more than 50 miles per week.

Tetrachoric Correlation Coefficient

When both variables are forced into dichotomies, the tetrachoric correlation coefficient is required. This technique would be appropriate for a study of the relationship of success as a high school coach, and college grade point average. It would be necessary to define successful and unsuccessful, and to force the grade point average into a dichotomy (e.g., below 3.0 and above 3.0) to perform this study.

Are you able to:
define correlation, correlation coefficient, and coefficient of determination?
construct a scattergram and interpret it?
determine the Spearman rank-difference correlation coefficient and interpret it?
determine the Pearson product-moment correlation coefficient and interpret it?

REVIEW PROBLEMS

1. Utilizing the rank-difference correlation coefficient method, determine the relationship between the height (inches) and weight (pounds) measurements of 20 individuals.

Student	Height	Weight	Student	Height	Weight
A	68	170	K	68	165
B	68	160	L	67	160
C	66	140	M	71	195
D	67	150	N	71	190
E	69	155	O	70	195
F	65	145	P	66	150
G	70	168	Q	69	170
H	71	182	R	66	148
I	74	208	S	65	140
J	65	144	T	76	210

2. Utilizing the product-moment correlation coefficient method, determine the relationship between a two-minute sit-up test and physical-fitness test scores. After you determine r, calculate the coefficient of determination and interpret the obtained value.

Student	Sit-up Scores	PF Scores	Student	Sit-up Scores	PF Scores
A	45	81	K	38	93
B	51	94	L	37	51
C	30	91	M	41	65
D	55	75	N	42	73
E	32	65	O	42	74
F	42	82	P	43	79
G	41	85	Q	38	42
H	52	65	R	39	65
I	61	73	S	45	54
J	39	85	T	43	63

TESTING FOR SIGNIFICANT DIFFERENCE BETWEEN TWO MEANS

As a physical educator you may have occasions when you would like to compare different methods of instruction or programs. You may wish to determine if a group has improved in skill, fitness or knowledge after participation in a particular program.

To illustrate, imagine you are the instructor at a fitness center, and you have 40 individuals of similar age in a cardiorespiratory fitness class. Rather than have all 40 individuals participate in the same program, you decide to randomly assign each person to one of two groups. One group will participate in aerobic dance, three times/week, for eight weeks. The other group will participate in a running program, three times/week, for eight weeks. There are other factors about the two programs that you would have to consider (e.g., intensity and duration of each session), but you want to know if one program will develop fitness better than the other.

At the conclusion of the eight weeks, you administer the same cardiorespiratory fitness test to the two groups and notice that the group means are different. Can you say that one program developed cardiorespiratory fitness better than the other? You cannot reach such a conclusion by merely observing the means. It is not unusual for the means to be different. In fact, if 1,000 random samples were drawn from a population and administered the same test, the sample means would approximate a normal curve. The question you must answer is: "Are the sample means significantly different?" To answer this question you must statistically analyze the scores.

The Null Hypothesis

In statistics, an hypothesis is a prediction about the relationship between two or more variables. The hypothesis that predicts there will be no statistical difference between the means of groups is the **null hypothesis**. The hypothesis that predicts there will be a difference is the **alternative hypothesis**. The hypotheses are written as:

Null hypothesis $\qquad\qquad\qquad\qquad\qquad H_0 : \overline{X}_1 = \overline{X}_2$

Alternative hypothesis $\qquad\qquad\qquad H_1 : \overline{X}_1 \neq \overline{X}_2$

This type of alternative hypothesis is used for a **two-tailed test**, meaning that the difference in means can be in either direction. If a statistical test of the null hypothesis presents no evidence that the hypothesis is false, you accept it and reject the alternative hypothesis. If the statistical test presents evidence that the null hypothesis is false (the mean for group I is larger or smaller than the mean for group II), you reject it and accept the alternative hypothesis.

It is acceptable to use an alternative hypothesis that is directional. This type of hypothesis is used for a **one-tailed test** and requires that the t distribution be used differently. The directional alternative hypothesis is written as:

$$H_1: \overline{X}_1 < \overline{X}_2 \text{ or } H_1: \overline{X}_1 > \overline{X}_2$$

For most studies, the nondirectional alternative hypothesis (two-tailed) is sufficient.

Degrees of Freedom

The **degrees of freedom (df)** concept is used in all statistical tests. For the statistical procedures used in this chapter, the degrees of freedom are calculated by subtracting 1 from N (N-1) for any set of scores. (The degrees of freedom are determined by the sample size.) The degrees of freedom indicate the number of scores in a distribution that are free to vary. For example, assume that you have determined the group mean for 20 scores. For this given mean, 19 scores could vary. Once the 19 scores are obtained, however, the 20th score must assume a fixed value if the mean is to remain the same. To convince yourself of this concept, work with five scores that have a mean of 10 (the sum of the five numbers is 50). Assign four scores any value from five to 12. If the mean is to remain 10, you will see that the fifth score cannot be just any value. Its value is determined by the values that you assigned to the first four scores. In the case of a t test where there are two groups, the degrees of freedom equal $(N_1 - 1) + (N_2 - 1) = N_1 + N_2 - 2$.

Level of Significance

The **level of significance** is the probability of rejecting a null hypothesis when it is true. The two most common levels of significance are .01 and .05. If you reject the null hypothesis at .01 level of significance, there is one chance in 100 that you are rejecting the null hypothesis when it is actually true. At .05 level, there are five chances in 100 that you are in error. The level of significance and the degrees of freedom are used together to determine the value that a statistical test must yield for you to reject the null hypothesis. Appendix B shows the t value for determining significance. To use the table in Appendix B, go down the df column to the degrees of freedom that you have determined and go across to the value (critical value) under the .05 and .01 columns. This value will determine if you reject or accept the null hypothesis. Notice that the greater the degrees of freedom, the smaller the value that determines if you reject or accept the null hypothesis.

Since the degrees of freedom are a result of the sample number, many studies attempt to have a large sample number.

Standard Error of the Mean

If a large number of equal size samples were randomly drawn from the same population and formed into a distribution, we would have a sampling distribution of means. From the sampling distribution of means, we can compute the standard deviation of the sampling distribution, called the **standard error of the mean (SEM)**. When the means are in close agreement, the value of the standard error of the mean is small. Also, we are more confident that any one mean is near the value of the population mean.

Since it is not practical to calculate the standard error of the mean from a sampling distribution of means, a formula has been derived to provide an estimate of the standard error. The formula is:

$$\text{SEM} = \frac{s}{\sqrt{N}} \quad \text{(s = standard deviation of sample scores)}$$

Standard Error of the Difference between Means

After calculating the standard error of the mean for each of the means, we can estimate the size difference to be expected between two sample means, randomly drawn from the same population. To determine this value, called the **standard error of the difference**, it is necessary to square the standard error of the mean of each group, add the results and then find the square root of the sum. The standard error of the difference represents the standard deviation of all the observed differences between pairs of sample means. The formula is:

$$S_{\bar{x} - \bar{x}} = \sqrt{\text{SEM}_1^2 + \text{SEM}_2^2}$$

t Test for Independent Groups

The **t test for independent groups** may be used to determine the significance of the difference between two independent sample means. When comparing the means of two independent samples, the following assumptions are made:

1. Initially the two sample groups come from the same population.
2. The population is normally distributed.
3. The two groups are representative samples, i.e., they have approximately equal variances.

To illustrate the steps involved in the use of the t test for independent groups, suppose you wanted to determine if running five days/week would develop cardiorespiratory endurance better than running three days/week. Your null hypothesis is that there will be no difference in the means of the two programs ($\bar{X}_1 = \bar{X}_2$). After randomly selecting the individuals for each group, you prescribe the same running program (intensity and duration for each day) for both groups. After 12 weeks of participation in the running program, you administer the Harvard Step Test to both groups. Table 2-11 shows the test scores and the necessary calculations for the t test. (For convenience, only 10 individuals will be in each group.) The steps for the calculations are:

1. Calculate the mean and standard deviations for each group.
2. Calculate the SEM for each group.
3. Calculate $S_{\bar{x}-\bar{x}}$.

Table 2-11. *t Test for Independent Groups: Harvard Step Test*

Group Running 3 days/week		Group Running 5 days/week	
X_1	$X_1{}^2$	X_2	$X_2{}^2$
80	6400	88	7744
79	6241	92	8464
81	6561	93	8649
80	6400	95	9025
82	6724	91	8281
81	6561	89	7921
80	6400	88	7744
82	6724	90	8100
81	6561	94	8836
83	6889	93	8649
$\Sigma X_1 = 809$	$\Sigma X_1{}^2 = 65461$	$\Sigma X_2 = 913$	$\Sigma X_2{}^2 = 83413$

$$\bar{X}_1 = 80.9 \qquad\qquad\qquad \bar{X}_2 = 91.3$$

$$s_1 = \sqrt{\frac{N\Sigma X^2 - (\Sigma X)^2}{N(N-1)}} \qquad\qquad s_2 = 2.50$$

$$= \sqrt{\frac{10(65461) - (809)^2}{10(9)}} \qquad\qquad SEM_2 = .79$$

$$= \sqrt{\frac{654610 - 654481}{90}}$$

$$= \sqrt{\frac{129}{90}}$$

$$s_1 = \sqrt{1.43} = 1.20$$

$$SEM_1 = \frac{s_1}{\sqrt{N_1}} = \frac{1.20}{\sqrt{10}} = \frac{1.20}{3.16} = 0.38$$

$$s_{\bar{x}-\bar{x}} = \sqrt{SEM_1{}^2 + SEM_1{}^2} \qquad\qquad t = \frac{\bar{X}_1 - \bar{X}_2}{s_{\bar{x}-\bar{x}}}$$

$$= \sqrt{(0.38)^2 + (0.79)^2}$$

$$= \sqrt{0.1444 + 0.6241} \qquad\qquad = \frac{80.9 - 91.3}{.87}$$

$$= \sqrt{0.7685} \qquad\qquad t = -11.95$$

$$s_{\bar{x}-\bar{x}} = 0.87$$

4. Calculate the t ratio by substituting the values in the formula:

$$t = \frac{\overline{X}_1 - \overline{X}_2}{s_{\overline{x} - \overline{x}}}$$

5. Determine the degrees of freedom (df). For this comparison, the
   degrees of freedom = 10 + 10 – 2 = 18.
6. Refer to the t values in Appendix B. If the computed t ratio is
   equal to or greater than the critical value in Appendix B, reject
   the null hypothesis. If the t ratio is less than the critical value,
   accept the null hypothesis. With 18 degrees of freedom, the t
   ratio of 11.95 is greater than the t of 2.101 needed for significance
   at the .05 level, and also greater than the 2.878 needed for significance at the .01 level.
   NOTE: The negative sign is ignored since it is the result of subtracting $\overline{X}_2$ from $\overline{X}_1$. If the group running five days/week had
   been designated as group 1, the result would have been positive.
   The important consideration is the size of t, not its sign.
7. Reject the null hypothesis; you may conclude that running five
   days/week develops cardiorespiratory endurance better than
   running three days/week.

t Test for Dependent Groups

If two groups are not independent but are related to each other, the
t test for dependent groups should be used. This test is also called
the t test for paired, related or correlated samples. The only changes in
the assumptions for the t test for dependent groups, as compared to
those for the t test for independent groups, are:

1. The paired differences are a random sample from a normal
   population.
2. The equal variances assumption is unnecessary, since you
   would be working with one group.

To illustrate the steps involved in the use of the t test for dependent
groups, imagine that you wish to determine if participation in a
basketball class will improve the scores of ninth-grade girls on a speed
spot shooting test. Your null hypothesis is that there will be no
difference in the means of the speed spot shooting pretest and posttest
($\overline{X}_1 = \overline{X}_2$). You administer the test the first day of the class and again at
the conclusion of the basketball unit. Table 2-12 shows the pairs of
scores and the necessary calculations for the t test. (Again, for
convenience, only 10 pairs of scores will be used.) The steps for the
calculations are:

1. List the pairs of scores so that you can subtract one from the
   other.
2. Label a column D and determine the difference for each pair of
   scores.
3. Label a column D^2, square each D and sum D^2 (ΣD^2).
4. Calculate the mean difference ($\overline{D}$).

5. Calculate the standard deviation of the difference. The formula is:

$$s_D = \sqrt{\frac{\Sigma D^2 - N(\overline{D}^2)}{N}}$$

6. Calculate the standard error of the difference ($s_{\overline{D}}$). The $s_{\overline{D}}$ is equivalent to the SEM and is obtained in a similar manner. The formula is:

$$s_{\overline{D}} = \frac{s_D}{\sqrt{N}}$$

7. Calculate the t ratio by substituting the values in the formula:

$$t = \frac{\overline{D}}{s_{\overline{D}}}$$

8. Determine the degrees of freedom. For this comparison the degrees of freedom = 10 – 1 = 9.
9. Refer to the t values in Appendix B. With 9 degrees of freedom the t ratio of 4.29 in is greater than the t value of 2.262 needed for

Table 2-12. *t Test for Dependent Groups: Speed Spot Shooting Test*

Pretest Scores	Posttest Scores	D	D²
10	12	2	4
12	15	3	9
9	10	1	1
11	10	–1	1
8	12	4	16
9	11	2	4
13	14	1	1
8	11	3	9
7	9	2	4
9	10	1	1
		$\Sigma D = 18$	$\Sigma D^2 = 50$

$\overline{D} = 1.8$

$$s_D = \sqrt{\frac{\Sigma D^2 - N(\overline{D}^2)}{N}}$$

$$= \sqrt{\frac{50 - 10(1.8^2)}{10}}$$

$$= \sqrt{\frac{50 - 10(3.24)}{10}}$$

$$= \sqrt{\frac{17.6}{10}}$$

$$s_D = \sqrt{1.76} = 1.33$$

$$s_{\overline{D}} = \frac{s_D}{\sqrt{N}}$$

$$= \frac{1.33}{\sqrt{10}}$$

$$s_{\overline{D}} = \frac{1.33}{3.16} = .42$$

$$t = \frac{\overline{D}}{s_{\overline{D}}}$$

$$t = \frac{1.8}{.42} = 4.29$$

significance at the .05 level of significance, and than the t value of 3.250 needed at the .01 level.

10. Reject the null hypothesis. You may conclude that participation in the basketball class improved performance on the speed spot shooting test.

Are you able to:
define null hypothesis, degrees of freedom, level of significance, standard error of the mean and standard error of the difference between means?
determine if there is a significant difference between two means through use of the appropriate t test?

REVIEW PROBLEMS

1. An instructor used different methods to teach a health unit to two classes. Use the appropriate t test to determine if the performances of the two classes on the knowledge test were significantly different.

Class 1	Class 2
88 93 91 82 85	82 86 89 88 91
87 90 86 92 89	92 89 85 89 92
94 88 87 87 90	92 93 94 89 94

2. Use the appropriate t test to determine if a group of 12 individuals experienced a significant change in percent body fat after participation in a 15-week exercise program.

Subject	Percent body fat before exercise program	Percent body fat after exercise program
A	26	21
B	17	15
C	18	16
D	20	16
E	21	18
F	25	21
G	19	16
H	21	18
I	27	23
J	21	17

TESTING FOR SIGNIFICANT DIFFERENCE
BETWEEN THREE OR MORE MEANS

The t test is a method for testing hypotheses about two sample means, but there may be occasions that require the testing of hypotheses about more than two means. For example, you may elect to compare the effects of three or more methods of teaching, cardiovascular fitness programs, weight-training programs or weight-reduction programs. **Analysis of variance** (ANOVA) is a method for comparing three or more means, or even at times to compare two means. For these reasons, ANOVA is used in research more than any other statistical technique.

Special Terms and Symbols

Before attempting to perform the steps of the new techniques, you should have an understanding of these terms:

N = number of scores

n = the number of scores in a group (number in each group does not have to be the same)

k = the number of groups

grand ΣX = sum of all scores in all groups

grand ΣX^2 = sum of the square of all squares in all groups

total sum of squares (SS_T) = the sum of the squared deviations of every score from the grand $\overline{X}$; represents the variability of each score in all groups from the grand $\overline{X}$

sum of squares within-groups (SS_W) = the sum of the squared deviations of each score from its group $\overline{X}$; also referred to as sum of squares for error

sum of squares between-groups (SS_B) = the sum of the squared deviations of each group $\overline{X}$ from the grand $\overline{X}$; also referred to as treatment sum of squares

mean square for the sum of squares within-groups (MS_W) = variance within groups

mean square for the sum of squares between-groups (MS_B) = variance between groups

F distribution = values required to reject null hypothesis

degrees of freedom within groups = $(N - k)$; total number of measures or scores(N) minus number of groups(k); degrees of freedom for denominator in F distribution

degrees of freedom between groups = $(k - 1)$; number of groups(k) minus 1; degrees of freedom for numerator in F distribution

Analysis of Variance for Independent Groups

The **analysis of variance for independent groups** is used when the sample groups are not related to each other. There are several assumptions for this ANOVA, but the basic assumptions are:

1. The samples are randomly drawn from a normally distributed population.
2. The variances of the samples are approximately equal.

To illustrate the steps involved in the analysis of variance for independent groups, suppose that a fitness instructor wishes to determine if there is a difference in three programs designed to improve trunk extension. The null hypothesis is that there will be no difference in the means of the three programs ($\overline{X}_1 = \overline{X}_2 = \overline{X}_3$). He randomly assigns the members of a fitness class to one of three groups, and each group participates in a different program to improve trunk extension, for 10 weeks. At the conclusion of the training period, the groups are given the same trunk extension test. Table 2-13 shows the scores and the necessary calculations for the analysis of variance. As with previous illustrations, the total number of scores is intentionally small. The steps for the calculations are:

1. Sum each group of scores to get ΣX_1, ΣX_2, and ΣX_3. Add the group sums to get a grand ΣX. $\Sigma X_1 + \Sigma X_2 + \Sigma X_3 =$ grand ΣX.
2. Square each score and sum the squared scores of each group (ΣX^2). Add the ΣX^2 for each group to get a grand ΣX^2. $\Sigma X_1^2 + \Sigma X_2^2 + \Sigma X_3^2 =$ grand ΣX^2.
3. Calculate the correction factor (C). C is necessary because raw scores are used rather than deviations of the scores from the mean.

$$C = \frac{(\text{grand } \Sigma X)^2}{\text{total N}}$$

4. Calculate the total sum of squares (SS_T).
$SS_T =$ grand $\Sigma X^2 - C$
5. Calculate the sum of squares between-groups (SS_B).

$$SS_B = \frac{(\Sigma X_1)^2}{n_1} + \frac{(\Sigma X_2)^2}{n_2} + \frac{(\Sigma X_3)^2}{n_3} - C$$

6. Calculate the sum of squares within-groups (SS_W).
$SS_W = SS_T - SS_B$
7. Calculate the mean square for the sum of squares between-groups.

$$MS_B = \frac{SS_B}{k-1}$$

8. Calculate the mean square for the sum of squares within-groups.

$$MS_W = \frac{SS_W}{N-k}$$

9. Calculate the F ratio.

$$F = \frac{MS_B}{MS_W}$$

10. Refer to the F distribution in Appendix C to determine if F is significant. To use the table in Appendix C, locate the appropriate column for the numerator degrees of freedom (degrees of freedom between groups, k-1). For the trunk extension study, there are 2 degrees of freedom between groups (3-1=2). We next find the row that corresponds to the degrees of freedom for the denominator (degrees of freedom within groups, N-k). We have 21 (24-3) degrees of freedom within groups. The F ratio of 8.57 is greater than the 3.47 table value at the .05 level, and the 5.78 value at the .01 level, so we reject the null hypothesis. The F ratio permits us to conclude that there is a significant difference in the three means; but, it does not indicate which mean is significantly superior, or if two means are significantly superior to one mean. There are tests to perform these functions (e.g., Tukey and Scheffé), but they will not be discussed in this book. Table 2-14 shows a summary of the ANOVA as it is usually reported in research publications.

Table 2-13. *ANOVA for Independent Groups: Trunk Extension Test*

Group I		Group II		Group III	
X_1	$X_1{}^2$	X_2	$X_2{}^2$	X_3	$X_3{}^2$
22	484	20	400	18	324
23	529	19	361	19	361
21	441	18	324	17	289
22	484	19	361	22	484
19	361	18	324	18	324
21	441	21	441	19	361
22	484	20	400	20	400
21	441	19	361	19	361
$\Sigma X_1 = 171$	$\Sigma X_1{}^2 = 3665$	$\Sigma X_2 = 154$	$\Sigma X_2{}^2 = 2972$	$\Sigma X_3 = 152$	$\Sigma X_3{}^2 = 2904$

- $\Sigma X_1 = 171$, $\Sigma X_2 = 154$, $\Sigma X_3 = 152$
  $\Sigma X_1{}^2 = 3665$, $\Sigma X_2{}^2 = 2972$, $\Sigma X_3{}^2 = 2904$

- grand $\Sigma X = 171 + 154 + 152 = 477$

- grand $\Sigma X^2 = 3665 + 2972 + 2904 = 9541$

- correction factor $\quad C = \dfrac{(\text{grand } \Sigma X)^2}{\text{total N}}$

$$C = \frac{(477)^2}{24} = \frac{227{,}529}{24} = 9480.38$$

- $SS_T = \text{grand } \Sigma X^2 - C$
  $SS_T = 9541 - 9480.38 = 60.62$

- $SS_B = \dfrac{(\Sigma X_1)^2}{n_1} + \dfrac{(\Sigma X_2)^2}{n_2} + \dfrac{(\Sigma X_3)^2}{n_3} - C$

$$= \frac{(171)^2}{8} + \frac{(154)^2}{8} + \frac{(152)^2}{8} - 9480.38$$
  $SS_B = 3655.13 + 2964.50 + 2888 - 9480.38 = 27.25$

- $SS_W = SS_T - SS_B$
  $SS_W = 60.62 - 27.25 = 33.37$

- $MS_B = \dfrac{SS_B}{k - 1} = \dfrac{27.25}{3 - 1} = 13.63$

- $MS_W = \dfrac{SS_W}{N - k} = \dfrac{33.37}{24 - 3} = 1.59$

- $F = \dfrac{MS_B}{MS_W} = \dfrac{13.63}{1.59} = 8.57$

Table 2-14. *Summary of ANOVA for Trunk Extension Test*

Source of variation	Sum of squares	df	Mean square	F
Between-groups	27.25	2	13.63	8.57*
Within-groups	33.37	21	1.59	
Total	60.62	23		

*Significant at the .01 level

Analysis of Variance for Repeated Measures

The **analysis of variance for repeated measures** is used when repeated measures are made on the same subjects. Basic assumptions are:

1. The samples are randomly selected from a normal population.
2. The variances for each measurement are approximately equal.

To illustrate this technique, we will assume that a basketball coach wishes to determine if loudness of sound is a factor in the making of foul shots. He arranges for the 10 members of the basketball team to shoot 15 foul shots under three different sound conditions (no sound, medium sound and loud sound). The null hypothesis is that the means of the three trials will be no different ($\overline{X}_1 = \overline{X}_2 = \overline{X}_3$). Table 2-15 shows the scores and the necessary calculations for the analysis of variance. (Note that in this technique N refers to the total number of measurements.) Ten subjects were measured three times, so N = 30. Also, k refers to the number of times that the group is measured. The steps for the calculations are:

1. Calculate the grand ΣX and grand ΣX_2 as in the ANOVA for independent groups.

   $\Sigma X_1 + \Sigma X_2 + \Sigma X_3 = $ grand ΣX
   $\Sigma X_1^2 + \Sigma X_2^2 + \Sigma X_3^2 = $ grand ΣX^2

2. Calculate the correction factor as before.

   $$C = \frac{(\text{grand } \Sigma X)^2}{N}$$

3. Calculate the total sum of squares (SS_T) as before.

   $SS_T = $ grand $\Sigma X^2 - C$

4. Calculate the sum of squares between-groups (SS_B) as before. Actually this is the sum of squares between-trials.

   $$SS_B = \frac{(\Sigma X_1)^2}{n_1} + \frac{(\Sigma X_2)^2}{n_2} + \frac{(\Sigma X_3)^2}{n_3}$$

5. Calculate the sum of squares to recognize the effects of the test-retest ($SS_{subjects}$). This is done by adding the scores of the three trials for each subject, squaring the sum, and then adding the squared sums for each subject. The sum of the squared sums for each subject is divided by k (the number of trials), and C is subtracted from the resulting value.

   $$SS_{subjects} = \frac{(X_{11}+X_{12}+X_{13})^2 + (X_{21}+X_{22}+X_{23})^2 + ...(X_{101}+X_{102}+X_{103})^2}{k} - C$$

Table 2-15. *ANOVA for Repeated Measures: Foul Shooting While Exposed to Different Sound Levels*

No Sound		Medium Sound		Loud Sound			
X_1	X_1^2	X_2	X_2^2	X_3	X_3^2	ΣRows	$(\Sigma$Rows$)^2$
11	121	12	144	10	100	33	1089
9	81	10	100	9	81	28	784
10	100	12	144	9	81	31	961
8	64	10	100	9	81	27	729
12	144	12	144	10	100	34	1156
10	100	11	121	9	81	30	900
12	144	13	169	11	121	36	1296
9	81	9	81	9	81	27	729
10	100	11	121	8	64	29	841
9	81	10	100	10	100	29	841

$\Sigma X_1 = 100$ $\Sigma X_2 = 110$ $\Sigma X_3 = 94$ grand $\Sigma X = 304$

$\Sigma X_1^2 = 1016$ $\Sigma X_2^2 = 1224$ $\Sigma X_3^2 = 890$ $(\Sigma$rows$)^2 = 9326$

- grand $\Sigma X = 304$; grand $\Sigma X^2 = 3130$

- correction factor $C = \dfrac{(\text{grand } \Sigma X)^2}{\text{total N}} = \dfrac{(304)^2}{30} = \dfrac{92416}{30} = 3080.53$

- $SS_T = $ grand $\Sigma X^2 - C = 3130 - 3080.53 = 49.47$

- $SS_B = \dfrac{(\Sigma X_1)^2}{n_1} + \dfrac{(\Sigma X_2)^2}{n_2} + \dfrac{(\Sigma X_3)^2}{n_3} - C$

  $= \dfrac{(100)^2}{10} + \dfrac{(110)^2}{10} + \dfrac{(94)^2}{10} - 3080.53$

  $SS_B = 3093.60 - 3080.53 = 13.07$

- $SS_{subjects} =$
  $$\dfrac{(X_{11}+X_{12}+X_{13})^2 + (X_{21}+X_{22}+X_{23})^2 + \ldots (X_{101}+X_{102}+X_{103})^2}{k} - C$$
  $$= \dfrac{(11+12+10)^2 + (9+10+9)^2 + \ldots (9+10+10)^2}{3} - 3080.53$$
  $SS_{subjects} = 3108.67 - 3080.53 = 28.14$

- $SS_E = SS_T - SS_B - SS_{subjects}$
  $SS_E = 49.47 - 13.07 - 28.14 = 8.26$

- $MS_B = \dfrac{SS_B}{k-1} = \dfrac{13.07}{2} = 6.54$

- $MS_{subjects} = \dfrac{SS_{subjects}}{r-1} = \dfrac{28.14}{10-1} = 3.13$

- $MS_E = \dfrac{SS_E}{(k-1)(r-1)} = \dfrac{8.26}{(2)(9)} = 0.46$

- F ratio $= \dfrac{MS_B}{MS_E} = \dfrac{6.54}{0.46} = 14.22$

6. Compute the sum of squares error. Since this sum of squares remains after SS_B and $SS_{subjects}$, it is easy to calculate.
$$SS_E = SS_T - SS_B - SS_{subjects}$$

7. Calculate the mean square for the sum of squares between-groups (trials).
$$MS_B = \frac{SS_B}{k - 1}$$

8. Calculate the mean square for the sum of squares subjects.
$$MS_{subjects} = \frac{SS_{subjects}}{r - 1}$$

9. Calculate the mean square for the sum of squares error.
$$MS_E = \frac{SS_E}{(k - 1)(r - 1)}$$

10. Calculate the F ratio.
$$F = \frac{MS_B}{MS_E}$$

11. Refer to the F distribution in Appendix C. The degrees of freedom for the numerator are: $(k-1)=(3-1)=2$. For the denominator, the degrees of freedom are: $(k-1)(r-1)=(3-1)(10-1)=18$. The F ratio of 14.22 is greater than the 6.01 value needed for significance at the .01 level, so we reject the null hypothesis. However, an additional test is needed to determine which means are significantly different. Possibly, there is no significant difference between the means of no sound and loud sound. Table 2-16 shows the analysis summary.

Table 2-16. *Summary of ANOVA for Foul Shooting While Exposed to Different Sound Levels*

Source of variation	Sum of squares	df	Mean square	F
Subjects (rows)	28.14	9	3.13	
Between-groups	13.07	2	6.54	14.22*
Error	8.26	18	0.46	
Total	49.47	29		

*Significant at the .01 level

The reliability, or consistency, of a test may be estimated through ANOVA. Test reliability will be discussed in Chapter 3. Through ANOVA the intraclass correlation coefficient (R) is computed. The Pearson product-moment correlation coefficient also can be used to estimate test reliability, but the intraclass correlation coefficient may be more accurate, for two reasons. First, product-moment correlation is limited to two trials. If more than two trials of a test are administered, it is necessary to reduce the scores to two sets, usually by averaging. Second, the Pearson product-moment correlation coefficient does not consider the variation of trial scores. It is possible that trial scores for the test performers may systematically increase or decrease, but the changes would not be detected if the product-moment correlation coefficient is used. Test reliability may be estimated as high, even though the scores systematically changed. Procedures for calculation of the intraclass correlation coefficient will not be described, but may be found in other statistical sources.

> Are you able to:
> define total sum of squares, sum of squares within-groups, sum of squares between-groups, mean square for the sum of squares within-groups, and mean square for the sum of squares between-groups?
> determine if there is a significant difference in two or more means through the appropriate one-way analysis of variance procedure?

THE MICROCOMPUTER

The use of the microcomputer now means that it is no longer necessary to have access to minicomputers or mainframe computers to statistically analyze data. With the appropriate computer program (software), it is now possible to determine measures of central tendency and variability, percentiles, correlational coefficients, significant differences between means and many other statistical procedures.

No detailed description of microcomputer hardware will be presented in this textbook, as microcomputer technology is constantly changing. However, since the microcomputer is easy to use and can aid you in the analysis of data, test construction and analysis, the storing and processing of data and in many other responsibilities you will perform as a physical educator, you should seek to develop microcomputer skills. On most college and university campuses there are several options that could aid you in acquiring this proficiency. Perhaps your major department offers a microcomputer applications course, or a campus microcomputer laboratory is available for student use. If these options are available, take advantage of them. Also, seek the help of other students who use the microcomputer. Microcomputer skills will enable you to perform your professional responsibilities in a more efficient manner.

Once you have the proficiency to utilize the microcomputer, you may wish to select a statistical software program. There are many such programs available. In selecting one, consider not only cost, but ease of use. Appendix D lists several statistical programs available.

This completes the discussion of statistics. If you have questions about any procedures presented in this chapter, study them again. Before reading Chapter 3, complete the following review problems.

REVIEW PROBLEMS

1. An elementary physical education teacher typically used two different methods to improve the agility of the students in her classes. Trying to determine if one program developed agility better than the other, she randomly assigned the students to one of two groups. After the students had been in the programs for 12 weeks, she administered the two groups the same agility test. Use the appropriate t test to determine if the group means are significantly different.

Scores for group I		Scores for group II	
13	12	14	13
13	11	12	15
10	8	10	12
11	14	11	10
12	10	13	14

2. A high school teacher was interested in determining if mental practice would improve badminton serving ability. He randomly selected 10 subjects from a population of students that had never played badminton, taught the correct way to serve, and administered a short-serve test to them. He gave the students instructions about mental practice and asked them to mentally practice the badminton short-serve 10 minutes/day for seven days. They were instructed not to practice badminton in any other way. He then tested the group again. Use the appropriate t test to determine if the group mean for the short-serve test improved after mental practice.

Subject	Pretest short-serve test scores	Posttest short-serve test scores
A	37	43
B	42	46
C	36	38
D	50	55
E	34	32
F	44	51
G	51	53
H	42	48
I	45	43
J	52	55

3. A physical fitness instructor was interested in comparing three cardiovascular fitness programs. After three groups participated in the programs, she measured the oxygen uptake (ml/kg/min) of all the subjects. Use the appropriate ANOVA technique to determine if the group means are significantly different.

Group I	Group II	Group III
46	47	49
46	50	51
48	50	50
47	48	49
50	49	52
48	47	53
47	51	49
51	50	52

4. A weight-training instructor was interested in determining the effects of external motivation on muscular strength. After a group of 10 individuals had participated in a weight-training class for 15 weeks, the instructor tested the group for maximum strength on three different occasions. During one test, no external motivation was provided. During the second test, only the instructor shouted encouragement, and during the third test, he arranged for several spectators to shout encouragement. Use the appropriate ANOVA technique to determine if there is a significant difference in the group means of the tests.

Subject	No external motivation	Instructor motivation	Spectator motivation
A	81	84	88
B	88	89	93
C	92	94	97
D	83	85	88
E	81	83	85
F	79	80	85
G	84	84	87
H	87	86	93
I	88	90	94
J	84	86	88

3

What Is a Good Test?

Upon completion of this chapter, you should be able to:
1. Describe criterion-referenced and norm-referenced measurement;
2. Define validity and the types of validity, give examples of each and describe how each may be estimated;
3. Define reliability and describe the four methods of estimating reliability;
4. Define objectivity and describe how it may be estimated; and
5. Describe the features related to administrative feasibility that should be considered when selecting or constructing a test.

As a physical educator you will often measure performances and attributes of individuals with a test, but it is irresponsible to randomly select a test. Before you select a test, or possibly construct your own test, consider: (1) if criterion-referenced measurement or norm-referenced measurement should be used, and (2) the criteria for determining a good test — validity, reliability, objectivity and administrative feasibility.

CRITERION-REFERENCED MEASUREMENT
Criterion-referenced measurement is used when individuals are expected to perform at a specific level of achievement. In this type of measurement one individual's performance is not compared with the performance of others; a minimum level of acceptable performance is described. Criterion-referenced measurement involves the use of behavioral objectives that describe the expected level of performance of the individual. Examples of criterion-referenced standards are:
- For successful completion of the running fitness class, the student must be able to run two miles in 14 minutes or less and correctly answer 80% or more of the fitness knowledge test questions.

65

- For successful completion of the badminton class, the student must correctly answer a minimum of 35 questions on the written test.

Again, with this type of measurement the student's performance is not compared with the performances of other students.

Criterion-referenced measurement also can be used to determine grades. For example, in a running fitness class the male grade standards might be:

"A": Run two miles in 13 minutes or less.
Correctly answer 90% or more of the fitness knowledge test questions.

"B": Run two miles in 13:01 to 13:30.
Correctly answer 80 to 89% of the fitness knowledge test questions.

"C": Run two miles in 13:31 to 14:00.
Correctly answer 70 to 79% of the fitness knowledge test questions.

Determining what performance earns an "A" or any other grade may be a problem. If you choose to use criterion-referenced measurement for grade purposes, the standards should be well-planned.

Criterion-referenced measurement has some limitations. When a pass/fail standard is used, it does not show how good or how poor a student's level of ability is. Additionally, it is too often that the standard for success is arbitrarily set by the teacher. Remember, we know that measurement may be used for several reasons, so there will be occasions when criterion-referenced measurement is appropriate.

NORM-REFERENCED MEASUREMENT

Norm-referenced measurement is used when you wish to interpret each student's performance on a test in comparison with other students' performances. This comparison is done using norms that enable the teacher to interpret a student's score in relation to the scores made by other individuals in the same population. Examples of norms are percentiles, z-scores and T-scores. Very often norm-referenced measurement is used to determine grades, but it may be used for other reasons, such as a way to establish appropriate levels of achievement for criterion-referenced standards. Norms for tests in physical education are usually reported by sex, weight, height and age or grade level. In selecting a test with norms, the following factors should be considered:

1. The sample size used to determine the norms — generally, more confidence can be placed in a large sample.
2. The population used to determine the norms — for example, if a basketball skills test has norms for 10th-grade students, only 10th-grade students should have been used to develop the norms. Varsity basketball players or students in other grades should not have been used.

3. The time the norms were established — norms should be updated periodically.

Both criterion-referenced measurement and norm-referenced measurement may be used in the measurement of student skills and knowledge. As a teacher you should recognize when it is appropriate to use each.

> Are you able to:
> define criterion-referenced and norm-referenced measurement?

VALIDITY

Validity, the most important criterion to consider when evaluating a test, refers to the degree to which a test actually measures what it claims to measure. If a test is designed to measure accuracy of placement in the badminton low, short-serve, it should accomplish that objective. In addition, validity is specific to a particular use. For example, even though cardiovascular fitness may be a factor in a long tennis match, a fitness test should not be used to determine tennis ability. A valid tennis test should be used to measure tennis skill.

Since the validity of tests varies, the selection of one test over another may depend on which test will best measure the desired trait. The validity coefficient indicates how well a test measures what it claims to measure, and as discussed in Chapter 2, the coefficient is determined through correlation techniques. The coefficient may range from –1.00 to +1.00, and the closer the coefficient is to +1.00, the more valid the test. A test being used as a substitute for another validated test should have a validity coefficient of about 0.80 or more. A test being used for predictive purposes may have a lower validity coefficient. Traditionally, predictive tests with validity coefficients of 0.50 have been accepted.

Validity of Norm-Referenced Tests

There are four types of validity for norm-referenced tests: content, predictive, concurrent and construct validity. The type of validity used depends on the nature of the test and how the test scores are to be utilized. A test that has a high degree of content validity may not be a valid test to predict future performance. It is important you understand the validity coefficient and the method used to find it when you select a standardized test or construct your own test. Some textbooks describe a fifth kind of validity, face validity. This term is used when a test obviously measures the desired skill or ability. For example, if a student is asked to run 50 yards as fast as possible, it is clear to the student that the purpose of the test is to measure running speed.

Content Validity: Content validity is related to how well a test measures all skills and subject matter that have been presented to the students. To have content validity, a test must measure the objectives for which the students are held responsible. As a teacher you should administer knowledge tests that sample the subject matter covered. This means that regardless of how long or short the test is, it should measure how well the students have mastered the objectives. More than likely you would have no problem constructing a test of 150 items which measures the students' knowledge of all the subject matter that has been presented, but such a test may be too long for them to complete. To have content validity, the test must be reduced to a realistic number of items (sample test) and still represent the total content of the longer test.

Content validity is expected of skills test also. The test should measure the skills that have been emphasized in class. Content validity for most teacher-made tests is a subjective judgment, but by asking yourself, "Does the test measure what the students have been taught in class?", you will be provided with a good estimate of content validity. It may help to ask your fellow teachers to assist you in answering this question. Content validity also may be found by administering the sample test to a group and administering the total test (referred to as universal content) a short time later. The two tests are then correlated (product-moment correlation) to determine the content validity of the sample test.

Predictive Validity: When you wish to estimate future performance, you are concerned with predictive validity. Generally, to estimate predictive validity, a predictor test is given and correlated with a criterion measure (obtained at a later date). In physical education, the later time is often after an instructional unit; in athletics, the later time could be after years of development.

The predictor test is the instrument used to measure the trait or ability of the students. A sports skills test is an example. The criterion measure is the variable that has been defined as indicating successful performance of a trait, but the definition of successful performance is sometimes difficult to determine. One method of determining successful performance is through a panel of experts. For example, a volleyball coach could administer a volleyball skills test to all team members. A panel of experts is asked to observe the team during games throughout the season and rate the players' performances. At the completion of the season, the coach would correlate (product-moment) the average of the experts' ratings (the criterion measurement) with the skills test administered at the beginning of the season to estimate the predictive validity of the test. College entrance examinations are used as predictor tests, with the criterion measure being success in college. Tests with predictive validity can be of value to you for the grouping of students when you know little about their level of skill, and you expect improvement in their performance during the instructional unit.

Concurrent Validity: Concurrent validity might be called immediate predictive validity. It indicates how well the individual currently performs a skill. To determine concurrent validity, test results are correlated with a current criterion measurement rather than future information; a test and the criterion measurement are administered at approximately the same time. This procedure is often used to estimate the validity (how well a test measures what it claims to measure) of a test. Concurrent validity may be established in several ways. A new test could be correlated (product-moment) with expert ratings, tournament play, or a previous validity test. These procedures are described in Chapter 4.

Concurrent validity is important if you wish to administer a test requiring less equipment or time than other tests. To illustrate: maximum oxygen consumption is best measured through gas analysis and performance on a treadmill (equipment and time). However, since the 12-minute run test correlates highly with the treadmill test, the run could be used to estimate the maximum oxygen consumption of an individual.

Construct Validity: Construct validity refers to the degree which the individual possesses a trait (construct) presumed to be reflected in the test performance. Anxiety, intelligence and motivation are constructs. These qualities cannot be seen with the human eye, yet an individual who possesses one of these characteristics is expected to behave in a certain way. Construct validity applies to testing in physical education. The term cardiovascular fitness may be classified as a construct. Cardiovascular fitness tests are often based on the constructs that differences in pulse rates or the ability to run a distance in a specified time reflects cardiovascular fitness. That is, the individual with good cardiovascular fitness will have a lower pulse rate after physical exertion and will perform better on a running test than the individual with poor cardiovascular fitness. Construct validity also applies to the measurement of sports skills. A tennis instructor assumes that when the student learns the skills of the serve, the forehand and backhand, the overhead smash and the volley, he will be able to put all the skills together and play tennis. These skills are constructs when referring to the total ability to play tennis. If a test includes items that measure these skills (constructs), it has construct validity.

Construct validity can be demonstrated by comparing higher skilled individuals with lesser skilled individuals. Again, consider a tennis skills test that is administered to both a tennis class and a varsity tennis team. With a test that has construct validity, the varsity players will most likely score higher than the members of the class.

Validity of Criterion-Referenced Tests

Criterion-referenced validity is related directly to predetermined behavioral objectives. The objectives should be stated in a clear, exact manner and be limited to small segments of the unit of instruction. To estimate the validity of a knowledge test, the items should be constructed to parallel the behavorial objectives, and there should be several items for each objective. The validity of each group of items is subjectively estimated by how well they measure the behavioral objective.

A second method requires testing prior to, and after instruction.

Validity is accepted if there is significant improvement after instruction or if the behavioral objectives are mastered by an acceptable number of students. This method may be used for knowledge and physical performance tests.

The success of criterion-referenced testing is dependent on the predetermined standard for success. The standard for success should be realistic, but high enough that the students are ready for the next level of instruction. If the students perform successfully at the next level, you may feel confident about the validity of a test.

Safrit (1986) describes procedures for estimating domain-referenced and decision validity for criterion-referenced tests. These methods will not be presented, but you may wish to refer to them.

Factors Affecting Validity

The validity of a test may be affected by several factors. Four of these factors are:

1. The student characteristics - A test is valid only for students of age, sex, and experience similar to those on whom the test was validated.
2. The criterion measure selected - Several measures have been presented for estimating the validity of a test. If each measure is correlated with the same set of scores, different correlation coefficients would be found.
3. Reliability - A test must be reliable to be valid. This concept is illustrated in the discussion of reliability later in this chapter.
4. Administrative procedures - If unclear directions are given, or if all students do not perform the test in the same way, the validity will be affected. Environmental factors (e.g., heat and humidity) also may affect validity.

Are you able to:
define validity and the types of validity for norm-referenced tests, and give examples of each?
describe the procedures for determining the types of norm-referenced validity?
describe the procedures for determining criterion-referenced validity?
list four factors that affect validity?

RELIABILITY

Reliability refers to the consistency of a test. A reliable test should obtain approximately the same results regardless of the number of times it is given. A test given to a group of students on one day should yield the same results if it is given to the same group on another day. Of course, some students may not obtain the same score on the second administration of a test, as fatigue, motivation, environmental conditions and measurement error may affect the scores. However, the order of the scores will be approximately the same if the test has reliability.

For a test to have a high degree of validity, it must have a high degree of reliability. If test scores are not reliable, the validity of a test is limited. Imagine administering a test that measures the ability to hit the golf ball for distance to a beginning golf class. Many students will have a good score on one attempt but a poor score on another attempt. This lack of consistency influences the validity of the test; though high reliability does not necessarily mean high validity. A test may be consistent, but it may not measure what it claims to measure.

There are several methods to determine reliability, and all are reported in terms of a correlation coefficient that ranges from –1.00 to +1.00. The closer the coefficient value is to +1.00 the greater the reliability of the test. Some tests will have greater reliability than others. Physical performance tests of running, jumping and throwing generally have high reliability coefficients, while tests such as the tennis serve, badminton serve and chip shot (in golf) usually have lower reliability coefficients. The lower coefficients are due to subjective judgment when declaring if an object landed within the marked boundaries.

Reliability of Norm-Referenced Tests

Four methods of estimating the reliability of norm-referenced tests will be presented: test-retest, parallel forms, split-half and Kuder-Richardson Formula 21.

Test-retest Method: The test-retest method requires two administrations of the same test to the same group of individuals, with the calculation of the correlation coefficient between the two sets of scores. The product-moment correlation method or analysis of variance (intraclass correlation coefficient) may be used to calculate the coefficient. Often the greatest source of error in the test-retest reliability estimate is caused by changes in the students themselves. If written tests are being administered, they are aware of the questions which will be asked on the retest and the answers they provided on the first test. The students also may have discussed the test. When a long interval of time elapses between the test and retest, maturational factors may influence the the results of the retest. This is especially true for physical performance tests. The appropriate time interval between administration of tests is sometimes difficult to determine. It could be as short as one day, or as long as several months, but if the test-retest method is used to estimate the reliability coefficient, the time interval must be considered.

Parallel Forms Method: The parallel forms method requires the administration of parallel or equivalent forms of a test to the same group, and the calculation of the correlation coefficient (product-moment or intraclass correlation coefficient) between the two sets of scores. Often both forms are administered during the same test period or in two sessions separated by a short time period. The primary problem associated with this method of estimating reliability is the difficulty of constructing two tests that are parallel in content and item characteristics.

If both tests are administered within a short time of each other, learning, motivation and testing conditions do not influence the correlation coefficient. The reliability of most standardized tests in education are estimated through this method.

Split-half Method: When using the split-half method, a test is split into halves and the scores of the two halves are correlated. This method requires only one administration of the test and does not require construction of a second test. A common practice is to correlate the odd-numbered items with the even-numbered items. (This method assumes that all individuals being tested will have time to complete the test, so it is not appropriate when speed of completion is a factor in the test.)

The reliability coefficient calculated by this method is for a test of only half the length of the original test. Since reliability usually increases as a test increases in length, the reliability for the full test needs to be estimated. The Spearman-Brown formula is often used for this purpose. The formula is:

$$\text{Reliability of full test} = \frac{2 \times \text{reliability on half test}}{1 + \text{reliability on half test}}$$

If the reliability between the two halves is found to be +.80, the reliability of the full test would be:

$$\text{Reliability of full test} = \frac{2 \times .80}{1 + .80} = \frac{1.60}{1.80} = .89$$

Though the split-half method may produce an inflated correlation coefficient, it is frequently used to estimate reliability coefficients for written tests. It also can be used for some skills tests in which the odd and even trials are correlated.

Kuder-Richardson Formula 21: There are many ways in which a test may be split in order to compute "half-test" scores for correlational purposes. For each split, however, a different reliability coefficient probably would be obtained. Kuder and Richardson developed a formula, K-R 20, that estimates the average correlation that might be obtained if all possible split-half combinations of a group of items were correlated. Two basic assumptions of the Kuder-Richardson formula are: (1) the test items can be scored "1" for correct and "0" for wrong and (2) the total score is the sum of the item scores. As was indicated with the split-half method, the Kuder-Richardson formula should not be used with a test in which speed of completion is a factor. Since K-R 20 requires much computation, the simpler formula, K-R 21, is often used to provide a rough approximation of K-R 20. The K-R 21 formula is:

$$r_{KR} = \frac{n}{n-1}\left(1 - \frac{\overline{X}(n - \overline{X})}{n(s^2)}\right)$$

$\underline{n}$ = number of items
$\overline{X}$ = test mean (average number of items correct)
s^2 = test variance (variance of items answered correctly)

To illustrate the use of this formula, assume that:

$$n = 50, \overline{X} = 40, \text{ and } s^2 = 25$$

$$r_{KR} = \frac{50}{49}\left(1 - \frac{40(50 - 40)}{50(25)}\right)$$

$$= \frac{50}{49}\left(1 - \frac{40(10)}{1000}\right)$$

$$r_{KR} = 1.02(1 - .40)$$

$$r_{KR} = 1.02(.60) = .61$$

Though K-R 21 is widely used, it gives a conservative estimate of reliability when the test items vary in difficulty as they often do.

Reliability of Criterion-Referenced Tests

The reliability of criterion-referenced tests is defined as consistency of classification, or how consistently the test classifies students as masters or nonmasters. Ebel (1979) states that the reliability of criterion-referenced tests can be determined in much the same way as the reliability of norm-referenced tests — that is, test-retest, parallel forms, split-half, or Kuder-Richardson formulas. One important difference, however, is that while norm-referenced reliability applies to the total test score, criterion-referenced reliability applies to a single cluster of items (each cluster is intended to measure the attainment of a different objective). In other words, several reliability coefficients, one for each cluster, will be estimated for a criterion-referenced test.

Safrit (1986) describes the proportion of agreement and kappa coefficient methods for estimating the reliability of criterion-referenced tests. These methods will not be presented but you may wish to refer to them.

Factors Affecting Reliability

The reliability of a test may be affected by many factors, including:

1. The method of scoring - As the need for accurate scoring increases, reliability decreases. This factor was described earlier in the text.
2. The heterogeneity of the group - Coefficients based on scores from 15-year-olds will probably be smaller than those based on a similar sized group that includes 14-, 15- and 16-year-olds. Therefore, when the reliability coefficient of a test is based on

test scores from a group ranging in abilities, it will be overestimated. If you wish a test to measure a particular skill of 15-year-olds, the reliability coefficient of the test should be based on 15-year-old individuals. When you read background information about a standardized test, note the heterogeneity of the group on which the reliability was estimated.

3. The length of the test - The longer the test, the greater the reliability. This is true of physical performance and written tests. Remember, we used the Spearman-Brown formula to demonstrate that the reliability coefficient for a whole test was larger than the reliability coefficient for one-half of the test.

4. Administrative procedures - The directions must be clear and all students must perform the test in the same way.

Are you able to:
define reliability?
determine reliability of a test through the test-retest, parallel forms, split-half and the Kuder-Richardson Formula 21 methods?
list three factors that affect the reliability of a test?

OBJECTIVITY

A test has high objectivity when two or more persons can administer the same test to the same group and obtain approximately the same results. Actually objectivity is a specific form of reliability, and may be determined by the test-retest (with different individuals administering the test) correlational procedure. Certain forms of measurement are more objective than others. True-false, multiple-choice and matching tests have high objectivity when scoring keys are available, while essay tests have very low objectivity. Measurement of jumping ability, free-throw shooting, throwing for distance and and success in archery are objective, but judgement of the quality of performance in gymnastics, diving and figure skating are not.

Objectivity is more likely to take place when the following factors are present:

1. Complete and clear instructions for administration and scoring of the test are given.
2. Trained testers administer the test. All testers must administer the test in the same way.
3. Simple measurement procedures are followed. If the measurements are complicated, mistakes are more likely to occur.
4. Appropriate, mechanical tools of measurement are used. This decreases the chances for measurement errors.
5. Results are expressed as numerical scores. Scores expressed in phrases or terms are less likely to reflect objectivity.

ADMINISTRATIVE FEASIBILITY

Administrative feasibility, along with validity, reliability and objectivity must be considered when selecting or constructing a test. In fact, if two tests are fairly equal in validity, reliability and objectivity, the following administrative considerations may determine which test you choose to use.

1. Cost - Does the test require expensive equipment that you do not have or cannot afford to purchase?

2. Time - Does the test take too much of your instructional time? Many authorities recommend that testing use no more than 10% of total instructional time. A test that requires several class meetings to administer may not be feasible to administer.

3. Ease of administration - (a) Do you need assistance in the administration of the test? If so, do you train student assistants or ask other teachers to assist you? The training of student testers usually requires much time, but it is essential that whoever administers the test be qualified to do so. (b) Are the instructions easy to follow? The students should be able to understand the directions and, regardless who administers the test, the results should be the same. (c) Is the test reasonable in the demands that are placed on the students? The students should not be ill or sore after taking the test.

4. Scoring - Will the services of another individual affect the objectivity of the scoring? In an effort to duplicate the actual activity, some tests require the services of another individual (e.g., in some tennis tests the ball is hit to the person being tested, in softball hitting the ball is pitched to the hitter). Tests such as these have a place in the measurement of skill, but the helper should be qualified to perform the services. The scoring of the test should not hinder the differentiation among the levels of ability.

5. Norms - Are norms available to compare your students with other students? If your students score well below published norms, you should attempt to determine the reason. When using published test norms, the factors described in the discussion of norm-referenced measurement should be considered. You may wish to establish local norms to reflect the progress the students have made in a particular program.

One final comment about a good test: when selecting a physical performance test, attempt to find a test that is similar to game performance. Students enjoy taking this type of test more than taking one that has no resemblance to the game skill for which they are being tested.

> Are you able to:
> describe the administrative criteria that should be considered in the selection and construction of tests?

You should feel capable of selecting good physical performance and written tests. Complete the review problems, and then we'll begin to prepare you to construct physical performance tests.

REVIEW PROBLEMS
1. Describe how you might use criterion-referenced measurement in a seventh-grade soccer class.
2. Select three sports skills tests and three other physical performance tests (e.g., agility, physical fitness, balance) described in this book and determine how well they meet test selection criteria.

4

Construction of Physical Performance Tests

Upon completion of this chapter, you should be able to:
1. Select physical performance tests that have been constructed properly; and
2. Construct single item tests that measure physical performance.

Though there are many adequate published tests for measurement of physical performance, there may be occasions when none of them meet the particular needs of your students; or, you feel that you are capable of devising a better test. The following guidelines will aid you in the construction of a good test. Since there is agreement on the techniques for estimation of the validity and reliability of norm-referenced tests, it probably would be best if you first developed this type of test.

KNOW WHAT IS REQUIRED OF A GOOD TEST

Prior to any attempt of constructing a physical performance test, you should be familiar with the criteria of a good test. Review the criteria in Chapter 3.

DEFINE THE PERFORMANCE TO BE MEASURED

The new test might be designed to measure a sports skill, a game situation, fitness, strength, flexibility or other related performances. You should define the exact performance you wish to measure and state the objective of the new test. Suppose you want to construct a new tennis serve test. Do you want to include the measurement of power in the test, or just measure the ability to serve the ball into the correct area? If it is to be a strength test, do you want to measure the strength of the leg, arm or another body part? It may be wise to name the muscles to be tested. If it is to be a flexibility test, you should identify the joint or body part to be measured. Also, include in your definition the group the test is to measure (i.e., sex and grade).

After you have identified and defined the performance to be measured, ask yourself:

1. Has the performance been included in the unit of instruction?
2. Can the performance be objectively measured?
3. Is there is no existing test that will meet my needs?

Once you are satisfied with your answers to these three questions, proceed to the next guideline.

ANALYZE THE PERFORMANCE

To construct a good test, it is essential that you analyze the performance to be measured; identify all components needed for a successful performance. (For example, performance in softball involves hitting, catching, throwing and running.) After you have identified the components, select the ones you want to measure. It is important that you give careful thought to this guideline. The components that you identify will determine the items you include in your test.

Suppose you want to construct a test to measure hitting ability. The skill of hitting may be broken down into four parts: grip, stance, swing and follow-through. Successful performance of the test should require the student to perform the fundamentals of these four parts in a mechanically sound way.

REVIEW THE LITERATURE

You should review tests that measure the same performance or related performance, and the research performed to develop the tests. This review will serve several purposes:

1. You will become more familar with the process of developing physical performance tests. You may find useful ideas that will aid you in your project.
2. You may choose to include previously published test items in your test.
3. You may find a previously validated test to use in establishing the validity of your test.
4. You will become more familiar with the components of the performance.

DEVISE THE TEST ITEMS

You now are ready to devise the item or items that will be included in your test. (You may also select published test items.) It is a good idea to develop more items than you actually plan to include in the test, and later select the best ones after analyzing all the items. Keep the following principles in mind:

1. Make the items as realistic as possible. If a sports skill is being measured, the item should be similar to the game situation. In addition, the items must be appropriate for the sex and age of the individuals being tested.
2. Make the items simple to perform. You do not want an item the students have difficulty remembering. If they hesitate or forget during test performance, the validity and reliability of the test will be affected.
3. Make the items practical. They should be inexpensive and require a minimum amount of time to administer.
4. Determine the test layout — dimensions and administrative order of items.
5. Make the scoring simple. Simplicity of scoring will aid objectivity, lessen the time required to train any assistants needed to administer the test and better enable the students to understand the scoring.

PREPARE THE DIRECTIONS

The directions must be clear and precise or the reliability and objectivity of the test will be affected. In addition, clear directions will prevent confusion among the students. When writing the directions, try to imagine questions that might be asked after the directions have been given to a group. Review the directions of tests found in this book and other textbooks to aid you in the wording.

HAVE THE TEST REVIEWED BY YOUR PEERS

This is not the time to be hesitant in asking for assistance in your project. Ask other instructors to study your test and offer constructive criticism. What may be clear or obvious to you, may not be to others. Asking for assistance now may prevent problems once you administer the test. Remember, when you ask for assistance, do not be over-sensitive if the other instructors are not in agreement with everything you have written. You do not have to accept all their suggestions; however, open-mindedness is important in constructing successful tests.

ADMINISTER THE TEST TO A SMALL GROUP
OF STUDENTS

At this point it would be wise to administer the test to a small group of students to determine if there are any problems with the directions, administration and scoring. Though not essential, having another instructor administer the test to a class while you observe and make notes of any problems, may be beneficial. The class must be representative of the group for which the test is designed. After the sample group has completed the test, make any necessary changes. If you administered more items than you plan to include in the final version of the test, you may wish to remove the items that appear to be troublesome.

DETERMINE THE VALIDITY, RELIABILITY AND OBJECTIVITY

Having completed the previous guidelines, you are ready to determine the validity, reliability and objectivity coefficients of your test by administering it to a large number of students. As with the small group, these students must be representative of the group for which the test is designed.

For norm-referenced tests, concurrent validity is usually desired. Concurrent validity can be estimated through one of the following methods.

1. If the test measures a sports skill, the scores can be correlated with tournament play. It is better to use a round-robin tournament since it provides the opportunity for the more skilled students to win. If the test is valid, the students who score well on the test will also place high in the tournament, and those who do poorly on the test will place low in the tournament.

2. The scores of your test can be correlated with the scores of a previously validated test. With this method it is necessary that you administer your test and the validated test; high correlation means that your test is valid. The obvious problem with this method is that you probably are devising your own test because the validated test is not acceptable (expense, time or some other reason). However, if a validated test is available, this is a good method.

3. The test scores can be correlated with the ratings of experts (individuals with a high degree of skill and/or knowledge in the sport). If using this method, it is necessary that you select or devise a rating scale. The rating scale should consist of numerical values accompanied by descriptive phrases. In other words, if 5 is the highest possible rating, there should be a phrase, or phrases, describing the skill the student must demonstrate to receive a rating of 5. An example of a rating scale for execution of the tennis forehand is found in Table 4-1. Prior to the experts rating the students, discuss the scale and be sure all experts are in agreement with the scale. If you elect to estimate the validity of your test through the use of expert ratings, review the discussion of rating scales in other sources before you attempt to construct a scale.

Reliability can be estimated through the methods of test-retest, parallel forms, split-half and the Kuder-Richardson formulas as described in Chapter 2. Use of the test-retest method will enable you to estimate reliability and objectivity coefficients at the same time.

DEVELOP NORMS

If you have constructed a norm-referenced test, a table of norms is needed. Review the calculation of z-scores, T-scores and percentiles described in Chapter 2; remember, norms are usually reported by age

Table 4-1. *Rating Scale for the Ability to Perform the Tennis Forehand*

5	Exceptional ability; ball consistently stroked with power; ball consistently lands close to base line
4	Above average ability; ball usually stroked with power; ball usually lands close to base line
3	Average ability; occasional power; capable of hitting ball deep but inconsistent in doing so
2	Below average ability; no power; ball consistently hit into opponent's forecourt
1	Inferior ability; ball is rarely hit over net

and sex. Since a large number of scores is required to develop the norms, it will be necessary that you test several classes. If this is not possible, you can accumulate test scores over a period of two or three years. You must administer the test the same way each time, however. Table 4-2 summarizes the guidelines for construction of physical performance tests.

INTERCORRELATIONS

This procedure is necessary only if your test includes several items (referred to as a test battery). When a test includes more than one item, all items should have high correlation with the criterion and low correlation with each other. The correlation of the items with each other is determined through a multiple correlation procedure. This procedure has been used with other statistical procedures to develop many of the physical fitness, motor ability and sports skills tests used in physical education programs. When constructing a test battery, all

Table 4-2. *Guidelines for construction of physical performance tests*

Review criteria of a good test
    validity, reliability, objectivity and administrative feasibility

Define the performance to be measured
    identify components for successful performance

Review the literature
    tests that measure the same performance or related performance

Devise the test items
    realistic, simple, practical, layout, scoring

Prepare directions
    clear and precise

Have test reviewed by peers
    open-minded

Administer test to small group
    representative of group for which test is designed

Determine validity, reliability and objectivity
    administer test to large group

Develop norms
    large number of scores required

items initially administered to the subjects are not expected to be included in the final test battery. When it is found that two items correlate highly with each other, the two items are considered to measure the same thing. The item that has the highest correlation with the criterion remains as part of the test while the other item is discarded. Since multiple correlation will not be discussed in this book, you should refer to a statistics book for the appropriate procedure.

Are you able to:
select a properly constructed physical performance test?
describe the procedures for construction of a physical performance test?

Your instruction for constructing physical performance tests is complete. Complete the review problem and then we will concentrate on the measure of knowledge and the construction of written tests.

REVIEW PROBLEM
1. Select three physical performance tests (at least one of them should have several items) described in this book and refer to the provided references for descriptions of their construction procedures. Note if the procedures are similar to the ones described for you. Also note how the validity and reliability of the tests were determined.

5

Construction of Written Tests

Upon completion of this chapter, you should be able to:
1. List and describe the steps for written test construction;
2. Construct a table of specifications and explain its use;
3. Define item analysis, item difficulty, and index of discrimination and conduct item analysis on test items;
4. Contrast the advantages and disadvantages of various test items; and
5. Construct true-false, multiple-choice, short answer, completion, matching and essay test items.

Since there are many good standardized physical performance tests available, it is possible that you will construct only a few of these tests while performing your responsibilities as a physical educator. The same cannot be said of written tests. If you enter the teaching profession, it is likely that you will construct many types of written tests throughout your career. If your responsibilities are in a fitness or wellness club, there probably will be occasions when you wish to determine the club members' knowledge of health-related matters. The information that you gather from the tests can aid you in determining the needs of the members and in the planning of appropriate programs.

As you gain experience in constructing written tests, you will find it less difficult to complete the task. However, at no time should you feel that a test can be constructed within a few minutes, or the night before it is to be administered. It takes time and planning to construct a good written test. You can expect only problems from a haphazard test. In addition, a poorly constructed test will not adequately fulfill the reasons for measurement, as described in Chapter 1.

STEPS IN CONSTRUCTION OF A TEST

There is more to test construction than writing the items. To construct a good test, five steps should be followed: test planning, test item construction, test administration, item analysis and item revision. Guidelines for these five steps, as well as construction of various types of objective items and essay items, will be covered in this chapter.

Test Planning

The first step in planning test items is consideration of content validity. The test should be representative of the instructional objectives and the content presented in the unit of instruction. The test should measure how well the students have fulfilled the objectives of the instructional unit.

With the unit objectives in mind, the next procedure is to develop a table of test specifications, which serves as an outline for construction of the test. Planning and adhering to a table of test specifications ensures that all material is covered and that the correct weight is given to each area. The table of test specifications indicates:

- kinds and number of test items
- kinds of tasks (thought processes) the items will present and the number of each kind of tasks
- content area and number of items in each area

(Some teachers also include an estimate of item difficulty.) Table 5-1 is an example of specifications for a volleyball test.

The most commonly used kinds of objective items are multiple-choice, true-false, matching and completion. The total number of items in a test is usually determined by the length of the class period, the length of the items, the difficulty of the items, the conditions under which the test is to be administered and the age of the students. Generally, most students should have time to try and answer all of the items, when working at a normal rate. You might estimate the slowest student able to answer multiple-choice items at the rate of one per minute and true-false items at the rate of two per minute. As you administer similar tests to similar groups your ability to estimate the time needed to complete a test will improve.

Several tasks, or thought processes, may be included on a test. In addition to knowledge (factual information), the test may require the students to demonstrate the ability to: comprehend, synthesize, evaluate, apply and analyze. You must decide if you only want a factual information test. Certainly it is easier to construct factual information items. If you attempt to construct the test items in a short period of time, you probably will put together this type of test. Though there is a need for items that measure knowledge, a good test will include various kinds of tasks. With adequate planning and practice you can develop the skill to write such a variety. When you plan the test specifications, plan for different kinds of tasks and the number of items for each task.

The content area deals with the areas covered during instruction. In a physical activity class, content might include such things as

Table 5-1. *Specifications for a 50-item Multiple-Choice Volleyball Test*

Content Area	Knowledge	Comprehension	Analysis	Application
		Task (number of questions and percentage of total)		
History	2(4%)			
Rules	5(10%)	5(10%)		5(10%)
Technique	2(4%)	5(10%)	8(16%)	
Offensive strategy	4(8%)			5(10%)
Defensive strategy	4(8%)			5(10%)

history, terminology, rules, equipment, technique or mechanical analysis, strategy and physiological benefits of participation. Before you begin construction of a test, plan the content areas and the number of items for each area. Too often physical education instructors spend only part of one class period describing the history of an activity and later administer a test that includes many historical questions. A good physical activity class test will include items dealing with rules, equipment, technique and strategy.

Item difficulty, which is the proportion of students who pass the item, should be related to the purpose for which the test is intended. It can be determined only after a test has been administered, and the ability to estimate it improves with experience. (Item difficulty is included in the section on item analysis.)

Observe Table 5-1 again. Notice that 15 items will be related to the rules of volleyball, but only five of the 15 items will be concerned directly with knowledge. The other 10 items cover comprehension and application of the rules. Development of test specifications makes you aware of the purpose of each item.

Test Item Construction

Regardless of the type of test item you construct, observe the following general guidelines:

1. Plan to allow enough time to complete the test construction. Put it aside after a few hours and work with it again a day or two later. It is rare that anyone is able to construct a good test without time to revise the items.

2. No item should be included on a test unless it covers an important fact, concept, principle or skill. Ask yourself three questions before you write the item: Why is the student responsible for this? What is the value of this point? What future benefit will it have?

3. Items should be independent of each other. This means that you should avoid items that provide answers to other items; correctly answering one item should not depend on correctly answering a previous item.

4. Write simply and clearly. Using correct grammar is essential, but try using terms and examples that the students understand. Avoid obvious, meaningless and ambiguous terms. Textbook

wording should be used rarely. The item should test the students' ability as related to the subject matter, not how well they interpret the item.

5. Be flexible. As a general rule the test should include more than one type of item. No one item is best for all situations or all types of material. Also, some students can better demonstrate their ability on certain types of items. (When using more than one type of item, place all items of a particular type together.)

6. Place easy items first. A test should have a difficulty of about 50 percent, but if easy items are to be part of the test place them at the beginning. When students have difficulty with the first few questions, they often are unable to concentrate on the remainder of the test. Easier items will build the confidence of the students.

7. As you construct the items, record the test number of each item in the table of test specifications. (For example, the numbers of the items that cover knowledge of history, application of rules, analysis of technique and other content areas and tasks are recorded in the appropriate row and column of the table.) You may find that you wish to change some of the specifications, but remember to monitor the content area and task of each item.

8. Prepare clear, concise and complete directions. Leave no doubt as to how the items are to be answered.

9. Ask other instructors to review the test. If they have problems with the wording of an item, it is likely the students will have problems also.

Test Administration

If you have correctly completed the above guidelines and also observe the following ones, you likely will have few problems during test administration.

1. Provide a typed copy of the test. It is annoying to have to interpret handwriting when taking a test.

2. Start the test on time. If you have constructed a test that requires approximately 50 minutes to complete, make sure the students have 50 minutes.

3. Be sure the test is administered under normal conditions. Whether you consider the test easy or difficult, it is not fair to the students to take the test under abnormal conditions.

4. Read the directions to the students. In their haste to begin the test, many students will begin before reading the directions.

Item Analysis

After you have administered and scored the test, you are ready to determine the quality of the items through a statistical procedure called **item analysis**. Item analysis serves to:
- indicate which items may be too easy or too difficult
- indicate which items may fail to discriminate clearly between

the better and poorer students for reasons other than item
difficulty
- indicate why an item has not functioned effectively and how it
  might be improved
- improve your skills in test construction

The exact procedures used in item analysis depend on the type of items
and test, the number of test-takers, the computational facilities
available and the purpose of analysis. More confidence can be placed
in item analysis when 100 or more tests are analyzed, but you can
obtain an indication of the quality of the items through analysis of a
smaller number of tests. Most item analyses are concerned with **item
difficulty, discrimination power** and **foil quality**. The first three
steps in item analysis are:

1. Arrange the scored tests in order from high score to low score.
2. Determine the upper 27% test scores and place them in one
   group. Do the same for the bottom 27% test scores. These groups
   are referred to as upper group (UG) and lower group (LG).
   Although upper and lower groups of 27% are considered the best
   for maximizing the difference between the two groups, any
   percentage between 25% and 33% may be used.
3. Tally the number of times the correct response to each item was
   chosen on the tests of each group.

Item difficulty: Item difficulty is defined as the proportion of
test-takers who answer an item correctly. If upper and lower groups
are not formed, the **difficulty index (p)** may be found by dividing the
number of test-takers correctly answering each item by the total
number taking the test.

$$p = \frac{\text{number answering correctly}}{\text{total number in group}}$$

If 50 students completed a test and 31 correctly answered an item, the
item difficulty would be .62.

$$p = \frac{31}{50} = .62$$

Another acceptable method for determining the difficulty index
requires use of upper and lower groups.

$$p = \frac{\text{number correct in UG} + \text{number correct in LG}}{\text{number in UG} + \text{number in LG}}$$

If the number correct in the upper group is 16, the number correct in the
lower group is 7 and the number in each group is 20, the item difficulty
is:

$$p = \frac{16 + 7}{20 + 20} = \frac{23}{40} = .58$$

Since it is necessary to separate the test scores into upper and lower
groups to determine the index of discrimination, you may prefer to use
the second method to determine item difficulty. You should note that
an easy item has a high index and a difficult item has a low index.

The typical norm-referenced test includes a range of difficulty, but the average test difficulty should be around 50%. The difficulty for criterion-referenced tests is established at the minimum proficiency level and, ideally, every student should pass every item at the end of the instructional unit. Since this is an unrealistic goal, however, items on criterion-referenced tests are usually constructed so that at least 80 to 85% of the students are expected to pass.

Interpretation of item difficulty is not always an easy task. The item may be easy because its construction makes the answer obvious or because the students have learned the material in the item. On the other hand, it may be difficult because it is constructed poorly, or because the students have not learned the material. You should consider all of these things if the item difficulty indicates the item is unacceptable, as it has been presented to the students. Table 5-2 shows the indices that may be used to evaluate item difficulty.

Table 5-2. *Evaluation of Item Difficulty*

Difficulty index	Item evaluation
.80 and higher	reject item
.71 – .79	may be accepted if index of discrimination is acceptable, but revise if discrimination is marginal
.30 – .70	good item
.20 – .29	may be accepted if index of discrimination is acceptable, but revise if discrimination is marginal
.19 and below	reject item

Item Discrimination: Item discrimination determines how well the item differentiates between the good student and the poor student. If the item discriminates, more students with high scores will answer the item correctly than will students with low scores. The index of discrimination is found by subtracting the number of the correct responses of the lower group from the number of correct responses of the upper group, and dividing the difference by the number of scores in each group. The formula is:

$$D = \frac{\text{number correct in UG - number correct in LG}}{\text{number in each group}}$$

With the same values that were used previously to determine an item difficulty of .58, the index of discrimination is:

$$D = \frac{16 - 7}{20} = \frac{9}{20} = .45$$

The index of discrimination can range from +1.00 to –1.00, but rarely do these extremes occur. A negative index indicates that more students in the lower group answered the item correctly than did in the upper group. An item with this negative index has no place in a test. Generally, an index of .40 or above on a norm-referenced test indicates that the item discriminates well. Table 5-3 lists the rules to consider when evaluating the index of discrimination for norm-referenced tests.

The usual item discrimination indices will not work for criterion-

Table 5-3. *Evaluation of Index of Discrimination**

Index of discrimination	Item evaluation
.40 and above	item discriminates
.30 – .39	reasonably good discrimination; may need improvement, particularly if item difficulty is marginal
.20 – .29	marginal discrimination, consider revision
below .20	reject item

*Ebel (1979)

referenced tests. One possible way to identify discriminating items for such tests is to administer the same item before instruction (pretest) and after instruction (posttest). Before instruction, few students should answer the item correctly, but after instruction most students should answer it correctly. If there is a large difference in the proportion of correct answers from pretest to posttest, the item discriminates.

A test item with a difficulty index between .30 and .70 has a good chance of being a discriminating item, but you should not assume this always to be true. Before you judge the quality of an item, consider the difficulty index and the index of discrimination.

Foil Quality: The choices for each item in a multiple-choice test are called foils, or alternatives. Ideally, in a multiple-choice test, each foil should be selected by some of the students. If a foil is not selected by any student, it has contributed nothing to the test. As a rule of thumb, a foil should be selected by at least 2 to 3% of the test-takers.

Another consideration is the pattern of incorrect responses by the upper and lower groups. For example, if an incorrect foil is selected by many students in the upper group but few in the lower group, it might suggest that the item needs revision. The item analysis of a multiple-choice test should include a record of the number that selected each foil as well as the item difficulty and index of discrimination. Table 5-4 shows the analysis of five multiple-choice items.

Item Revision

After completing the item analysis, you are ready to perform any necessary revision. Revision usually involves discarding or rewording some items, changing foils and changing items to different types (for example, changing multiple-choice items to true-false items). If you will perform the above steps the first time you administer a test, and analyze and revise the test after at least one additional administration of the test to a similar group, you will have a good test.

Are you able to:
describe the five steps in constructing written tests?
construct a table of test specifications and explain its use?
define item analysis, item difficulty, index of discrimination and conduct item analysis on test items?

Table 5-4. *Example of Item Analysis for Multiple-Choice Test*

60 students completed the test
Groups of 27% (16 test scores in each group)

Item		Foils				D	
		A	**B**	C	D	.50	.63
1	Upper Group	1	**13**	2	0		
	Lower Group	4	**3**	5	4		
		A	B	**C**	D		
2	Upper Group	0	1	**12**	3	.53	.44
	Lower Group	3	4	**5**	4		
		A	**B**	C	D		
3	Upper Group	0	**8**	0	8	.50	.00
	Lower Group	1	**8**	0	7		
		A	B	C	D		
4	Upper Group	**11**	3	2	0		
	Lower Group	**4**	10	2	0	.47	.44
		A	B	C	**D**		
5	Upper Group	2	4	3	**7**	.25	.38
	Lower Group	7	4	4	**1**		

Item 1. All foils considered, difficulty and discrimination good. Retain item.

Item 2. All foils considered, difficulty and discrimination good. Retain item.

Item 3. Foil C not considered and foil A considered only once, no discrimination. Reject item.

Item 4. Foil D not considered, difficulty and discrimination acceptable. Retain item but replace foil D.

Item 5. All foils considered, difficulty marginal and discrimination could be improved. Revise item.

OBJECTIVE TEST ITEMS

Many individuals often claim that objective test items permit correct responses on the basis of simple recognition, rote memory or association, and do not measure the thought processes of comprehension, analysis and application. These same individuals also believe that only essay tests can truly measure these thought processes. Objective items can measure different kinds of thought processes, but it takes time and effort to construct the items.

True-False Items

The true-false item is a declarative statement, and the test-taker must decide if the statement is correct or incorrect. The true-false item is widely used in teacher-made tests because items can be written rapidly and scored with ease.

Many teachers limit true-false items to factual content, but they can be used to test applications and principles. In addition, knowledge in the form of propositions can be measured. The following tennis items are examples of propositions:

T F   If the score is 15-30, the server is ahead in points.
T F   If the score is 15-30, the serve should be to the receiver's left service court.

Another excellent way to use the true-false item is to describe a situation, and then ask the students to respond to items about the situation. Game situations and strategy are very appropriate for this approach.

Advantages of true-false items are:
1. A wide range of material may be covered in a single testing period. The response time required by a true-false item is less than that required by multiple-choice or completion items, so more items may be included on a test.
2. The scoring is easy.
3. Ease of construction is given as an advantage, and generally this is true. However, if the true-false items are to measure thought processes other than simple knowledge, they will require some time to construct.

Disadvantages of true-false items are:
1. Since there are only two possible answers, random guessing could produce a score of 50 percent correct. Realizing this, many students do not study as they should.
2. Since the students have a 50% chance of guessing the correct answers, the reliability of the test items tend to be lower.
3. The correct answer often depends on one word.

Guidelines for Writing True-False Items: True-false items can be used effectively if you will adhere to the following guidelines.
1. Avoid the use of specific determiners. Words such as all, always, never, no and none are clues that the item is probably false. Words such as sometimes, usually and typically suggest that the item is probably true.
2. Include an equal number of true and false items, or include more false items than true ones. False items tend to discriminate more than true items.
3. Avoid the exact language of the textbook.
4. Avoid trick items. For example, using the wrong first name of an individual to make an item false is not a good practice.
5. Avoid negative and double negative terms. The inclusion of double negatives may confuse the students and does not contribute to testing their ability. If you feel that negative statements should be used, *underline* the negative term(s).
6. Avoid ambiguous statements. There should be no doubt the statement is completely true or completely false.
7. All items should be of the same approximate length. Some teachers have a tendency to make true statements longer than false statements.
8. Limit each item to a single concept. Items that include more than one concept are often confusing to the students.

One final comment about true-false items: An alternate format for the true-false item is to require the students to correct false statements. The major disadvantage of this technique is that often the item can be corrected in several ways. A better technique is to have the students identify only the false element in the item.

Examples of True-False Items: For each of the following statements, print a T in the blank in front of the statement if you believe it to be true, and an F if you believe it to be false. Each item has a value of 3 points.

_____ 1. If the standard deviation of a group of scores increases, the variability increases.

_____ 2. A T-score of 60 is located one standard deviation above the mean.

_____ 3. A correlation coefficient of +.60 is twice as significant as a correlation coefficient of +.30.

_____ 4. If the tail of a distribution curve is to the right, the skew is negative.

Read the described tennis situation and the statements that follow. If you believe the statement to be true, print a T in the blank in front of the statement. If you believe the statement to be false, print an F. Each item has a value of 3 points.

Player A makes a good serve and player B successfully returns it. Either player will now lose a point if:

_____ 1. the ball bounces twice on his side of the court.

_____ 2. he hits the ball and it touches the net before it lands in the opponent's court.

_____ 3. after hitting the ball, his racket slips out of his hand.

_____ 4. he hits the ball before it crosses the net.

Multiple-Choice Items

The multiple-choice item consists of two main components: the stem, and three to five foils. The foils also can be called alternatives; the incorrect alternatives can be referred to as distractors. The stem may be more than one sentence long, but it is usually a direct question or an incomplete statement. It should present the problem in enough detail so there is no ambiguity about what is being asked. There are several advantages of the multiple-choice items:

1. They can measure almost any understanding or ability. However, as with other test items, they will measure different abilities only if they are designed to do so. Too often multiple-choice items are constructed to measure only rote memory.
2. They can be used to test most types of material.
3. The chances of guessing the correct answer are much less than for true-false items.
4. They can be scored easily.

The disadvantages are:

1. They are more difficult to construct than other objective tests. Considerable time is required to develop good items that include at least four foils for each item.
2. They sometimes encourage memorization of facts rather than the understanding of concepts. As noted earlier, this can be corrected if the items are well planned.

3. Since fewer items can be asked than with true-false items (time element), less material can be covered.

Guidelines for Writing Multiple-Choice Items: Multiple-choice items are not easy to construct, but the following guidelines will aid you in the task.

1. The stem should be concise, easy to read and understand, and contain the central issue of the item. A properly constructed stem has meaning by itself so the good student knows the correct answer before reading all the foils. If the stem is an incomplete sentence or question, make the foil complete the stem.

2. All foils should be plausible, but there should be only one correct foil. Ridiculous or obvious foils have no place in the test. The student who does not immediately know the correct foil after reading the stem should have to consider all foils. If distractors are not chosen by some of the students, they should be eliminated from the test.

3. Use at least four foils for each item. If you can think of five good foils, use them. This keeps the guessing factor at .20. However, if you can think of only three acceptable foils for an item, use just three.

4. All foils should be grammatically consistent, homogeneous in content and approximately the same length. If the stem is singular, all foils should be singular. If some foils begin with a vowel while other foils in the same item do not, use "a(n)." Avoid the tendency to include more information in the correct foil than in the incorrect foils. This occurs when the stem is worded so the correct foil needs to be qualified.

5. Avoid negative wording; state the stem in the positive. If it is necessary to use negative words, capitalize each letter or *underline* them.

6. If the items are numbered, use A, B, C, D and E to designate the foils. Also, unless limited by the number of pages, the foils are easier to read if they are placed in vertical order rather than horizontal order.

7. Avoid patterns in the positions of the correct foils. Make a point to place the correct foil in each position approximately an equal number of times, i.e., use A, B, C, D and E equally.

8. Use the foil "none of the above" or "all of the above" with care. If you use "none of the above" all options must be clearly wrong, or one must be clearly correct. If the student has only four foils to consider, the use of "all of the above" reduces the student's discrimination task to three foils. It would probably be best to include a plausible fourth foil rather than use "all of the above."

9. When possible, list the foils in a logical or sequential order. When variables or dates are arranged in sequence the correct

foil should occasionally be the first or last in the sequence. This helps the student to overcome the tendency to disregard the extremes of the sequence as probably not correct.

10. If the item is testing the definition, or meaning, of a word, the word to be defined should be in the stem and the foils should consist of alternative definitions or meanings.

11. Although not mandatory, it sometimes helps the student if the stem begins with a "w" word such as which, why, where, what, when, who. This introduces the stem with the main point of the item.

12. Do not word the stem so that you are asking the student's opinion. If this is done, you may have difficulty defending one correct answer.

Examples of Multiple-Choice Items: Print the letter of the one correct answer on the blank line to the left of the item number. Each item has a value of 2 points.

_____ 1. For a knowledge test, a score of 55 has a percentile rank of 40. What does this indicate?
    A. 40 students answered 55 percent of the test correctly
    B. 40 percent of the students had a score of 55 or less
    C. 55 percent of the students had a score of 40 or less
    D. 40 percent of the students had a score of 55 or more

_____ 2. If the correlation coefficient between two variables is -.80:
    A. the relationship is quite small
    B. the relationship does not always exist
    C. the two variables are significantly unrelated
    D. the value of one variable decreases, as the value of the other variable decreases
    E. the value of one variable increases, as the value of the other variable decreases

_____ 3. Which muscle extends the lower leg and flexes the upper leg?
    A. quadriceps femoris   C. gluteus maximus
    B. biceps femoris   D. gastrocnemius

_____ 4. What is the approximate maximum heart rate of a 20-year old individual?
    A. 180   C. 200
    B. 190   D. 210

Short-Answer and Completion Items

The distinction between a short-answer and completion item is primarily the length and format of response. A short-answer item requires the student to respond to a question in a word, phrase, or a sentence or two. In a completion item, the simplest short-answer form, one to several words are omitted from a sentence, and the student is asked to provide the missing information. Both items are suited to measure factual knowledge, comprehension of principles and the ability to identify and define concepts. Identification items also are a form of short-answer items.

The advantages of short-answer and completion items are:
1. They are affected much less by guessing than are true-false or multiple-choice items.
2. They come closer to assessing recall, as contrasted with recognition, than does any other type of objective test item. This usually requires intensive study on the part of the student.
3. They are valuable when steps or procedures are to be learned.
4. They are easy to construct.

The disadvantages of these items are:
1. Scoring takes longer than for choice-type items, especially when only correct spelling is accepted.
2. Often, unless extreme care is taken in the construction of each item, a number of answers might be wholly or partially correct. The scorer has to decide which responses are acceptable and how much credit to give for each variation. This usually means that only the test constructor is able to score the tests.
3. They encourage rote learning; however, there are occasions when recall and memorization are appropriate (first aid and cardiopulmonary resuscitation [CPR], for example).

Guidelines for Writing Short-Answer and Completion Items: Though short-answer and completion items are easier to construct than other objective test items, these guidelines should be observed when constructing the items.
1. Be sure the item can be answered with a unique word, phrase or number, and there is only one correct answer.
2. Be sure the students know what type of response is required. Indicate also how precise the response should be. (This is especially true when computation of fractions or decimals is involved.)
3. Think of the answer first. Then try to write an item to which that answer is the only appropriate answer. By doing this you can avoid constructing items that have multiple correct answers.
4. With completion items, try to place the blank near the end of the sentence. This usually will make the intent of the item clearer and avoid the possibility of multiple answers.
5. Use no more that two blanks in an item. Too many blanks can make the item confusing to the student.
6. Avoid lifting items directly from the textbook. One sentence taken out of context from a paragraph may fail to adequately present the concept of the entire paragraph.
7. Make the actual blanks for the responses the same length. Varying the length of the blank according to the length of the expected answer provides clues for the students. (For ease of scoring, provide short blank lines in the item and blank lines of

appropriate length in a column to the right or left of the items for the student to write the responses.)

Examples of Short-Answer Items: Answer the following questions. They have a value of 3 points each.

1. What are the three measures of central tendency?
2. In a study of leg strength and hand grip, a correlation of -.90 was found. Interpret this correlation.
3. In a distribution of scores, the mean is 22 and the standard deviation is 2. What percent of the scores are between the scores of 16 and 28?

Examples of Completion Items: Complete the items by writing the correct answer on the blank line to the left of each item. Each item has a value of 2 points.

_____ 1. The _____ is usually the most reliable measure of variability.
_____ 2. A T-score of 75 is found ____ standard deviations above the mean.
_____ 3. In a T-scale, the mean is assigned a T-score of _____ .

Matching Items

The matching test usually consists of a column of items (stimulus words or phrases) on the left-hand side of a page and a column of options (alternatives) on the right. The student's task is to select the option that is correctly associated with the item. Matching items are similar to multiple-choice items in that the options serve as alternatives for all the items. They also are similar to short-answer items since they usually are limited to specific factual information (names, dates, labels).

The advantages of matching items are:

1. They are easy to construct and score.
2. They provide many scoreable responses per test page or per unit of testing time.
3. They motivate students to integrate their knowledge and to consider relations among the items.
4. The odds of guessing the correct answer are low.

The disadvantages are:

1. They are time-consuming to take.
2. They usually test only factual information.
3. They are limited to association tasks.

Guidelines for Writing Matching Items: To construct an effective and fair matching item test, use the following guidelines.

1. Include only homogeneous material in each matching exercise.
2. The basis for matching each item and option should be clear in the directions. The directions should inform the students if an

option can be used more than once, if each item has only one correct answer and how the marking is to be done.

3. The sets of items should be relatively short (five or six in the lower grades, and 10 to 15 in the upper grades). The shorter lists enable the students to respond more rapidly. If more matches are desired, arrange for several matching groups within a single test. Ideally, each group of matching items will involve a different topic.

4. All items and options for a matching exercise should be on one page. This arrangement enables the students to complete the exercise in a shorter time and reduces the likelihood of errors being made as a result of turning pages back and forth.

5. Use an appropriate format. Usually it is best to list the homogeneous items on the left and the options on the right. For ease of scoring, leave a blank space beside each numbered item for the letter of the matched option.

6. Arrange the responses in alphabetical or logical order. This will reduce the time required for the student to find the correct answer.

7. Develop more options than items. By having two or three more options, guessing will be reduced.

Examples of Matching Items: Select the letter of one option from Column II that best associates with a term in Column I. Print your answer on the appropriate line. Each response has a value of 3 points.

Column I	Column II
_____1. Turnverein	A. Sargent
_____2. Royal Central Institute of Gymnastics	B. Jahn
_____3. vertical jump	C. Naismith
_____4. physical education costume for women	D. Ling
_____5. basketball	E. Williams
	F. Bloomer
	G. Hitchcock

ESSAY TEST ITEMS

All the test items we have covered are considered objective items. The final item to be discussed is the essay item, which is evaluated subjectively. These items are designed to measure the students' ability to use higher mental processes — identify, interpret, integrate, organize and synthesize — and to express themselves by writing.

The advantages of the essay items are:

1. They are easily constructed, as several items can be constructed in a few minutes.

2. They can measure complex concepts, thinking ability, and problem-solving skills.

3. They encourage students to learn how to effectively organize and express their own ideas.

4. Guessing is minimized.

The disadvantages are:
1. They usually are very time-consuming to score.
2. The scoring requires some decision making on the part of the scorer; thus reliability may be decreased.
3. Since they take longer to answer, only a few items can be answered during one class period. This covers a limited field of knowledge.

Guidelines for Writing Essay Items

Though essay items seem the easiest test items to construct, there are guidelines which should be followed when preparing them.

1. They should require the students to demonstrate a command of essential knowledge. Too often essay items call only for reproduction of materials presented in the textbook or class lectures.
2. Each item should be phrased so there is only one correct answer. When items have more than one correct answer, it is difficult to evaluate the student's level of achievement.
3. Indicate the scope and direction of the required answer. Vague phrasing will lead to a wide variation of responses and make the task of evaluating the items even more difficult.
4. Require all students to answer the same items. If students answer different items, the basis for comparing the scores is limited. When students choose the items they can answer best, the range of test scores will probably be smaller, decreasing the reliability of the scores.
5. Indicate the approximate amount of time for the students to devote to each item, and the point value of each item. Many students need guidelines in how to budget their working time. Additionally, stating the amount of time that should be devoted to each item gives a clue as to the detail expected on a given item.
6. Generally it is best to use a reasonable number of short essay items than a few longer ones. Short essay items are likely to be less ambiguous to the student and easier to score.
7. Write the ideal answer to the item. This will give you a better idea of the item's reason, and will aid you in scoring the items.

Guidelines for Scoring Essay Items

Since essay items can be difficult to evaluate, these guidelines are provided.

1. Develop a method for scoring the tests. Some teachers identify essential points that should be included. Other teachers may rank each item according to the quality of response.
2. Evaluate the same item on all the students' papers before going on to the next item. It is also wise to occasionally check your consistency by reviewing how you evaluated an item on the first few papers you scored.

3. Try to conceal the name of the student whose test you are evaluating. Not knowing whose paper is being evaluated prevents the influence of any biases you may have toward students.

Examples of Essay Items

Read each item carefully and answer each one as completely as possible. The approximate amount of time that you should spend on each item and the point value of each item are indicated in parentheses.

1. Define correlation, and contrast the Spearman rank-difference correlation coefficient and the Pearson product-moment correlation coefficient. (10 minutes, 20 points)
2. Define standard scores and contrast T-scores, z-scores, and percentiles. (10 minutes, 20 points)
3. A teacher is interested in determining if her new teaching method is effective. Describe how she can determine its effectiveness. Include in your discussion:
   1. the testing procedures she should use
   2. when she should test
   3. the statistical analysis she should use (15 minutes, 30 points)

Are you able to:
contrast the advantages and disadvantages of the objective and essay items described in the text?
construct true-false, multiple-choice, short answer and completion, matching and essay test items?

You have completed your study of written test items. As you now know, there is much work required for construction of a good test, and using the different types of test items has advantages and disadvantages. All test items, however, can serve to measure the achievement of the students if the items are well constructed. Complete the review problems that are provided, and we'll move on to determining grades for students.

REVIEW PROBLEMS

1. Construct a written test for a high school tennis class. The test should include 30 multiple-choice items and 20 true-false items. Ask a friend to take the test and provide comments about any items that might need to be rephrased and about any foils that are obviously incorrect or correct.
2. A physical education teacher administered a 50-item knowledge test to her 200 ninth-grade students. After scoring the tests she determined the upper 27% and the lower 27% of the scores. She tabulated the following results for the first five items:

Item	Group	# Correct Answers
1.	Upper	44
	Lower	8
2.	Upper	45
	Lower	39
3.	Upper	35
	Lower	28
4.	Upper	14
	Lower	2
5.	Upper	37
	Lower	14

What are the item difficulty and index of discrimination of each item? Interpret your findings for each item.

6

Grading The Students

Upon completion of this chapter, you should be able to:
1. List and describe the use of grades;
2. List the three behavior areas and factors commonly graded in these areas, and state why some factors should not be graded;
3. List and describe the criteria for grades;
4. Define norm-referenced grading and the grading methods of natural breaks, standard deviation, percentage and norm, then describe the advantages and disadvantages of these methods;
5. Define criterion-referenced grading and the grading methods of contract and percentage-correct, then describe the advantages and disadvantages of these methods;
6. Define the weighting of factors and describe a method for performing this technique;
7. Describe four methods for reporting term grades; and
8. Describe your grading philosophy and develop a grading method that could be used in a teaching assignment.

Before we begin the discussion of grading in physical education, think back to your junior and senior high school days. Do you remember the grades you received in your physical education classes? Do you remember the factors that were used to determine your grades? Did you and the other students feel you were graded fairly? Hopefully, your instructors explained the factors that would be used to determine the grades and that all students were evaluated objectively, but too often this is not the case. Too many physical education instructors merely base grades on attendance, participation and effort. Students that miss some classes, fail to always take part in class activities and appear to be giving less than their best effort do not receive high grades. In other words, the instructor subjectively categorizes the students. There is nothing wrong with rewarding students for effort, but grades earned in physical education classes should involve more than participation and effort.

Proponents of grades based on participation argue that if objective grading is used, some students earn low grades and lose interest in physical education. It is possible that a few students who do not earn high grades will be upset, but they will not lose interest in a class because of grades. They lose interest when effective teaching does not take place. Effective teaching includes fair and objective grading.

Grades are recognized as symbols which denote progress and achievement toward established criterion-referenced or norm-referenced course objectives. As the teacher you will decide if the course objectives are criterion-referenced or norm-referenced, but grades should always be related to the objectives. There are different acceptable methods that can be used to determine grades, and the choice is yours. It is essential, however, that you be consistent and fair.

USE OF GRADES

If you enter the teaching profession, you will have the responsibility of reporting grades for every one of your students, each term. Grades may be reported differently, but they have important uses for four groups: students, parents, teachers and administrators. You should be prepared to discuss your grading policies and how you determined the students' grades with the four different groups.

Students

Grades inform the students of their achievement levels. When students have been informed of the course objectives, the evaluation methods, and the grade standards, they usually are not surprised by the grades they earn. However, most students like to be informed of their achievement levels by the teacher, and certain students will be challenged to work for higher marks. This motivation is more likely to occur if you have provided feedback to the students throughout the term, and if the students feel that you have a sincere interest in them. Unfortunately, for some students a good grade, rather than the attainment of course objectives, becomes the primary goal. Though it is difficult to prevent, you should attempt to counsel the students about this type of attitude.

Parents

Grades inform the parents of the progress and achievement of their children. Displeased when their children do not get the grades hoped for, some parents will ask you why their son or daughter did not receive a better grade in physical education. You will have a difficult time with many of these parents if you explain that their children did not have a good attitude, did not work hard enough in the class, and therefore did not deserve a better grade. On the other hand, if you explain the objectives of the instructional unit and how you evaluated the students, and provide the scores their children earned, your task will be less difficult. Do not expect all parents to agree with your methods of evaluation, but at least they will understand and probably appreciate the seriousness with which you consider grades. You may avoid such disagreements by sending the parents information about the purposes and objectives of physical education, and your grading philosophy, at the beginning of the school year.

Teachers

To determine the students' grades, it will be necessary that you do a comprehensive evaluation of all students. This evaluation will enable you to better know the strengths and weaknesses of the students. In addition, after evaluating the accomplishments of the students, you will be able to evaluate the effectiveness of your teaching and the efficiency of the program. If many students are failing to complete the objectives of the program, you need to examine your teaching methodology and the expectations of the program. It may be necessary to make changes in both.

The students' grades from previous physical education classes may be beneficial to you at the beginning of each school year. If the grades indicate the students' level of skill, you can readily identify the higher-skilled students, and if necessary, group the students. However, since different factors often are used to determine grades in physical education, you should assume that the grades indicate the skill level of the students only if you are familiar with the grading philosophy of the previous teacher.

Administrators

School administrators use grades to make decisions related to promotion, graduation, academic honors, athletic eligibility and guidance. They also use grades to determine if students have fulfilled educational objectives. Further, administrators place grades in every student's permanent record, which can have a positive or negative influence when the student applies for a job or admission to college.

Are you able to:
list and describe the uses of grades?

FACTORS USED IN GRADING

Many different factors are used by physical educators to determine the grades of students. All factors can be grouped under the three behavior areas of affective, cognitive, and motor.

Affective Factors

It is desirable that participation in a physical education program influence the affective behavior (attitudes and feelings) of students. Let's examine the factors that are usually considered to reflect affective behavior. (Affective behavior measurement is covered in Chapter 18.)

Sportsmanship: You always should insist that the students play fairly. They should exhibit good sportsmanship as winners or losers in a game or event. Those who do not should be disciplined. But, can you expect students who exhibit poor sportsmanship at the beginning of the term to change after participation in your class? Usually, poor sportsmanship is due to emotional problems other than those that arise during a game situation, and requires more than grades to improve these behaviors. When sportsmanship is used in determining the grade, students are likely to interpret it as a penalty for misbehavior rather than as something that is earned.

Perhaps the best method for dealing with sportsmanship problems is to insist upon it during class participation, and to individually counsel students about their behavior. This method will require that you keep written records of incidents of poor sportsmanship. Try this approach, and your students may realize that you have a sincere interest in their personal development.

Attendance, Participation and Showering: Skill development takes place through proper instruction, participation and practice of fundamentals. Students who fail to attend class regularly, and who have poor skills, usually do not improve or fulfill other course objectives. If grades are related to the extent the students fulfill course objectives, these students will not earn good grades. A teacher may not have an attendance policy, but these students have been penalized by their poor attendance.

On the other hand, there may be highly skilled students who are able to complete the course objectives at a satisfactory level, or better, without regular attendance. Should you lower the grades of these students? Since most school systems have attendance policies, problems related to attendance should be handled by the principal, not by the teacher. Base your grades on completion of course objectives, not attendance.

Perhaps more of a problem occurs when students attend class, but do not dress out for some reason. Again, it is best not to use the grade as a threat, but to attempt to make the class enjoyable and challenging for the students. If you are successful in developing this type of class atmosphere, the students will want to participate.

Similar to these two factors is the practice of grading the students on showering. Though the students should be instructed in the importance of showering after physical activity, there may be reasons that some students do not wish to shower. For example, the showers may not permit privacy for the students who desire it. Or, the instructor may not allow enough time to cool down before showering. Even if these are not the reasons students avoid showering, grading for showering is not a good practice. Advise and encourage, but do not reward students for showering, nor penalize them for failing to shower.

Effort: Effort is difficult to evaluate objectively. A poorly-skilled individual may appear to be putting forth much effort, while a highly-skilled individual appears to be putting forth little effort. Should the highly-skilled student be penalized? If effort is graded, it is possible that the poorly-skilled individual will receive the same grade as the highly-skilled individual. Is this fair? Some teachers argue that when effort is graded the students are motivated to try harder. Perhaps this is true, but as a teacher you have the responsibility to promote inner motivation. Even though it sounds idealistic, the students' desire to excel should come from within, not from external rewards.

If you wish to include effort as a course requirement, seek to develop an objective method for evaluating it. You could develop realistic grade standards, so that anyone who puts forth the effort will at least be able to meet the minimum standards for the class.

Cognitive Factors

There is general agreement that grading in physical education should include mental factors. Though many teachers limit the mental evaluation to knowledge of rules, history and fundamentals, the student also should be required to demonstrate the ability to understand, and apply and analyze rules, strategy and technique. As stated in Chapter 5, it takes time to construct tests that will properly measure these factors, but the teacher has the responsibility to do so.

Motor Factors

Most physical educators grade the motor skill of students. The degree of emphasis will vary, but teachers usually grade skill in the activity, game performance and fitness.

Skill in the Activity: Two aspects of skill are generally used when grading the skill in an activity: achievement and improvement. Grading for achievement consists of measuring the skill of the students at the conclusion of an instructional unit and assigning the appropriate grades. As with any cognitive or motor skill the levels of ability will vary; unless the standards for skill are very low, only a portion of the students usually earn high grades.

Perhaps the most important consideration when grading skill achievement is to establish realistic norm-referenced or criterion-referenced objectives. If a school system has a coordinated physical education program, it is less difficult to plan realistic objectives because teachers are aware of the students' movement backgrounds. Knowing the physical education objectives for the previous years, and the skills the students were expected to develop, enables a teacher to plan the appropriate objectives.

When a class has a variety of students with limited movement backgrounds, and some students with good movement backgrounds, it is difficult to establish fair objectives. The skill objective may be too low for the students with good movement backgrounds, and too difficult for other students. (The availability of beginning and advanced classes will help prevent this problem, but such classes are not always possible in many school programs.) When this dilemma does occur, the approach of some teachers is to homogeneously group the students in a class and use different grading standards for each group. However, if this method is used, problems can add up: (1) some students with better than average skill may deliberately seek to be placed in the lower-skilled group, in an attempt to assure a good grade, and (2) if the student's record does not indicate beginning or advanced class, what do the grades for the different groups mean? Does the grade of "B" earned by a student in the lower-skilled group mean the same as a "B" earned by a student in the higher-skilled group? For these reasons, many physical education teachers agree that the level of achievement should be evaluated in the same way for all students in a particular class.

Some physical educators believe that students should be graded on skill improvement. It is desirable that all students improve their skill through participation in a physical education instructional unit, but is it fair to all students to grade on improvement? In addition, can improvement be measured accurately? Usually, improvement is measured by administering a test at the beginning and at the end of an instructional unit, and subtracting the pretest score from the posttest score. The difference in the scores is interpreted as the improvement score. There are several problems associated with this technique.

1. When students know that improvement is a factor in grading, some may deliberately score low on the pretest to show much improvement on the posttest.
2. Testing some skills before a minimum level of proficiency has been developed can be dangerous (gymnastics and wrestling, for example). In addition, fitness testing should not be done on poorly-conditioned individuals.
3. With some activities, the instructional term may not be long enough to provide students adequate time to practice and show improvement. Also, if the instructional term is too long, the improvement of some students may be due to physical maturity rather than ability.
4. If all students perform at their best on the pretest, the low-skilled students may have an advantage in the earning of high grades because they have greater potential for improvement. The high-skilled students will probably improve very little. To correct for this inequity, a scale for improvement must be developed for each skill level. Several hundred scores should be collected and analyzed to develop such a scale. The students with high skill should not be expected to improve as much as the students with low skill.
5. Subject areas such as math, English, science and history do not grade on improvement. If physical education is to be accepted in the same way as other subjects, grades should not be based on improvement.

You can see the disadvantages of grading on improvement appear to far outweigh any advantages. If you feel that it is important to report improvement, do so with a form separate from the grade report.

Game Performance: Grading game performance for individual activities may be done through tournament play. Tournaments should be double elimination or round-robin play, however. It is usually necessary to grade game performance in team activities through subjective evaluation. The individual should be graded on contributions to the team, as well as individual accomplishments.

Fitness: Though the educational objective of physical fitness is unique to physical education, many physical educators do not include it in the grading process of all activities. It may be that it is not practical to provide class time in all instructional units for fitness activities, but after a fitness unit has been completed, the students should be expected to maintain a specified level of physical fitness throughout the school term.

Are you able to:
list the three behavior areas and the factors commonly graded in these areas, and state the reasons why some of these factors should not be graded?

CRITERIA FOR GRADES

As you now are aware, many factors can be considered in the grading of students. Some factors can be accurately and fairly graded, while other factors are best served by reporting them directly to the students and parents (rather than including them in the reported grade.) Barrow and McGee (1979) provide the following criteria for grades. If observed, you will have a grading process that is educationally sound and fair to the students.

1. Grades should be **related to the educational objectives**. If a factor has not been included as an instructional objective, it should not be graded.
2. The grades should have **validity, reliability and objectivity**. Grades should indicate achievement of the factors that they purportedly represent. The validity of a grading method is low when the grades are not related to the instructional objectives.

    A grading system should be consistent. It should yield the same grade for the same performance, regardless of the number of times the grade is calculated. In addition, unless modifications are made, it should yield the same results for the same performance year-to-year.

    Though it may be necessary to grade some factors subjectively (e.g., gymnastics), a grading system should be as objective as possible. A grading system has high objectivity if several teachers can perform the same measurements on students and arrive at the same final grade. If some factors can only be measured subjectively, checklists or rating scales should be used.

Grades that are determined subjectively are usually unreliable and difficult to defend if challenged.

3. The **weight** (the percentage or proportion of the total grade) of each graded factor should be related to the emphasis placed on the factor during the instructional unit. It is possible, but unlikely, that all graded factors will have equal weight. An illustration of the weights of factors is provided in Table 6-5.

4. The weights of the factors and the method with which the final grade is determined should be **understandable** to the students and parents. Each student should be able to determine the earned grade before it is provided by the teacher. The technique for determining grades should not be a secret to the students and parents, and neither should it be so complicated that they do not understand it.

5. Whether grades are norm-referenced or criterion-referenced, they should **discriminate** the good student from the poor student. Students who perform at a high level should receive better grades than students who perform at a lower level. As in other subject areas, physical education grades should discriminate between the levels of attainment.

6. The grades should have **administrative economy**. An educationally sound grading system should be used, but the system should be feasible in terms of time, cost and personnel. Remember, clerical help for the teacher is limited, and grades must be prepared in a short time period. If the grading system requires so much time that other teaching responsibilities suffer, it is not practical. Microcomputers are now being used to record and determine grades, giving teachers more instructional time.

Are you able to:
list and describe grading criteria?

METHODS OF GRADING

There are many different grading methods used by physical education teachers. Regretably, not all are good. Grading systems are classified as either norm-referenced or criterion-referenced, and both include very good methods of grading.

Norm-Referenced Grading

The norm-referenced system of grading is based on the normal probability curve that was described in Chapter 2. Norm-referenced standards compare the performance of the students with each other. Levels of performance that discriminate among ability groups are developed. The levels of ability may range from high to low; the appropriate grade is used to indicate the attained ability. There are many different methods of norm-referenced gradings, not all of which are acceptable. Several methods follow.

Natural Breaks Method: Generally, when test scores are ranked, gaps occur in the distribution. These breaks may be used as cut-off points for letter grades. Though quick and convenient for the teacher, this method is not recommended. A student's grade depends only on where the gaps occur, and there certainly is no consistency from one term to another. A numerical grade may be a "B" one term, but an "A" another term. Table 6-1 shows how this method may be used.

Table 6-1. *Grades Assigned by Natural Breaks Method*

95		79	
95		77	
93		77	
93		76	
92		76	
91		75	
91	A	73	
....		73	
88		72	
87		72	C
87		....	
86		69	
85		68	
85		66	
83		64	
82	B	63	D
....		....	
		57	
		55	F
		....	

Standard Deviation Method: This method assumes that the scores are normally distributed, and that the standard deviation can be used to determine the grades. So, the first thing you must do is to calculate the mean and the standard deviation of a distribution of scores. You then have several choices for arranging the distribution into sections for grade purposes. Table 6-2 shows three arrangements. For illustration purposes, look at a sample written test that has a mean of 74 and a standard deviation of 6. The arrangement in Example 3 is used.

The "C" range is determined first since its range affects the "B" and "D" ranges.

$$C = \overline{X} \pm 0.5s$$
$$= 74 \pm (.5)6$$
$$= 74 \pm 3$$
$$C = 71 \text{ to } 77$$

The upper limit of the "B" range is:

$$B = \overline{X} + 1.5s$$
$$= 74 + (1.5)6$$
$$B = 83$$

The lower limit of the "D" range is:

D $= \overline{X} - 1.5s$

$\quad = 74 - (1.5)6$

D $= 65$

The ranges for the grades are:

A = above 83

B = 78 to 83

C = 71 to 77

D = 65 to 70

F = below 65

If this method is used with a small class, the percentage of scores for each grade is not likely to be exactly the same as presented in Table 6-2. (A distribution for a small number of scores does not usually result in a normal distribution.) The standard deviation method of grading is best when scores are collected for several classes and grouped into one distribution. It may be necessary to collect the scores over a period of two or more years, but the larger set of scores will result in an approximately normal distribution. Once you have established a grade range based on a large distribution of test scores, you can convert subsequent scores for the test into letter grades. Used in this manner, the standard deviation method is an acceptable norm-referenced grading system.

Percentage Method: Using the percentage method, the teacher decides what percentage of the class is to receive each letter grade, lists

Table 6-2. *Grades Assigned by Standard Deviation Method*

		Example 1	
Grade	Standard Deviation Range	Percent	
A	2.0s or more above mean	2	
B	Between +1.0s and +2.0s	14	
C	Between +1.0s and –1.0s	68	
D	Between –1.0s and –2.0s	14	
F	2.0s or more below mean	2	

		Example 2	
Grade	Standard Deviation Range	Percent	
A	1.75s or more above mean	4	
B	Between +0.75s and +1.75s	19	
C	Between +0.75s and –0.75s	54	
D	Between –0.75s and –1.75s	19	
F	1.75s or more below mean	4	

		Example 3	
Grade	Standard Deviation Range	Percent	
A	1.5s or more above mean	7	
B	Between +0.5s and +1.5s	24	
C	Between +0.5s and –0.5s	38	
D	Between –0.5s and –1.5s	24	
F	1.5s or more below mean	7	

the grades in order and assigns the grades. For example, suppose a teacher has a class of 30 students. Table 6-3 shows how many students would receive each letter grade with three different groups of percentages.

Examples 1 and 3 of Table 6-3 also show one of the problems encountered with this method. The selected percentage may require the rounding of numbers, which results in a different total than the actual number of students. Example 1 totals 29 and example 3 totals 31. When this occurs the teacher must decide which letter grade is to be received by more or less students than indicated by the percentage.

There is another problem with this method. Suppose in Example 2, when the scores are listed in order, the highest five are:

94
92
91
91
91

Only the highest three scores should receive the grade of "A", but scores 3, 4, and 5 are the same. The teacher must decide if only the highest two scores receive an "A," or the highest five. If only two scores receive the grade of "A," more than six students will be given a "B." If five scores are given the grade of "A," less scores will be given a "B." This problem could occur anywhere in the distribution and with any percentage group.

Table 6-3. *Grades Assigned by Percentage Method (class of 30 students)*

	Example 1		Example 2		Example 3	
Grade	% of Students	# of Students*	% of Students	# of Students	% of Students	# of Students*
A	7	2	10	3	15	5
B	24	7	20	6	20	6
C	38	11	40	12	30	9
D	24	7	20	6	20	6
F	7	2	10	3	15	5

*Will not total 30 due to rounding of numbers.

There are other disadvantages with this method. Average-ability students will receive higher grades in a class with low-ability students, than in a class with high-ability students. Also, consider if the class is homogeneous in ability. Though all students are approximately equal in ability, some students will receive high grades and some will receive low grades. Finally, there is no consistency with this method. A particular score may vary from term to term in the grade assigned to it.

The disadvantages of the percentage method can be overcome if it is used in the same way as the standard deviation method. A large number of scores should be collected before the percentage groups are designated. Once the percentage groups ("A," "B," "C," "D," "F") have been determined with a large number of scores for a particular test, subsequent test scores can be assigned the appropriate letter grade. The problems of the percentage method still may occur, but only during the initial determination of the letter grades. Once the letter grades have been assigned to the scores, these problems will be eliminated. Used specifically in this manner, the percentage method is acceptable for norm-referenced grading.

Norms Method: Norms are performance standards based on analysis of scores. They are developed by collecting scores for a large number of individuals of similar sex, age, experience, ability and other such characteristics. Norms may be developed at the national, state or local level. At any of these levels, several hundred scores should be collected and analyzed before the norms are accepted. Percentiles, T-scores and z-scores are forms of norms.

The norms method is an excellent system for norm-referenced grading for several reasons. The norms may be used for several years before new norms need to be developed. Also, they are unaffected by the group being tested since all students in the group could excel in performance and earn a high grade. Finally, they have consistency in that the grade for a given performance will be the same for a group during any school term. (The procedures for developing norms are described in Chapter 2.)

Criterion-Referenced Grading

Criterion-referenced standards are clearly defined; the students know exactly what is expected of them. Standards may be developed for each grade that can be earned, or the standards may be pass-fail. When standards are developed for each grade, the students choose to work for a particular grade, and they are not in competition with each other. If pass-fail, the standards represent the level of ability that most students should be able to achieve during the instructional unit.

Contract Method: The contract grading method can be used with a class or with each student. With the class contract, the quality, amount and type of work to be performed to earn the various grades are the same for all members of the class. For example, in a 10th-grade softball class, the "A" grade standards for each girl might be:

- Score 19 or above on overhand throw for accuracy
- Score 19 or above on the fielding test
- Score 90 or above on the written test
- Write a one-page report on the technique of bunting
- Write a one-page report on the technique of fielding a ground ball in the outfield and throwing to home plate

Other standards would be written for the remaining grades. The teacher may or may not permit the class to assist in the developing of the contract. With the individual contract, the teacher and student agree upon the type, amount and quality of work the student must do to earn a particular grade. Each student could have a different contract, and every student could earn an "A" grade.

This method of grading allows for individual differences in ability and for successful performance, as defined by the student. Too often when this method is used, however, the emphasis is on the quantity of work, rather than the quality of work. If quality standards can be designed, this system is acceptable for criterion-referenced grading.

Percentage-Correct Method: Teachers often use the percentage-correct method for grading. With this method, the student is advised what percentage of attempts must be correct to earn the various grades. Table 6-4 shows four examples of this method. The percentage-correct method also can be used with physical performance scores, but there will be no maximum score for performances such as throwing and jumping events. In these events the grade of "A" or "A+" would be any score greater than a specified score. The standards for the grades should be based on previous test scores which have been analyzed, not standards the teacher arbitrarily selects.

When using the percentage-correct method, it is sometimes difficult to compare different tests, since the level of difficulty for the tests will not always be the same. A grade of 85 on one written test may be a better score than a grade of 85 on another test, depending on the test difficulty. (This problem could occur with physical performance tests also.) When one test is considered more difficult than another, different weights should be assigned to the tests.

Table 6-4. *Grades Assigned by Percentage-Correct Method*

	Grade	Example 1	Example 2
	A	90 to 100	93 to 100
	B	80 to 89	85 to 92
	C	70 to 79	77 to 84
	D	60 to 69	70 to 76
	F	below 60	below 70
		Example 3	Example 4
	A+	98 to 100	98 to 100
	A	94 to 97	95 to 97
	A–	90 to 93	93 to 94
	B+	87 to 89	91 to 92
	B	83 to 86	87 to 90
	B–	80 to 82	85 to 86
	C+	77 to 79	83 to 84
	C	73 to 76	79 to 82
	C–	70 to 72	77 to 78
	D+	67 to 69	75 to 76
	D	63 to 66	72 to 74
	D–	60 to 62	70 to 71
	F	below 60	below 70

The percentage-method is an acceptable criterion-referenced grading system if the grade standards are determined as objectively as possible. It is a better system when the instructor assigns weights to factors or tests, with different degrees of difficulty. There are no limits on the number of students who may earn high grades, and the students know exactly what they must do to earn a particular grade.

WHICH METHOD OF GRADING IS BEST?

Only a few of the grading methods used in physical education have been presented in this chapter. These, and many others, are not without faults. As teachers gain experience, they develop a method that suits them best. However, all teachers, beginning and experienced, should use a grading system that fulfills the grading criteria previously described, and one they agree with philosophically. If you teach, a major decision will be whether to use criterion-referenced grading or norm-referenced grading. Since both have a place in the grading process, you should be prepared to use either, depending which best serves the needs of the students and the teacher.

THE WEIGHTING OF FACTORS

Usually a teacher places more emphasis on certain factors in a teaching unit, meaning those factors have more value in determining the unit grade. To reflect the importance of these factors, weights are assigned to them. If evaluation scores for all factors are averaged without the assigning of weights, all scores will have equal value. As previously stated the use of weights should be considered with knowledge and physical performance tests, as well as when one test is more difficult than another. Table 6-5 shows how weights might be used with a tennis unit. Note that the motor area has a weight three

Table 6-5. *Use of Weights in Determining Grade for Tennis*

Area	Weighting of Area	Factor	Weighting of Factor	Grade	Points
Motor	6	Skill test	3	B+	27
		Game performance	1	B+	9
		Tournament standing	2	A+	24
Cognitive	2	Written test	2	A–	20
TOTALS	8		8		80
COMMENTS:	Grade = 10 (A–)				

times greater than the cognitive area. Also note that game performance has the least weight in the motor area. This is done because the grade for game performance is determined through subjective evaluation, whereas the skill test and tournament standing grades are determined objectively. If letter grades are assigned for these factors, a numerical table for conversion of letter grades, as shown in Table 6-6, should be available.

Table 6-6. *Numerical Conversion Table for Letter Grades*

A+ = 12	B+ = 9	C+ = 6	D+ = 3	F = 0
A = 11	B = 8	C = 5	D = 2	
A- = 10	B- = 7	C- = 4	D- = 1	

Are you able to:
define the weighting of factors and describe a method for performing this technique?

REPORTING OF FINAL GRADES

Teachers may have a choice in a grading method, but they usually do not have a choice in how the grades are to be reported. All teachers within a school, or school system, are required to report grades in the same way.

Letter - The letter grades "A," "B," "C," "D," and "F" are most commonly used. Some school systems use + and–with the grades, "A+," "A," and "A-." Often this requires the teacher to convert numerical grades into letter grades, so a system, as shown in Table 6-4, is needed.

Numerical - The numerical average is reported rather than a letter grade. The grade may be the average of the actual scores or of the percentage correct. Though letter grades are not reported with this method, some schools equate the numerical ranges with letter grades: "A" = 93 to 100, "B" = 85 to 92, and so forth.

Pass - fail - The grade indicates only if the student has been successful or unsuccessful in completing the course objectives.

Descripters - Words, terms and phrases are used to describe the student's performance. Examples are: excellent, above average, average, below average, working at near capacity, making moderate use of ability, working substantially below ability, outstanding progress, appropriate progress, progress below capabilities, little or no progress.

Are you able to:
describe four methods for reporting grades?

Grading is not always an enjoyable task, but it is a necessary one. It is not a responsibility that is to be taken lightly. A grading system should be fair, consistent, related to the educational objectives and as objective as possible. Teachers who arbitrarily devise grading systems are failing in their responsibilities to the students, parents and administration. Complete this review problem and we'll begin to study the administration of physical performance tests, and many of the tests that are available for use.

REVIEW PROBLEM

1. Imagine that you have accepted a teaching position in a junior high school. You have been asked by the principal to provide your grading philosophy and a grading system for a tennis unit. Include the use of weight factors in your grading system.

7

Testing Physical Performance

Upon completion of this chapter, you should be able to:
1. Describe the proper procedures for administration of physical performance tests;
2. Properly administer physical performance tests; and
3. Define motor ability, motor capacity and motor educability.

Do you remember taking physical performance tests during your junior and senior high school physical education classes? When the students arrived for class were the instructors prepared to administer the tests, or were they rushing to complete test preparations? Were they familiar with the test items, or did they appear to be unsure as to how the items should be administered? Did they require all students to perform the items correctly, or did they permit some students to perform the items incorrectly? Did they interpret the test results to the class, or were the students informed of the test results only through a grade? These questions illustrate the many responsibilities associated with the administration of physical performance tests. This chapter will teach you to properly administer such tests.

TEST ADMINISTRATION RESPONSIBILITIES

The administration of physical performance tests requires pretest, testing and posttest responsibilities. If a test is to be effective and the purposes of testing are to be fulfilled, the responsibilities in all three areas must be completed. The following testing responsibilities are described for (1) a school environment and (2) as if the test has more than one item. These responsibilities are basically the same, however, regardless of what type group is tested or how many items are included in a test.

Pretest Responsibilities

Pretest responsibilities include anything that is to be done before the students arrive to take the test. Those responsibilities are:

117

1. Provide opportunities for the students to practice the test items, or activities similar to the items. Through practice the students will know how to perform the items and know exactly what is expected during the testing. The purpose of the test also should be described.
2. Prepare the scorecards. The scorecards should be easy to follow and to use. If scorecards are not to be used, be prepared to score the results in another manner.
3. Train all test assistants and make sure they are familiar with their responsibilities. They should know how to administer the test, and be aware of all safety precautions. In addition, they should be prepared to deal with any unplanned developments that may occur during testing.
4. Know exactly how the test instructions are to be given to the group. Practice giving the instructions. If the instructions are rather involved, it may be wise to write them on paper.
5. If smaller groups are needed, plan how they are to be formed. If the absence of several students could affect your method for forming groups, plan more than one method.
6. Review all safety precautions. No one should be injured while performing the test because you failed to take safety precautions.
7. Provide all necessary equipment and floor or court markings. Test the equipment for safety and make sure nothing is on the field or court that is unsafe.

Testing Responsibilities

When all pretest responsibilities are completed, the testing responsibilities are easier to perform. The essential responsibilities are:
1. Organize the group for instructions. The purpose of the test should have been discussed during a previous class meeting, but if it has not, do so at this time.
2. Give test instructions. Always face the group and speak clearly. Do not attempt to give the instructions or demonstrate the items with your back to the group.
3. Demonstrate test items. If more appropriate, items may be demonstrated after smaller groups are formed. Whenever possible, have someone demonstrate the items while you describe them.
4. If test assistants are available, form smaller groups. The number of groups formed may depend on the number of items on the test.
5. Administer the test items. Insist that all individuals perform the items correctly. Remember that the validity and reliability of the test are affected if all students are not required to perform the items in the same way.
6. If time allows, gather the group for reaction to the test and any beneficial discussion.

Posttest Responsibilities

If the test is to have meaning to the students, the following posttest responsibilities should be completed.

1. Score all test items. Scoring the test may require the use of norms. If norms (standardized or local) are available, this is a simple task. If they are not available, develop your own. Whether the test is norm-referenced or criterion-referenced, you should calculate the mean, mode, median, deciles and standard deviation of the test. These values will be useful in reporting the test results to the class and in comparing classes.

2. If you are testing for grading purposes, determine the grade for each student.

3. Interpret the test results to the students. This should be done immediately after the test has been taken, and it should involve more than just reporting the students' grades. If some students did not perform well on the test, discuss the possible reasons with them. Also, if criterion-referenced standards are used, students still would like to know how the class did as a group.

4. Evaluate the test. Did the test fulfill your reasons for testing? Was it a learning experience for the students? Did the pretest, testing and posttest responsibilities go well? Make notes of any changes you should make in your responsibilities for the next administration of the test.

These are the major responsibilities for physical performance testing. Test administration becomes easier with experience, but you should never take test responsibilities lightly.

> Are you able to:
> describe the proper procedures for administration of physical performance tests?

TYPES OF PHYSICAL PERFORMANCE TESTS

During the first half of the 20th century there was much interest in measuring the motor ability of students. This included the innate and acquired ability of an individual to perform motor skills of a general nature, exclusive of highly specialized sports or gymnastic skills. For three reasons, however, the measurement of motor ability is no longer popular. First of all, many physical educators question the existence of a general motor ability. They feel that abilities are highly specific to the performance task. Secondly, the construct validity of motor ability test batteries has never been established. Lastly, there is no common agreement on what the components of motor ability are.

During the same time period that motor ability testing was popular, tests were designed to measure motor capacity (the individual's potential ability to perform motor skills) and motor educability (the individual's ability to learn new motor skills). These tests also are no longer popular. It now appears that many physical educators measure the physical performance qualities of agility, balance, circulorespiratory endurance, flexibility, muscular strength and muscular endurance. Though there is no common agreement on the basic qualities that underlie physical performance, it cannot be disputed that individuals with poor abilities in these qualities are less likely to succeed in sports and other physical activities. Tests often are used to identify these individuals so appropriate activities may be prescribed to improve their weak abilities. In addition, due to the current emphasis on well-being and health fitness, physical educators employed in schools and fitness centers are measuring the components of health fitness (cardiorespiratory fitness, flexibility, muscular strength, muscular endurance and body composition).

Conducted since the early 1900s, sports skills measurement is very popular today. Sports skills measurement is popular because most, if not all, junior and senior high physical education programs include the development of sports skills as a major objective. It is important that valid, reliable and objective tests be used to measure these skills. To assure that such tests are available, the AAHPERD in 1959 began a project to revise existing skills tests, to develop new ones for some sports and to determine new standards in 15 sports. The project has not been completed as this text goes to press, but new standards have been developed for several sports skills tests. Other than the AAHPERD project, very few new sports skills tests or norms have been developed in recent years.

8

Agility

Upon completion of this chapter, you should be able to:
1. Define and measure agility;
2. State why agility should be measured; and
3. Prescribe activities to improve agility.

Agility, sometimes referred to as the maneuverability of the body, is the ability to rapidly change the position and direction of the body, or body parts. Heredity is a major factor in an individual's level of agility, but it also depends on strength, speed, coordination and dynamic balance. In fact, many individuals are able to improve agility by increasing their ability in these variables. Agility also can be improved through instruction, training and practice of agility drills.

Agility is important in all activities and sports. Individual and team sports involve quick starts and stops, rapid change of direction, efficient footwork and quick adjustments of the body, or body parts. Individuals with good agility have a better chance of success in physical activity than individuals with poor agility. Agility test items are usually of three types: (1) change in running direction, (2) change in body position, and (3) change in body part direction. Examples of the three types are the dodge or obstacle run (running direction), squat thrusts (change in body position) and a test that requires a change in the position of the hands or feet (change in body part direction). Agility tests that require only movement of the hands or feet are rarely used in physical education. Agility may be specific to an activity or sport, but most valid agility tests serve to identify individuals with poor agility. You should not expect, however, each individual to do equally well on all agility tests.

WHY MEASURE AGILITY?

Improvement in agility is an acceptable objective for a physical education class. So, as an objective, agility improvement should be determined through measurement. It is doubtful, however, that the agility levels of the students should be used in determining grades. It is questionable as to how much improvement in agility will occur in the amount of time spent on agility instruction in the school environment. But, if agility is an important factor in the performance of sports, and if you grade sports skills, agility is actually graded. Agility tests are sometimes used to classify students for a particular activity or sport, but a test that measures the skill within the activity or sport should be used for classification purposes.

Agility tests are best used for diagnostic purposes, to determine which individuals have poor agility. When testing for diagnostic purposes, criterion-referenced measurement is more appropriate than norm-referenced measurement. A predetermined score should be used to place students into acceptable and unacceptable agility groups, and activities designed to improve agility should be prescribed for the individuals placed in the unacceptable group. It is the instructor's responsibility to determine the appropriate activities. Individuals with unacceptable agility may need strength, speed, coordination and dynamic balance development exercises; or simple agility drills may serve the purpose, depending on the individual. After completion of the prescribed activities or drills, improvement in agility can be determined by the administration of the same agility test.

Are you able to:
define agility and state why it should be measured?

TESTS OF AGILITY

The agility tests selected for review are practical, inexpensive to administer and satisfactory for both sexes. Objectivity coefficients and norms are not reported for all the tests. Norms can be developed to meet your local needs. You may wish to develop local norms for the tests for which norms are reported. Your primary purpose in developing norms should be to establish a criterion-referenced standard for the test(s) that you choose to use.

To obtain consistency and comparability of results, agility tests should be performed on a nonslip surface, and all students should wear shoes that provide good traction. Additionally, the students should practice performing the agility test(s), and be familiar with the performance requirements.

RIGHT-BOOMERANG RUN (Gates and Sheffield 1940)
Test Objective. To measure running agility.
Age Level. 10 through college.
Equipment. Stopwatch, tape measure, a chair or similar object for center station and four cone markers or Indian clubs for outside points.
Validity. Using the sum of T-scores for a 15-item agility battery as the test criterion, a validity coefficient of .72 has been reported for females. With a similar 16-item battery, coefficients ranging from .78 to .87 have been reported for junior high males.
Reliability. .93 for females and .92 for males.
Norms. Table 8-1 reports norms for boys in seventh and eighth grades.

Administration and Directions. A chair is placed 17 feet from the starting line and a cone marker is placed 15 feet on each side of the center point. On the signal, "Go," the student runs to the center station, makes a quarter turn right, runs around the outside station and returns to the center, makes another quarter turn, and completes the course as shown in Figure 8-1. The student should be instructed to run as fast as possible through the course and not to touch the chair and cones.

Scoring. The score is the time to the nearest one-tenth of a second to complete the course. A penalty of one-tenth second is deducted from the score for each time chairs or markers are touched.

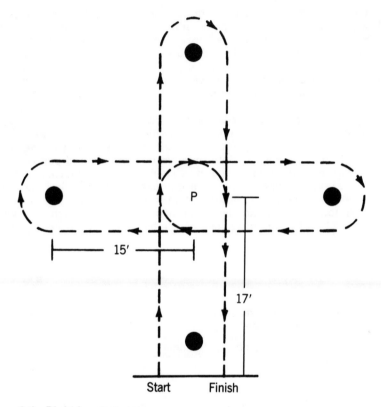

Figure 8-1. *Right boomerang run.*

Table 8-1. *Norms in Seconds for Right-Boomerang Run for Seventh and Eighth Grade Males**

PERFORMANCE LEVEL	Score
Above Average	12.9 and below
Average (42 to 69%)	13.9 to 13.0
Below Average	14.0 and above

*Adapted from B. L. Johnson and J. K. Nelson, *Practical measurements for evaluation in physical education*, 4th ed., Edina, Minnesota: Burgess Publishing, 1986.

SQUAT THRUST (BURPEE TEST)

Test Objective. To measure how rapidly body position can be changed.
Age Level. 10 through college.
Equipment. Stopwatch.
Validity. .34 for females and .55 for males with the criterion of general athletic ability.
Reliability. .92.
Objectivity. .99 (Johnson and Nelson 1986).
Norms. Table 8-2 reports norms for elementary through senior high school age. (Johnson and Nelson [1986] also provide norms for males and females in high school and college.)
Administration and Directions. On the command, "Go," the student is to complete as many squat thrusts as possible in 10 seconds. The squat thrust sequence is: (1) from a standing position, squat and place the hands in front of the feet; (2) thrust the legs backward and take a front leaning rest position (push-up position); (3) return to a squat position; and (4) rise to a standing position (Figure 8-2). Students may be arranged in pairs to count for each other, but they should be cautioned about counting only correct performances of the squat thrust.
Scoring. Each completed squat thrust is scored as one. Scores for a partial squat thrust are: one-fourth for touching the hands to the floor, one-half for thrusting the legs backward, and three-fourths for returning to the squat position. The final score is the total number of complete and partial squat thrusts performed in 10 seconds. There is a one-point penalty for each occasion the following faults occurs: (1) the feet are thrust backward before the hands touch the floor; (2) the feet are not thrust back, so that the body is in a front leaning position; (3) the hands leave the floor before the return to a squat position; and (4) in the standing position the body is not erect and the head up.

Table 8-2. *Norms for 10-Second Squat Thrust Test for Grades Elementary through Senior High**

PERFORMANCE LEVEL	Elementary School	Jr HS	Sr HS
	MALES		
Above Average	6¾ and above	7 and above	7½ and above
Average	5½ to 6½ (42 to 69%)	6 to 6¾ (49 to 69%)	6¾ to 7¼ (46 to 62%)
Below Average	0 to 5¼	0 to 5¾	0 to 6½
	FEMALES		
Above Average	6¾ and above	6¼ and above	6 and above
Average	5½ to 6½ (42 to 66%)	5½ to 6 (38 to 66%)	5¼ to 5¾ (34 to 62%)
Below Average	0 to 5¼	0 to 5¼	0 to 5

*Adapted from C. H. McCloy and N. D. Young, *Tests and measurements in health and physical education*, 3rd ed., New York: Appleton-Century-Crofts, 1954.

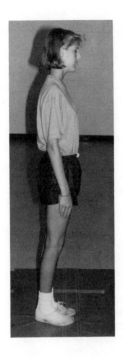
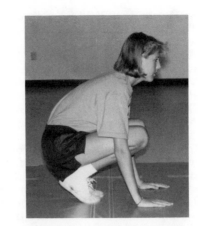
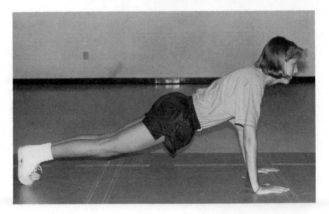
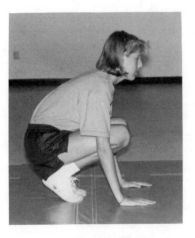
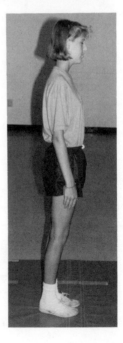

Figure 8-2. *Squat thrust sequence.*

SEMO AGILITY TEST (Kirby 1971)

Test Objective. To measure agility while moving the body forward, backward and sideward.

Age Level. High school and college.

Equipment. Four cone markers and a stopwatch.

Validity. .63 when correlated with the AAHPERD shuttle run test.

Reliability. .88 for high school and college males.

Objectivity. .97

Norms. Kirby provided norms for college males.

Administration and Directions. Cones are placed in each corner of the free-throw lane of a basketball court or in the corners of a 12 x 19 feet rectangle which is on a good running surface (Figure 8-3). Beginning at Point A facing the free-throw line, on the signal, Go, the test performer: (1) side steps to outside of Point B; (2) backpedals from B to D, passing inside D to be in a position facing A; (3) sprints to A, passing around the cone; (4) backpedals from A to C, passing inside C to be in a position facing B; (5) sprints to B, passing around the cone; and (6) side steps from B to finish line at A.

Scoring. Two trials are permitted, with the better time recorded to the nearest one-tenth of a second accepted as the score. Practice trials should be given before the test is administered. Do not permit crossover steps when the side step is performed. Also require the student to keep the back perpendicular to an imaginary line connecting the corner cones, when performing the backpedal. If the student performs any part of the test incorrectly, the test is invalid. The test should be administered until the student performs one trial correctly. With Kirby's norms, if a college male requires more than 13.02 seconds to complete the course, he is classified as an advanced beginner. Johnson and Nelson (1986) report that a college female who requires more than 14.50 seconds also is classified as an advanced beginner.

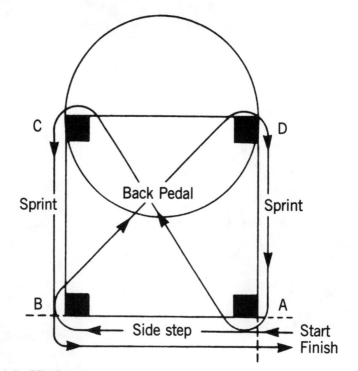

Figure 8-3. *SEMO agility test.*

AAHPERD SHUTTLE RUN (AAHPERD 1976)

Test Objective. To measure agility while running and changing direction.
Age Level. 9 through college.
Equipment. Stopwatch, measuring tape, marking tape, and two blocks of wood (2″ x 2″ x 4″).
Validity. Not reported by AAHPERD.
Reliability. Not reported by AAHPERD.
Norms. The AAHPERD test manual includes percentile norms for males and females, ages 9 through 17+. Table 8-3 provides the quartile norms.
Administration and Directions. Lines are placed 30 feet apart with marking tape. The two blocks are placed adjacent to and outside of the line not being used as the starting line. On the signal, "Go," the test performer: (1) runs from the starting line to the blocks and picks up one; (2) returns to the starting line and places the block behind the line; (3) runs to pick up the second block; and (4) returns to the starting line and places the second block behind the line.
Scoring. Two trials are permitted with the better time to the nearest one-tenth second accepted as the score. Rest should be allowed between trials. The student is not permitted to throw or drop the blocks. To eliminate this problem, the test is sometimes administered without the blocks; the student is instructed to touch behind the line.

Table 8-3. *Norms in Seconds for AAHPERD Shuttle Run for Ages 9 through 17+* *

	AGE							
	9–10	11	12	13	14	15	16	17+
MALES								
PERCENTILE								
95	10.0	9.7	9.6	9.3	8.9	8.9	8.6	8.6
75	10.6	10.4	10.2	10.0	9.6	9.4	9.3	9.2
50	11.2	10.9	10.7	10.4	10.1	9.9	9.9	9.8
25	12.0	11.5	11.4	11.0	10.7	10.4	10.5	10.4
0	17.0	20.0	22.0	16.0	18.6	14.7	15.0	15.7
FEMALES								
95	10.2	10.0	9.9	9.9	9.7	9.9	10.0	9.6
75	11.1	10.8	10.8	10.5	10.3	10.4	10.6	10.4
50	11.8	11.5	11.4	11.2	11.0	11.0	11.2	11.1
25	12.5	12.1	12.0	12.0	12.0	11.8	12.0	12.0
0	18.0	20.0	15.3	16.5	19.2	18.5	24.9	17.0

*Adapted from *AAHPERD youth fitness test manual*, Reston, Virginia, AAHPERD, 1976.

BARROW ZIGZAG RUN (Barrow 1979)

Test Objective. To measure agility while running and changing direction.
Age level. Junior high through college. (Though this test was originally designed for males, it may be satisfactorily used with junior high through college age females.)
Equipment. Stopwatch, five standards that are used for high jump, volleyball or badminton. Cones also may be used.
Validity. .74, with the total score for 29 test items measuring eight factors.
Reliability. .80.
Objectivity. .99.
Norms. Table 8-4 reports norms for males in grades seven through 11.

Table 8-4. *Norms in Seconds for Barrow's Zigzag Run for 7th through 11th Grade Males**

PERFORMANCE LEVEL	GRADE				
	7	8	9	10	11
Above Average	25.2 and below	24.5 and below	24.6 and below	25.8 and below	25.8 and below
Average (T-score 45 to 55)	29.0 to 25.3	29.5 to 24.6	27.9 to 24.7	28.9 to 25.9	28.9 to 25.9
Below Average	29.1 and above	29.6 and above	28.0 and above	29.0 and above	29.0 and above

*Adapted from H. M. Barrow and R. McGee, *A practical approach to measurement in physical education*, 3rd ed., Philadelphia: Lea & Febiger, 1979.

Administration and Directions. The course is designed as shown in Figure 8-4. On the signal, "Go," the test performer runs, as fast as possible, the prescribed course in a figure-eight fashion for three complete laps. The standards should not be touched in any manner. If a foul is committed or the course is run improperly, the student is required to run the course again. The validity and reliability of the test would probably be affected minimally if you chose to require the students to run only two laps.

Scoring. The score is the time to the nearest one-tenth second required to complete the course three times.

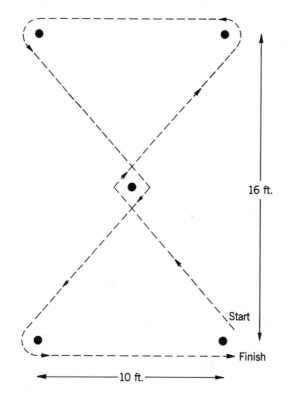

Figure 8-4. *Barrow zigzag run.*

ACTIVITIES TO DEVELOP AGILITY

If you diagnose some students to have poor agility, you should attempt to improve this agility. McClenaghan and Gallahue (1978) suggest the following activities for the development of agility in young children. These activities, or modifications of them, also may be used for junior and senior high students with poor agility.

Changes in the Height of the Body

1. alternate jumping maximum and minimum heights
2. alternate fast and slow jumping
3. jump, and toss an object to yourself
4. hop on one foot
5. hop two to four times on one foot, then the same number of times on the other foot
6. jump over a stationary rope
7. jump over a swinging rope
8. jump over a turning rope
9. jump over a rope you are turning
10. jump rope with a partner

Changes in Distance

1. jump as far as you can
2. jump as near as you can
3. jump and land with your feet in different positions
4. jump backward
5. walk backward
6. run backward or sideward
7. leap over objects
8. jump different heights
9. jump and land lightly
10. jump and land on different surfaces

Changes in Direction

1. jump and turn (quarter, half, three-quarter, full turn)
2. jump forward, then sideward, then backward
3. jump in a circle, square, triangle and so forth
4. run between chairs
5. run forward and change direction quickly, on command
6. slide sideways and change direction quickly, on command
7. jump over a turning rope and change your body position
8. move forward, sideward or backward while jumping over a rope you are turning
9. run through a series of tires (laid flat on the ground)
10. do tumbling tricks requiring your body to roll in various ways (log rolls, forward rolls, backward rolls and so on)

CONDITIONING AND AGILITY ACTIVITIES

Side-straddle Hop
Stand erect with arms at sides and feet together; jump, spreading the legs to the side and at the same time bring the arms overhead; jump and return to starting position; attempt to perform in a smooth and continous action. One side-straddle hop is counted each time you return to the starting position.

Heel Touch
Stand erect with hands at the sides; jump and touch both heels with the fingers. Each jump is counted as one.

Squat thrust
See squat thrust test.

Treadmill
Assume push-up position with one leg forward; keep hands in place while alternately bringing one leg forward and extending the other leg in a running position. One treadmill is counted each time the right leg is forward.

Zigzag Run
Arrange chairs in a position to provide a zigzag course; run as fast as possible in a zigzag course around the chairs.

REVIEW PROBLEMS

1. Review additional agility tests found in other textbooks. Note the groups for whom the tests are intended and the validity, reliability and objectivity coefficients.
2. Administer one of the tests described in this chapter to several of your fellow students. Ask them to provide constructive criticism of your test administration.
3. An elementary physical education teacher administered the 10-second squat thrust and the AAHPERD shuttle run tests to 15 10-year-old boys. Determine the relationship of the two groups of scores. Interpret the correlation coefficient.

Student	10-second squat thrust (number)	AAHPERD shuttle run (seconds)
A	7.00	9.8
B	6.50	10.8
C	5.50	11.4
D	7.50	9.6
E	5.25	12.0
F	6.50	10.4
G	6.75	10.5
H	6.00	11.0
I	5.75	11.4
J	5.00	12.5
K	6.00	11.3
L	6.75	10.3
M	5.75	11.2
N	6.50	10.7
O	5.75	11.5

9

Balance

Upon completion of this chapter, you should be able to:
1. Define and measure static and dynamic balance;
2. State why balance should be measured; and
3. Prescribe activities to improve balance.

Balance is the ability to maintain equilibrium against the force of gravity. The balance center (semicircular canal) in the inner ear, the kinesthetic sense in the muscles and joints ("feel" of an activity) and visual perception contribute to balance. In certain positions, balance also is affected by strength. If the supporting muscles cannot hold the body weight, body parts or an external weight firmly in position, balance is limited. For some individuals, increased strength results in improved balance.

Basically, there are two types of balance: static and dynamic. The recovery of balance, after the body's balance has been disturbed, may also be considered a type of balance. Static balance, the ability to maintain equilibrium while stationary, is often thought of as steadiness. To maintain static balance, the center of gravity must be over the base of support. Assuming a position to shoot a rifle, looking through a microscope and posing for a photographer are examples of static balance.

Dynamic balance is the ability to maintain equilibrium while in motion or to move the body or parts of the body from one point to another and maintain equilibrium. Dancing, walking, driving a golf ball and bowling are examples of dynamic balance. Static and dynamic balance are necessary for successful performance in physical activity, but the ability to recover balance is also essential in many activities. Running, kicking, hopping, dismounting from gymnastics apparatus, performing gymnastic floor exercises and wrestling are examples of such activities. In fact, all human motion occurs as a result of the disturbance of the body's balance.

WHY MEASURE BALANCE?

Balance is necessary not only in sports and related physical activities, but also in our usual, everyday activities. Individuals with

133

poor balance are at a disadvantage in efficiently performing most physical activities. Though heredity may be a factor, an individual's ability to maintain balance can be improved through appropriate physical activities. Thus, since performance of any physical skill requires some degree of balance and since balance can be improved, balance tests should be used to determine those individuals with poor balance. Activities then should be prescribed to improve their balance. However, as balance is specific to a body part and may be specific to a sport or physical activity, different types of balance tests should be used for diagnostic purposes. Also, different types of activities designed to improve balance should be prescribed.

As with agility, it is recommended that a specific improvement in balance not be used to determine grades. If balance is an important component of a physical activity, the student's performance in that activity will be affected by the degree of balance skill. Through the assigning of grades for performance in an activity, balance has been graded.

> Are you able to:
> define balance and state why it should be measured by the physical educator?

TESTS OF BALANCE

Balance tests are classified as static or dynamic. The tests selected for review are practical, inexpensive to administer and satisfactory for both sexes. Reliability and objectivity coefficients are not available for all the tests, and regrettably, the published norms are primarily for college-age individuals. It will be necessary that you develop local elementary, junior high or senior high norms for your use. It is recommended that balance test norms be used in the same manner as suggested for agility norms, to develop criterion-referenced standards. Though not a factor in all balance tests, fatigue may influence the performance of some students. For this reason, it is best not to administer balance tests after any strenuous activity. So the test performers will be familiar with the test, permit them to practice the test. The practice will enable many of the students to score better.

Static Balance Tests

STORK STAND
Test Objective. To measure stationary balance while the body weight is supported on the ball of the foot of the dominant leg.
Age Level. 10 through college.
Equipment. Stopwatch.
Validity. Face validity.
Reliability. Coefficients of .85 and .87 have been reported using the test-retest method.

Objectivity. Johnson and Nelson (1986) report a study which found an objective coefficient of .99.

Norms. Table 9-1 reports norms for college students.

Administration and Directions. Individuals may be tested in pairs. The test performer stands on the foot of the dominant leg, places the other foot against the inside of the supporting knee, and places the hands on the hips as shown in Figure 9-1. On the signal, "Go," the performer raises the heel of the dominant foot from the floor and attempts to maintain balance as long as possible. The test administrator counts aloud the seconds. The partner of the test performer records the number of seconds the performer is able to maintain balance. The trial is ended when the hands are moved from the hips, when the ball of the dominant foot moves from its original position or when the heel touches the floor. Three trials are administered.

Scoring. The best time, in seconds, of the three trials is the score. Since there is no time limit, and some individuals may be able to maintain their balance for some time, you may choose to halt the performance of those individuals who exceed the norm for above average.

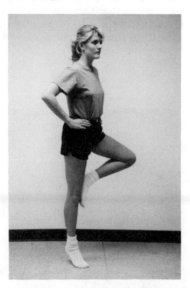

Figure 9-1. *Stork stand.*

Table 9-1. *Norms in Seconds for Stork Stand, Bass Stick Test (Lengthwise), and Bass Stick Test (Crosswise) for College Students**

	Stork Stand	Bass Stick (LW)	Bass Stick (CW)
PERFORMANCE	**MALES**		
LEVEL			
Above Average	37 and above	306 and above	165 and above
Average	15 to 36	221 to 305	65 to 164
Below Average	14 and below	220 and below	64 and below
	FEMALES		
Above Average	23 and above	301 and above	140 and above
Average	8 to 22	206 to 300	60 to 139
Below Average	7 and below	205 and below	59 and below

*Adapted from B. L. Johnson and J. K. Nelson, *Practical measurements for evaluation in physical education*, 4th ed., Edina, Minnesota: Burgess Publishing, 1986.

BASS STICK TEST (Lengthwise) (Bass 1939)

Test Objective. To measure stationary balance while the weight of the body is supported on a small base of support on the ball of the foot.

Age Level. 10 through college.

Equipment. Sticks 1″ x 1″ x 12″ (you may test one-half of the class at the same time if you have enough sticks), stopwatch and adhesive tape.

Validity. Face validity is accepted.

Reliability. .90.

Norms. Table 9-1 reports norms for college students.

Administration and Directions. All sticks should be taped to the floor. Individuals may be tested in pairs. The test performer places a foot lengthwise on the stick (ball of the foot and heel should be in contact with the stick). On the signal, "Go," the performer lifts the opposite foot from the floor and attempts to hold this position for a maximum of 60 seconds (Figure 9-2). The test administrator counts aloud the seconds while the partner of the performer records the number of seconds the performer is able to maintain balance. The trial is ended when any part of either foot touches the floor. Three trials are taken on each foot. If any performers lose their balance within the first three seconds of a trial, the trial is not considered an attempt.

Scoring. The score is the total time in seconds for all six trials.

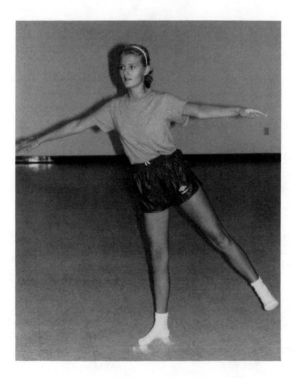

Figure 9-2. *Bass lengthwise stick test.*

BASS STICK TEST (Crosswise) (Bass 1939)

This test is the same as the lengthwise test except that the ball of the foot is placed crosswise on the stick. Table 9-1 includes norms for college students.

You will find additional static balance tests directly related to gymnastics performance in other measurement textbooks. Head balance, head and forearm balance, and handstand are examples of such tests.

Dynamic Balance Tests

JOHNSON MODIFICATION OF THE BASS TEST OF DYNAMIC BALANCE (Johnson and Nelson 1986)

Test Objective. To measure the ability to maintain balance during movement and upon landing from a leap.

Age Level. High school through college.

Equipment. Stopwatch, tape measure and floor tape.

Validity. Face validity; .46 when correlated with Bass Test of Dynamic Balance.

Reliability. .75 using test-retest.

Objectivity. .97.

Norms. Norms for college women are available (Johnson and Nelson 1986).

Administration and Directions. Eleven pieces of tape (1″ x 3/4″) are placed in the pattern as shown in Figure 9-3. The test performer (1) stands with the right foot placed on the starting mark; (2) leaps to the first tape mark, lands on the ball of the left foot and attempts to hold for five seconds; (3) leaps to the second tape mark, lands on the ball of the right foot and attempts to hold for five seconds; and (4) continues to the other tape marks, alternating feet and attempting to hold a steady position for five seconds. The ball of the foot must completely cover the tape. The test administrator should count aloud the seconds of each balance.

Scoring. The test scoring is:

five points for landing successfully on the tape mark (tape completely covered)

one point (up to five seconds) for each second the steady position is held on the tape marks

A maximum of 10 points per tape mark, and 100 points for the test may be earned.

The test performer is penalized five points for any of the following landing errors:

- failure to stop upon landing

- touching the floor with any part of the body other than the ball of the landing foot

- failure to completely cover the tape mark with the ball of the foot

If the test performer makes a landing error, the correct balance position may be assumed and held for a maximum of five seconds.

If the test performer lands successfully on the tape mark, but commits any of the following errors prior to the completion of the five-second count, a penalty of one point is given.

- touching the floor with any part of the body other than the ball of the landing foot

- failure to hold the landing foot steady while in the steady position

If balance is lost, the test performer must return to the proper mark, and leap to the next mark.

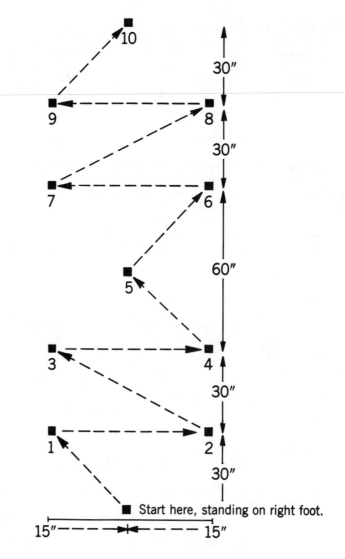

Figure 9-3. *Floor pattern for modified Bass dynamic balance test.*

BALANCE BEAM WALK (Jensen and Hirst 1980)

Test Objective. To measure balance while walking on a balance beam.

Age Level. 9 through college.

Equipment. Regulation balance beam and stopwatch.

Validity. Face validity.

Norms. No norms reported.

Administration and Directions. Standing on one end of the beam, the test performer slowly walks the full length of the beam, pauses for five seconds, turns around and walks back to the starting point. Three trials are allowed.

Scoring. Pass-fail. Since there is no time limit for this beam walk, the test could require much class time to administer. You may wish to shorten the time for test administration, or to increase the difficulty of the test by limiting the amount of time permitted to complete the test. The test difficulty may also be increased through the use of a two-inch balance beam.

MODIFIED SIDEWARD LEAP (Scott and French 1959; Safrit 1986)

Test Objective. To measure the ability to maintain balance during movement and upon landing from a leap.

Age Level. Junior high through college.

Equipment. Stopwatch, tape measure and floor tape.

Validity. Face validity.

Reliability. .66 to .88 at differing age levels.

Norms. No norms reported.

Administration and Directions. Place three one-inch square spots in a straight line, 18 inches apart as shown in Figure 9-4. Place additional spots at right angles to the line. These spots should be three inches apart and range in distance from Spot A (24 to 40 inches), according to height of the test performers. Generally, three or four spots properly placed will cover the range in height. Place a small cork (may be the bottom of an old badminton bird) or other light object on Spot B.

The test performer (1) places the left foot on Mark X with the right side toward Spot A (the correct spot for each individual may be determined through practice); (2) leaps sideward and lands on the ball of right foot on Spot A (the leap should require both feet to be off the floor at the same time, but it should not require extensive effort); (3) immediately leans forward and, using only one hand, pushes the cork off Spot B (the floor should not be touched with either hand); and (4) holds a balanced position for five seconds (the position may be either forward or erect). Four trials are administered: two as above, and two with the student placing the right foot on Mark X, landing on the ball of the left foot, and leaning forward to Spot C.

Scoring. The maximum number of points for each trial is 15:

1. Five points for landing correctly on Spot A
2. Five points for leaning and pushing object off Spot B or C
3. One point for each second that balance is held on Spot A, up to five seconds

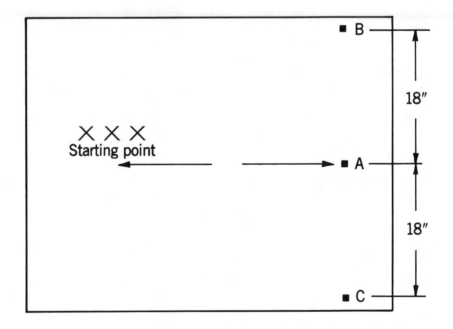

Figure 9-4. *Floor marking for the modified sideward leap test.*

ACTIVITIES TO DEVELOP BALANCE

Balance can be improved through extensive practice of activities that place individuals (1) in balanced positions which they attempt to maintain and (2) in balanced positions which help them develop a "feel" (kinesthetic sense) for such positions. Balance also can be improved through activities that place individuals in a state of imbalance, forcing them to attempt to recover balance. Nichols, Arsenault, and Giuffre (1980) recommend the following activities for the teaching of balance to elementary students, but the activities, or modifications of them, may be practiced at any level of instruction.

Static Balance Activities

Knee balance: In a kneeling position, attempt to balance on one knee while the arms are to the side. The position is held for 10 to 15 seconds, then the other knee is used.

Stork stand: While in the same position as stork stand test, attempt to hold the position for 10 to 20 seconds.

Swan stand: Lean forward at the hips and lift the right foot off the floor. While balancing on the left foot, lift the right leg behind, and as high as possible. Hold for 10 to 15 seconds. Repeat on the other foot.

V-sit: Sit on the floor and lift the arms and legs into the air while balancing on the buttocks. Hold for 10 to 20 seconds.

Dynamic Balance Activities

Tape line: Tape a line on the floor, then (1) walk forward, backward and sideways; (2) walk while balancing a book or bean bag on the head; and (3) run, hop or skip in different directions.

Hopping: Try to (1) hop over objects using the left foot and then the right; (2) hop with the eyes closed; (3) hop while holding on to different objects; or (4) hop in and out of tires.

Rug twister: Place a rug sample so that the rubber backing faces upward. Stand on the rug and twist back and forth to move around the floor.

Hop leap: Place tape marks on the floor approximately one yard apart. Leap from mark to mark, alternating the landing foot. Maintain a one foot static balance on each mark for five seconds.

Recapturing Balance Activities

1. Jump off a low bench landing with both feet inside a hoop.
2. Jump forward off a chair and clap the hands above the head while in midair.
3. Jump forward off a chair with one foot going forward and the other backward, and land with the legs back together.
4. Jump forward off a low bench, make a half turn in midair and land facing the bench.
5. Jump sideways off a low bench. Jump backward.
6. Jump forward off a chair and catch a ball in midair.

The balance beam and walking boards can be used to provide many types of balance activities. The boards should be different widths, heights and inclines to provide challenges that increase in difficulty. Initially, when using the balance beam, it may be best to have it at a low height. As the students gain confidence, the height can be increased.

REVIEW PROBLEMS
1. Review additional balance tests found in other textbooks. Note the groups for whom the tests are intended and the validity, reliability and objectivity coefficients.
2. Administer one static balance test and one dynamic balance test described in this chapter to several of your fellow students. Ask them to provide constructive criticism of your test administration.

10

Cardiorespiratory Fitness

Upon completion of this chapter, you should be able to:
1. Define and measure cardiorespiratory fitness;
2. State why cardiorespiratory fitness should be measured; and
3. Prescribe activities and exercises to develop cardiorespiratory fitness.

Cardiorespiratory fitness is the ability to perform large muscle, whole body physical activity of moderate to high intensity for relatively long periods of time. It is the ability of the circulatory and respiratory systems to adjust to vigorous exercise, and to recover from the effect of such exercise. It involves the functioning of the heart and lungs, the blood and its capacity to carry oxygen, the blood vessels and capillaries supplying blood to all parts of the body and the muscle cells, which use the oxygen to provide the energy necessary for endurance exercise. Activities such as aerobic dance, distance running, brisk walking, swimming, bicycling and cross-country skiing are associated with cardiovascular fitness. Terms such as aerobic power, aerobic fitness, cardiovascular endurance and cardiorespiratory endurance essentially mean cardiorespiratory fitness.

Cardiorespiratory fitness indicates a high state of efficiency of the circulatory and respiratory systems in supplying oxygen to the working muscles. The more oxygen you are able to take in and utilize, the longer you are able to work (exercise) before fatigue or exhaustion occurs. Generally, the more intense the work or performance of an activity, the greater the amount of oxygen processed by the body (oxygen uptake). The greatest rate at which oxygen can be taken in and utilized during exercise is referred to as maximum oxygen consumption (VO_2 max). Maximum VO_2 is also termed maximum oxygen intake, maximum oxygen uptake or aerobic capacity. Since oxygen consumption is related to body weight, VO_2 max is usually reported in terms of the volume of oxygen consumed, per kilogram of

143

body weight, per minute of work (ml/kg/min). The maximum VO_2 an individual can attain measures the effectiveness of the heart, lungs and vascular system in the delivery of oxygen during heavy work, and the ability of the working cells to extract it. The higher the VO_2 max attained, the more effective are the circulatory and respiratory systems. VO_2 max in untrained college males generally ranges from 42 to 45 ml/kg/min of work, while values for females are 3 to 4 milliliters lower at the same level of fitness. Many endurance athletes have been able to achieve values as high as 65 to 80 ml/kg/min.

WHY MEASURE CARDIORESPIRATORY FITNESS?

As flexibility, muscular strength and muscular endurance exercises may reduce the frequency of musculoskeletal problems and other health problems, they should be included in an exercise program. However, the most important aspect of an exercise program is cardiorespiratory conditioning. Performed with the correct intensity, duration and frequency, cardiorespiratory conditioning activities serve to:

1. increase physical working capacity at all ages
2. decrease the risk of developing obesity and problems associated with obesity
3. decrease the risk of coronary heart disease
4. aid in the management of both stress and depression
5. enable most people to feel better, physically and mentally

These health benefits are very important. As a physical educator, you should be prepared to assist individuals in the attainment of them. Through measurement you may identify individuals who have poor cardiorespiratory fitness, and then prescribe the appropriate activities for them. Some individuals are motivated when taking the test to adopt or to continue an active and healthful lifestyle. In addition, cardiorespiratory tests may be used to screen individuals for other activities. However, the screening test should not take the place of a medical examination, and maximal effort should not be required unless the test is conducted under proper conditions (emergency care equipment available, with qualified personnel to use the equipment).

Cardiorespiratory fitness testing is often performed before and after participation in physical conditioning activities, to measure changes in fitness. Sometimes, in the school environment, the cardiorespiratory test results may be included in the determination of a unit grade. Unless prohibited due to medical problems, all individuals can experience change in cardiorespiratory fitness through proper conditioning activities. However, if a score on a cardiorespiratory test is to be used in the grading process, reasonable objectives should be stated at the beginning of the unit and an appropriate amount of time (weeks) should be provided for the attainment of the objectives.

TESTS OF CARDIORESPIRATORY FITNESS

The best single measure of cardiorespiratory fitness is VO_2 max, but performing this measurement requires expensive equipment (a treadmill or bicycle ergometer and gas analysis equipment) and trained personnel. Because of these requirements, VO_2 max tests are rarely performed in physical education classes or fitness centers. Cardiorespiratory fitness tests that require inexpensive equipment and that can be administered to large groups are presented here. However, validity, reliability and objectivity coefficients are not available for all the tests presented.

We know that oxygen consumption has a direct linear relationship to heart rate; so, cardiorespiratory fitness can be estimated by measurement of the heart rate during and after testing. Though electronical measurement of the heart rate is preferred for accuracy, it is not practical or feasible in the testing of groups. In group testing, the heart rate is usually measured by counting the pulse rate at the radial artery in the wrist, or at the carotid artery in the neck (lightly place first two fingers at these sites). As counting errors affect the validity of the test, it is essential that those individuals who are responsible for counting the pulse rate practice the procedure several times before the test is administered. Running tests (the timing of running a specified distance, or the distance an individual can run in a stated time) also correlate highly with maximum oxygen consumption. Scoring accuracy is greater with running tests since it is necessary only to count the number of laps around a particular course, or to record the time for running a specified distance.

Regardless of the type cardiorespiratory test administered, many variables can influence cardiorespiratory functions. It has been found that exercise, age, sex, environmental temperature, humidity, altitude, digestion, loss of sleep, changes in body position, emotional and nervous conditions, body fatness, running efficiency and motivation can influence cardiorespiratory testing. It is not possible to control all of these variables, but you should be aware of them and recognize their influence on the tests. Also, all performers should be medically approved to take a cardiorespiratory fitness test, and you should recognize that good judgment may mean the postponement of cardiorespiratory testing when the influence of any of these variables could jeopardize the health of the test performer.

12-MINUTE AND 9-MINUTE RUN (AAHPERD 1980)
Test Objective. To measure cardiorespiratory fitness.
Age Level. Junior high through adult for 12-minute run and ages five-18 for 9-minute run.

Equipment. A stopwatch, whistle and any flat, measured area. As sharp turns usually slow the runner, it is best if the running course does not have them. If sharp turns are unavoidable, however, do not compare the running times for the course with a course that has no sharp turns. Different norms should be prepared for the course with sharp turns.

Validity. A validity coefficient of .90 has been reported when maximum oxygen consumption was used as the criterion.

Reliability. Using the test-retest method, a coefficient of .94 has been reported.

Norms. Tables 10-1 and 10-2 report norms for both runs. Cooper (1982) provides norms for ages 13 through 60+ for the 12-minute run.

Administration and Directions. All test performers should practice distance running and understand the advantage of maintaining a constant pace before attempting the test. The runners should be motivated to give their best effort, or the validity of the test will be affected. The running course should be marked so the test administrator is able to determine with ease and promptness the exact distance in yards covered by the runner. Placing markers every 10 to 25 yards will facilitate the scoring process. In addition, assigning a spotter to each runner will make the scoring process more efficient. After the test performers have warmed-up, they gather behind a line, and on the starting signal they run (walking is permitted) as many laps as possible around the course. The spotters count the number of laps for the runner, and when the signal (whistle) to stop is given, they run to the spot of the runner. The runners should be instructed to keep moving until they have cooled down.

Scoring. Both runs are scored to the nearest 10 yards. The importance of accurate counting of laps should be emphasized to the spotters.

1-MILE AND 1.5-MILE RUNS

Test Objective. To measure cardiorespiratory fitness.

Age Level. Five through adult for 1-mile run and 13 through adult for 1.5-mile run.

Equipment. Stopwatch and a flat, measured area.

Validity and Reliability. Both runs are valid tests because they are related to maximum oxygen consumption. As with other distance runs, these runs have acceptable reliability when administered to properly prepared performers.

Norms. Table 10-3 reports norms for the 1-mile run, and Table 10-1 reports norms for the 1.5-mile run. Cooper (1982) also provides norms for ages 13 through 60+ for the 1.5-mile run.

Administration and Directions. Again, all performers should practice distance running and understand the advantage of maintaining a constant pace before attempting the test. Assigning a partner, or spotter to each runner will aid in the recording of the scores. After the runners have warmed-up, they

Table 10-1. *Norms for 12-Minute Run (Yards) and 1.5-Mile Run (Minutes and Seconds) for Ages 13 through 18**

| | **MALES** | | **FEMALES** | |
| | 12-Minute Run | 1.5 Mile Run | 12-Minute Run | 1.5 Mile Run |
PERCENTILE	Yards	Time	Yards	Time
95	3297	8:37	2448	12:17
75	2879	10:19	2100	15:03
50	2592	11:29	1861	16:57
25	2305	12:39	1622	18:50
5	1888	14:20	1274	21:36

*Adapted from *AAHPERD youth fitness test manual*, Reston, Virginia: AAHPERD, 1976.

Table 10-2. Norms in Yards for 9-Minute Run for Ages Five through College

PERCENTILE	5	6	7	8	9	10	11	Age 12	13	14	15	16	17+	College
						MALES								
95	1760	1750	2020	2200	2175	2250	2250	2400	2402	2473	2544	2615	2615	2640
75	1320	1469	1683	1810	1835	1910	1925	1975	2096	2167	2238	2309	2380	2349
50	1170	1280	1440	1595	1660	1690	1725	1760	1885	1956	2027	2098	2169	2200
25	990	1090	1243	1380	1440	1487	1540	1500	1674	1745	1816	1887	1958	1945
5	600	816	990	1053	1104	1110	1170	1000	1368	1439	1510	1581	1652	1652
						FEMALES								
95	1540	1700	1900	1860	2050	2067	2000	2175	2085	2123	2161	2199	2237	2230
75	1300	1440	1540	1540	1650	1650	1723	1760	1785	1823	1861	1899	1937	1870
50	1140	1208	1344	1358	1425	1460	1480	1590	1577	1615	1653	1691	1729	1755
25	950	1017	1150	1225	1243	1250	1345	1356	1369	1407	1445	1483	1521	1460
5	700	750	860	970	960	940	904	1000	1069	1107	1145	1183	1221	1101

*Adapted from *Health related physical fitness test manual*, Reston, Virginia: AAHPERD, 1980; and R. R. Pate, *Norms for college students: health related physical fitness test*, Reston, Virginia: AAHPERD, 1985.

Table 10-3. Norms in Minutes and Seconds for 1-Mile Run for Ages Five through College*

PERCENTILE	5	6	7	8	9	10	11	Age 12	13	14	15	16	17+	College
						MALES								
95	9:02	9:06	8:06	7:58	7:17	6:56	6:50	6:27	6:11	5:51	6:01	5:48	6:01	5:30
75	11:32	10:55	9:37	9:14	8:36	8:10	8:00	7:24	6:52	6:36	6:35	6:28	6:36	6:12
50	13:46	12:29	11:25	11:00	9:56	9:19	9:06	8:20	7:27	7:10	7:14	7:11	7:25	6:49
25	16:05	15:10	14:02	13:29	12:00	11:05	11:31	10:00	8:35	8:02	8:04	8:07	8:26	7:32
5	18:25	17:38	17:17	16:19	15:44	14:28	15:25	13:41	10:23	10:32	10:37	10:40	10:56	9:47
						FEMALES								
95	9:45	9:18	8:48	8:45	8:24	7:59	7:46	7:26	7:10	7:18	7:39	7:07	7:26	7:02
75	13:09	11:24	10:55	10:35	9:58	9:30	9:12	8:36	8:18	8:13	8:42	9:00	9:03	8:15
50	15:08	13:48	12:30	12:00	11:12	11:06	10:27	9:47	9:27	9:35	10:05	10:45	9:47	9:22
25	17:59	15:27	14:30	14:16	13:18	12:54	12:10	11:35	10:56	11:43	12:21	13:00	11:28	10:41
5	19:00	18:50	17:44	16:58	16:42	17:00	16:56	14:46	14:55	16:59	16:22	15:30	15:24	12:43

*Adapted from *Health related physical fitness test manual*, Reston, Virginia: AAHPERD, 1980; and R. R. Pate, *Norms for college students: health related physical fitness test*, Reston, Virginia: AAHPERD, 1985.

gather behind a starting line, and on the signal to start, they run (walking is permitted) the distance as fast as possible. The partner of each runner is at the finish line and records the test time of the runner. The test administrator calls out the times as the runners cross the finish line.

Scoring. The score is the time in minutes and seconds to complete the run.

3-MILE WALKING TEST (NO RUNNING) (Cooper 1982)

Test Objective. To measure cardiorespiratory fitness through walking.

Age Level. 13 through 60+.

Equipment. Flat, measured surface and stopwatch.

Norms. Cooper provides fitness standards for male and female age groups, age 13 through 60+. Table 10-4 reports the "good" classification standards for the 3-mile walking test. Lower times will place the test performers in the excellent classification and higher times will place them in the fair to very poor classifications.

Administration and Directions. All test performers should practice walking for speed and endurance before attempting the test. After warming up, the test performers gather behind the starting line. On the signal to start, they attempt to cover three miles in the fastest time possible, without running. A partner for each walker is at the finish line to record the finishing time, as the test administrator calls it out.

Scoring. The time in minutes and seconds to walk the three miles is the score.

12-MINUTE SWIMMING TEST (Cooper 1982)

Test Objective. To measure cardiorespiratory fitness through swimming.

Age Level. 13 through 60+.

Equipment. Swimming pool, stopwatch and whistle.

Norms. Cooper provides fitness standards for male and female age groups, age 13 through 60+. Table 10-4 reports the "good" classification standards. Greater distances will place the test performers in the excellent classification, and lesser distances will place them in the fair to very poor classification.

Administration and Directions. All test performers should practice cycling for distance and pacing before attempting the test. The cycling course performers gather at one end of the pool. Each performer is instructed to swim in an individual lane. On the signal to start, they push off from the side and swim as far as possible in 12 minutes, using any stroke and resting when necessary. A test partner counts the laps and observes where the swimmer is when the signal to stop is given. The swimmer continues to swim to cool down.

Scoring. The distance in yards swum is the score.

12-MINUTE CYCLING TEST (Cooper 1982)

Test Objective. To measure cardiorespiratory fitness through cycling.

Age Level. 13 through 60+.

Equipment. A bicycle with no more than three gears and a flat, measured distance.

Norms. Cooper provides fitness standards for male and female age groups, age 13 through 60+. Table 10-4 reports the "good" classification standards. Greater distances will place the test performers in the excellent classification, and lesser distances will place them in the fair to very poor classifications.

Administration and Directions. All test performers should practice cycling for distance and pacing before attempting the test. The cycling course should be on a hard, flat surface in an area where traffic is not a problem. Every quarter-mile should be marked. On the day of the test the wind should be less than 10 mph. After warming-up, the test performers gather at the starting line, and on the signal to start they attempt to cycle as far as possible in 12 minutes. A test partner spots the position of the cyclist when the signal to stop is given. All cyclists should continue to move until they have cooled down.

Scoring. The score is the distance in miles cycled.

Table 10-4. Standards for Classification of Good Fitness for 3-Mile Walk, 12-Minute Swimming, and 12-Minute Cycling Tests for Ages 13 through 60+*

TEST	13–19	20–29	Age 30–39	40–49	50–59	60+
			MALES			
3-mile walking (minutes & seconds)	33:00 to 37:30	34:00 to 38:30	35:00 to 40:00	36:30 to 42:00	39:00 to 45:00	41:00 to 48:00
12-minute swimming (yards)	700 to 799	600 to 699	550 to 649	500 to 599	450 to 549	400 to 499
12-minute cycling (miles)	4.75 to 5.74	4.50 to 5.49	4.25 to 5.24	4.00 to 4.99	3.50 to 4.49	3.00 to 3.99
			FEMALES			
3-mile walking (minutes & seconds)	35:00 to 39:30	36:00 to 40:30	37:30 to 42:00	39:00 to 44:00	42:00 to 47:00	45:00 to 51:00
12-minute swimming (yards)	600 to 699	500 to 599	450 to 549	400 to 499	350 to 449	300 to 399
12-minute cycling (miles)	3.75 to 4.74	3.50 to 4.49	3.25 to 4.24	3.00 to 3.99	2.50 to 3.49	2.00 to 2.99

*Adapted from K. H. Cooper, The aerobics program for total well-being, New York: M. Evans and Company, 1982.
[a]Lower times or greater distances place the individual in the excellent fitness category and higher times or lesser distances place the individual in the fair–very poor fitness categories.

QUEENS COLLEGE STEP TEST (Katch and McArdle 1977; McArdle et al. 1972)

Test Objective. To measure cardiorespiratory fitness with a submaximal step test.

Age Level. College.

Equipment. Gymnasium bleachers and a metronome. To facilitate testing, record the instructions and commands (cadence) on tape. It is helpful to the test performers if the cadence is maintained through the commands "up, up, down, down," rather than through the metronome. Recording the instructions and commands standardizes the administration of the test and permits you to circulate among the performers during the test.

Validity. Using VO_2 max as the criterion, correlation coefficients of -.75 and -.72 were found for college-age women and men, respectively.

Reliability. Coefficients of .92 and .89 were found for college-age women and men, respectively.

Norms. Table 10-5 reports norms.

Administration and Directions. Before administration of the test provide all participants ample time to practice measuring the pulse rate by palpating the carotid artery for 15-second intervals. Test performers should have a partner to count the pulse rate. Since the test cadence is different for males and females, pair a male with a female, then you can test the males as a group and the females as a group. Demonstrate the test and allow the test performers a brief practice period (15 to 20 seconds) to learn the cadence. After the practice period, permit the participants to rest. To perform the test, all participants step up and down on the bleacher for three minutes. The cadence for males is 24 steps/minute (metronome set at 96 beats/minute), and the cadence for females is 22 steps/minute (metronome set at 88 beats/minute). At the end of three minutes, the test performers remain standing while the partners count their pulse rate for 15 seconds, beginning five seconds after the completion of the test. (Pulse count should be completed 20 seconds after test performer has completed test.)

Scoring. Multiply the 15-second pulse rate by four to obtain the performer's score in beats/minute. Katch and McArdle also developed regression equations to predict VO_2 max from heart rate per minute. They are included in Table 10-5.

Table 10-5. *Norms for the Queens College Step Test for College Students**

PERCENTILE	MALES Heart Rate	VO_2	FEMALES Heart Rate	VO_2
95	124	59.3	140	40.0
75	144	50.9	158	36.6
50	156	45.8	166	35.1
25	168	40.8	176	33.3
5	184	34.1	196	29.6

Equations for predicting VO_2 max
Males: VO_2 max (ml/kg/min) = 111.33 − .42(pulse rate beats/min)
Females: VO_2 max (ml/kg/min) = 65.81 − .42(pulse rate beats/min)

*Adapted from F. I. Katch and W. D. McArdle, *Nutrition, weight control, and exercise*, Boston: Houghton Mifflin, 1977.

HARVARD STEP TEST (Brouha 1943)

NOTE: This is a strenuous test, and should not be used on older individuals.

Test Objective. To estimate the capacity of the body to adjust to and recover from hard muscular work.

Age Level. College males.

Equipment. A bench or platform 20 inches high, a stopwatch and a metronome. Recording the commands "up, up, down, down" assists the performers in maintaining the cadence and permits you to circulate among them.

Validity. Studies on Harvard undergraduates showed that athletes scored higher than nonathletes, and the scores of the athletes increased with more training and decreased after they stopped training.

Norms. Classification standards are given in the discussion of Scoring.

Administration and Directions. Permit the test performers to practice counting their pulse at the radial or carotid artery. Pair up the test performers. The test performer steps up and down on a bench 30 times/minute for five minutes, unless he must stop earlier because of fatigue. The body should be erect each time he steps onto the bench and the lead foot may be changed during the test. As soon as he stops performing the test, he sits down and remains sitting throughout the pulse count. There are two forms of the test. Using the long form, the pulse is counted for 30 seconds on three occasions: one minute after exercise (1 to 1½ minutes), two minutes after exercise (2 to 2½ minutes), and three minutes after exercise (3 to 3½ minutes). In the short form, the pulse is counted only for 30 seconds, one minute after exercise (1 to 1½ minutes).

Scoring. In the long form, a physical efficiency index (PEI) is computed with the formula:

$$PEI = \frac{\text{duration of exercise in seconds x 100}}{2 \text{ x sum of pulse counts in recovery}}$$

The PEI standards for the long form are:

    below 55   — poor
    55 to 64   — low average
    65 to 79   — high average
    80 to 89   — good
    above 89   — excellent

For individuals who do not complete the five-minute test, the following scoring standards may be used:

Duration	Score
less than 2 minutes	25
from 2 to 3 minutes	38
from 3 to 3½ minutes	48
from 3½ to 4 minutes	52
from 4 to 4½ minutes	55
from 4½ to 5 minutes	59

In the short form, the scoring formula is:

$$PEI = \frac{\text{duration of exercise in seconds x 100}}{5.5 \text{ x pulse count for 1 to 1½ minutes after exercise}}$$

The PEI standards for the short form are:

    below 50   — poor
    50 to 80   — average
    above 80   — good

Modifications of Harvard Step Test

Modifications of the Harvard Step Test have been made so it may be used on both sexes, in elementary grades through college. The modified tests, described below, are reported to perform the same functions as the original Harvard Step Test; they will test cardiorespiratory fitness and discriminate between individuals in good and in poor physical condition.

Junior and Senior High Males (Gallagher and Brouha 1943)

Males 12 through 18 years of age with a body surface area (based on height and weight) less than 1.85 use an 18-inch bench; while males of the same age with a surface area of 1.85 or more use a 20-inch bench. A nomogram for estimating body surface is provided in the reference. Both groups perform 30 steps/minute for four minutes. The sequence of pulse counts and the formula for scoring are the same as those used for college males. The classification standards for this test are:

50 or less — very poor
51 to 60 — poor
61 to 70 — fair
71 to 80 — good
81 to 90 — excellent
91 or more — superior

Junior High, Senior High and College Females (Skubic and Hodgkins 1963)

For this test the bench is 18 inches high, the sequence is 24 steps/minute, the duration of exercise is three minutes and only one 30-second pulse count is taken one minute after exercise (1 to 1½ minutes). The cardiovascular efficiency score (CES) is determined through the formula:

$$CES = \frac{\text{No. of seconds completed x 100}}{\text{recovery pulse x 5.6}}$$

Norms for the three female groups are reported in Table 10-6.

Elementary School Males and Females (Brouha and Ball 1952)

For this test the bench is 14 inches high and the cadence is 30 steps/minute. The duration of the exercise is adjusted by ages: three minutes for ages eight through 12 and two minutes for age seven. The pulse count, scoring formula and classification standards are the same as those used for the original Harvard Step Test.

Table 10-6. *Norms for Cardiovascular Efficiency Test (Step Test) for Junior High, Senior High and College Females*

Rating	Junior High*		Senior High*		College**	
	Cardiovascular Efficiency Score	30-Second Recovery Rate	Cardiovascular Efficiency Score	30-Second Recovery Rate	Cardiovascular Efficiency Score	30-Second Recovery Rate
Excellent	72–100	44 or less	71–100	45 or less	71–100	45 or less
Very Good	62–71	45–52	60–70	46–54	60–70	46–54
Good	51–61	53–63	49–59	55–66	49–59	55–66
Fair	41–50	64–79	40–48	67–80	39–48	67–83
Poor	31–40	80–92	31–39	81–96	28–38	84–116
Very Poor	0–30	93 & above	0–30	96 & above	0–27	117–120

*V. Skubic and J. Hodgkins, Cardiovascular efficiency test scores for junior and senior high school girls in the United States, *Research Quarterly* 35: 184–192, 1964.
**J. Hodgkins and V. Skubic, Cardiovascular efficiency test scores for college women in the United States, *Research Quarterly* 34: 454–461, 1963.

DEVELOPMENT OF CARDIORESPIRATORY FITNESS

Cardiorespiratory fitness is developed through aerobic activities, such as running, walking, swimming, cross-country skiing or bicycling for a relatively long distance, or jumping rope for an extended period at an appropriate intensity. Individuals should select an aerobic activity or activities they enjoy and to which they can make a commitment to continue. Running is the most convenient aerobic activity for development and maintenance of cardiorespiratory fitness, though some people find it tedious. In addition, individuals with joint problems (in the back, knees and ankles) and foot disorders are unable to run for an extended period. Though some sports activities and forms of training require intense effort for short periods of time, they are inappropriate for development of cardiorespiratory fitness because they are not aerobic. These activities can, however, provide other exercise benefits and are highly recommended for these benefits.

An exercise program designed to develop cardiorespiratory fitness should be performed a minimum of three to four (nonconsecutive) days/week, but five to six days/week is preferable. Many individuals exercise five to seven days/week but prefer to modify the intensity or the duration on alternate days. They exercise with greater intensity or for a longer period every other day. The exercise sessions for the other days consist of light, rhythmic movement. The avoidance of two consecutive days of intense or long exercise sessions prevents chronic fatigue for most individuals.

Determining the intensity at which one should exercise is critical; however, if training effects are to occur, the principle of overload must be observed. Overload is a gradual increase in the intensity of the physical activity. For the cardiovascular and respiratory systems (or any other physiologic components of fitness) to improve, they must work harder than they are used to working. Stress must be imposed upon them so that over a period of time they will be able to accommodate the additional stress. Sedentary persons who initiate an exercise program should begin at a relatively low intensity and gradually increase the level of exertion. With great expectations of physical development, many individuals undertake a program, but mistakenly begin their activity at an intensity that is too high for them. Their efforts result in soreness and discomfort, which hinder continuation of the program. Also, upon recovery from the soreness, these individuals have no desire to resume the exercise program.

Monitoring the heart rate is the easiest method of determining the intensity of exercise. Unless advised differently by a qualified physician, most individuals should exercise at 60 to 75% of their maximum heart rate range. This range may be found by completing the following steps:

1. estimate the maximum heart rate (220 minus age)
2. subtract the resting heart rate from value found in step 1
3. multiply value found in step 2 by .60
4. add the value found in step 3 to the resting heart rate (this value is minimum target heart rate)
5. multiply value found in step 2 by .75 and add to resting heart rate (this value is maximum target heart rate)

Sedentary individuals should begin an exercise program at 50 to 60% of their maximum heart rate range and increase the percentage as cardiorespiratory fitness improves.

The exercise period should include five to 10 minutes of flexibility exercises and a minimum of 20 minutes of aerobic activities. As the level of fitness improves, the duration of the exercise period can be increased.

REVIEW PROBLEMS

1. Review additional step tests found in other textbooks. Note the groups for whom the tests are intended and the validity and reliability coefficients.
2. Administer one step test and one running test described in this chapter to several of your fellow students. Ask them to provide constructive criticism of your test administration.
3. If possible, observe the administration of cardiorespiratory fitness tests at the health and fitness clubs in your community. Observe how the instructions are given, how the results are interpreted to the group and what safety precautions are followed.

11

Flexibility

Upon completion of this chapter, you should be able to:
1. Define and measure flexibility;
2. State why flexibility should be measured; and
3. Prescribe activities to improve flexibility.

Flexibility is the ability to move the body joints through a maximum range of motion, without undue strain. It is not a general factor, but it is specific to given joints and to particular sports or physical activities. An individual with good flexibility in the shoulders may not have good flexibility in the lower back or posterior upper legs. Flexibility is more dependent on the soft tissues (ligaments, tendons and muscles) of a joint than on the bony structure of the joint itself. However, the bony structures of certain joints do place limitations on flexibility, as illustrated by extension of the elbow or knee, and hyperextension and abduction of the spinal column.

Flexibility also is related to body size, sex, age and physical activity. Any increase in body fat usually decreases flexibility. Generally, females are more flexible than males. Anatomical distinctions or differences in regular physical activity may account for these flexibility differences. During the early school years flexibility increases, but a leveling off or decrease begins in early adolescence. The dramatic loss of flexibility in the aging process is probably due to failure to maintain an active program of movement.

Generally, active individuals are more flexible than inactive individuals. The soft tissues and joints tend to shrink, losing extensibility when the muscles are maintained in a shortened position. Habitual postures and chronic heavy work through restricted ranges of motion also can lead to adaptive shortening of muscles. Physical activity with wide ranges of movement helps prevent this loss of extensibility. Generally then, flexibility is more related to habitual movement patterns for each individual and for each joint, than to age or to sex.

WHY MEASURE FLEXIBILITY?

Flexibility is an important component of health related fitness, and the lack of it can create functional problems or disorders for many

155

individuals. Medical records indicate that low back pain is one of the most prevalent health complaints in our nation, and many low back disorders are caused by poor muscle tone, poor flexibility of the lower back and inadequate abdominal muscle tone. Additionally, anyone with a stiff spinal column is at a disadvantage in many physical activities and also fails to get full value from the shock-absorbing arrangement of the spine when walking, running or jumping. Lack of flexibility in the back can be responsible for bad posture, compression of peripheral nerves, painful menstruation and other ailments. Furthermore, short muscles limit work efficiency. They become sore when they perform physical exertion, and, without a good range of movement, the individual is more likely to incur torn ligaments and muscles during physical activities.

Since individuals with good flexibility have greater ease of movement, less stiffness of muscles, enhancement of skill and less chance of injury during movement, the measurement of flexibility should be included in all physical education and wellness programs. Individuals with poor flexibility should be identified, with the appropriate exercises and activities prescribed for them. Flexibility tests are usually administered to identify individuals with too little range of joint movement, but they also can be administered to determine if individuals have too much flexibility in certain joints. It is possible that too much range of movement may result in joint instability and increase the possibility of injury.

Though the measurement of flexibility is usually performed for diagnostic purposes, many physical educators believe it is acceptable to grade flexibility performance. However, since the degree of flexibility most desirable for health purposes has not been determined, the grading of flexibility is questionable. If flexibility performance is graded, the standards should be reasonable, and the students should be informed of the standards at the beginning of the unit.

Are you able to:
define flexibility and state why it should be measured?

TESTS OF FLEXIBILITY

For clinical assessment of flexibility, devices such as the Leighton Flexometer, the electrogoniometer, and the goniometer are used. There also are many valid, practical tests that may be used in physical education and wellness programs, and that may be administered to both sexes. Such tests are covered in this chapter. All of the described tests pose no risk of injury to the performer.

There are two types of flexibility tests. Relative flexibility tests are designed to be relative to the length or width of a specific body part. In these tests, the movement and the length, or width, of an influencing body part are measured. Absolute flexibility tests are designed to measure only the movement in relation to an absolute performance goal. Both types of tests are presented.

Since the test performers will be stretching to their maximum, they should warm-up prior to taking the flexibility tests. Also, warm-up exercises improve flexibility performance, thus improving the reliability of the scores. The warm-up should include slow sustained static stretching of all joints to be tested.

AAHPERD SIT-AND-REACH TEST (AAHPERD 1980)

NOTE: Though a description of the AAHPERD Sit-and-Reach Test is provided, other similar sit-and-reach tests are acceptable. A bench that is a few inches higher or lower than the test apparatus described in the AAHPERD Test Manual may be used without affecting the validity and reliability of the test.

Test Objective. To measure the flexibility of the lower back and posterior thighs.

Age Level. Five through adulthood.

Equipment. The AAHPERD Test Manual (1980) provides detailed instructions for construction of test apparatus with a measuring scale in which nine inches (23 centimeters) is set at the level of the feet. If the AAHPERD norms are applied, the specially constructed box, or benches which are only 12 inches high, should be used when administering this test. If local norms are established, benches turned on their sides, or the bottom row of bleachers that are a few inches higher than 12 inches, may be used. Rulers may be taped to the benches or bleachers so that several students can be measured at the same time.

Validity. Logical validity has been claimed. The AAHPERD sit-and-reach test has been validated against several other tests and coefficients ranging between 0.80 and 0.90 have been found.

Reliability. .70 or higher.

Objectivity. Not reported.

Norms. Table 11-1 includes norms for ages five through college. The AAHPERD test manuals provide percentile norms.

Administration and Directions. The test apparatus should be prevented from slipping (may be placed against a wall) and the test performer should not be wearing shoes. The performer (1) sits at the test apparatus with the knees fully extended and the feet shoulder-width apart, flat against the end of the board; (2) with the palms down and hands placed on top of each other, extends the arms forward; and (3) reaches directly forward four times and holds the position of the maximum reach on the fourth trial for one second (Figure 11-1).

Scoring. The score is the most distant point reached on the fourth trial, measured to the nearest one-quarter inch or centimeter. The test administrator should be in a position to note the most distant line touched by the fingertips of both hands. If the hands reach unevenly, the position is not held for one second or the knees bend, the test should be readministered. You should be aware that it is normal for many boys and girls not to reach the nine-inch level during the pre-adolescent and adolescent growth spurt (ages 10 through 14). It is not unusual for the legs to become proportionately longer in relation to the trunk during this period. Flexibility exercises should be prescribed for individuals who score below P_{50}, as any score below this percentile represents poor flexibility in the posterior thigh, lower back or posterior hip. Individuals who score below P_{25} have a critical lack of flexibility.

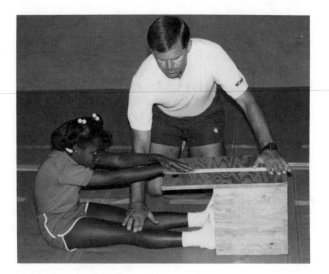

Figure 11-1. *Sit-and-reach test.*

TRUNK-AND-NECK EXTENSION (Johnson and Nelson 1986)
Test Objective. To measure the ability to extend the trunk.
Age Level. Six through college.
Equipment. Mat and yardstick, or tape measure.
Validity. Face validity.
Reliability. .90 through test-retest.
Objectivity. .99.
Norms. Table 11-2 reports norms for college students.
Administration and Directions. The test performer should sit in a hard chair, and the test administrator should measure to the nearest one-quarter inch the distance from the tip of the performer's nose, to the seat of the chair in which the performer is sitting. (The chin must be level when the distance is measured.) The test performer then assumes a prone position on a mat, placing both hands on the lower back. With a partner holding the hips against the mat, the performer raises the trunk as high as possible from the mat. The distance from the tip of the nose to the mat is measured (Figure 11-2).
Scoring. The best of three lifts is subtracted from the trunk and neck length score. The closer the trunk lift is to the trunk and neck length, the better the score.

TRUNK EXTENSION
The trunk extension test is very similar to the trunk-and-neck extension previously described. The difference is this test measures absolute flexibility and does not require measurement of any body parts.
Age Level. Six through college.
Equipment. Mat and yardstick, or tape measure.
Validity. Face validity.
Reliability and Objectivity. Not reported.
Norms. Table 11-2 reports norms for college students.
Administration and Directions. The test performer lies prone on a mat with a partner holding the hips against the mat. With the fingers interlocked behind the neck, the chest and head are raised off the mat as far as possible. The distance in inches is measured from the mat to the chin (Figure 11-3).
Scoring. The best of three lifts is the score.

Table 11-1. *Norms in Inches for AAHPERD Sit-And-Reach Test for Ages Five through College**

PERCENTILE	Age													
	5	6	7	8	9	10	11	12	13	14	15	16	17+	College
MALES														
95	12.50	13.50	13.00	13.50	13.50	13.00	13.50	13.75	14.25	15.50	16.25	16.50	17.75	17.75
75	11.50	11.50	11.00	11.50	11.50	11.00	11.50	11.50	12.00	13.00	13.50	14.25	15.75	15.50
50	10.00	10.25	10.00	10.00	10.00	10.00	10.00	10.25	10.25	11.00	12.00	12.00	13.50	13.50
25	8.75	8.75	8.75	8.75	8.75	8.00	8.25	8.25	8.00	9.00	9.50	10.00	11.00	11.50
5	6.75	6.25	6.25	6.25	4.75	4.75	5.25	4.75	4.75	6.00	5.25	4.50	6.00	7.50
FEMALES														
95	13.50	13.50	13.50	14.25	13.75	13.75	14.50	15.75	17.00	17.50	18.25	18.25	17.50	18.50
75	12.00	12.00	12.25	12.25	12.25	12.25	12.50	13.50	14.25	15.00	16.25	15.50	15.75	16.25
50	10.75	10.75	10.75	11.00	11.00	11.00	11.50	12.00	12.25	13.00	14.25	13.50	13.75	14.50
25	9.00	9.00	9.50	9.00	9.00	9.50	9.50	10.00	9.50	11.00	12.25	12.00	12.25	12.50
5	7.00	7.00	6.25	6.75	6.75	6.25	6.25	6.00	6.75	7.00	7.50	5.50	8.75	9.50

*Adapted from *Health related physical fitness test manual*, Reston, Virginia: AAHPERD, 1980; and R. R. Pate, *Norms for college students: health related physical fitness test*, Reston, Virginia: AAHPERD, 1985.

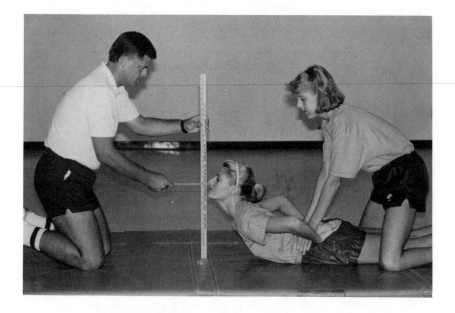

Figure 11-2. *Trunk-and-neck extension test.*

Table 11-2. *Norms in Inches for Trunk-And-Neck Extension and Trunk Extension Tests for College Students**

	Trunk and Neck Extension	Trunk Extension
PERFORMANCE LEVEL	**MALES**	
Above Average	6 to 0	20 and above
Average	8 to 6¼	18 to 19
Below Average	8¼ and above	17 and less
	FEMALES	
Above Average	5¾ to 0	17 and above
Average	7¾ to 6	15 to 16
Below Average	8 and above	14 and less

*Adapted from B. L. Johnson and J. K. Nelson, *Practical measurements for evaluation in physical education,* 4th ed., Edina, Minnesota: Burgess Publishing, 1986; and D. K. Miller and T. E. Allen, *Fitness: a lifetime commitment,* 3rd ed., Edina, Minnesota: Burgess Publishing, 1986.

SHOULDER-AND-WRIST ELEVATION (Johnson and Nelson 1986)
Test Objective. To measure shoulder and wrist flexibility.
Age Level. Six through college.
Equipment. Mat and two yardsticks, or one yardstick and a tape measure.
Validity. Face validity.
Reliability. .93 through test-retest.
Objectivity. .99.
Norms. Norms for college students are reported in Table 11-3.
Administration and Directions. The arm length of the test performer should be measured from the acromion process to the middle fingertip, as the

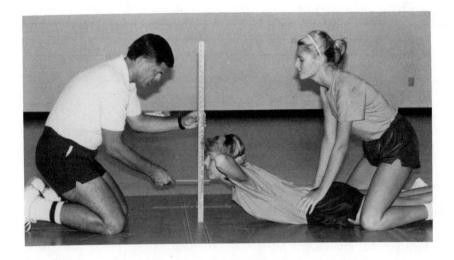

Figure 11-3. *Trunk extension test.*

arm hangs down. The test performer then assumes a prone position with the arms extended forward directly in front of the shoulders and holds a yardstick, with the hands about shoulder-width apart. The yardstick is raised upward as far as possible, while keeping the chin on the floor. As it is difficult to elevate the shoulders without extending the wrists, the movement of the two joints are combined for the test score. When the highest point is reached, the distance is measured to the nearest one-quarter inch. Though some individuals are extremely flexible and they can move the yardstick beyond the highest vertical point, the measurement is still taken at the highest vertical point.

Scoring. The score is the best of three trials subtracted from the arm length. The closer the lift is to the arm measurement, the better the score.

Table 11-3. *Norms in Inches for Shoulder-And-Wrist Elevation and Shoulder Lift for College Students**

PERFORMANCE LEVEL	Shoulder-and-Wrist Elevation	Shoulder Lift
	MALES	
Above Average	8¼ to 0	23 and above
Average	11½ to 8½	20 to 22
Below Average	11¾ and above	19 and less
	FEMALES	
Above Average	7½ to 0	21 and above
Average	10¾ to 7¾	18 to 20
Below Average	11 and above	17 and less

*Adapted from B. L. Johnson and J. K. Nelson, *Practical measurements for evaluation in physical education,* 4th ed., Edina, Minnesota: Burgess Publishing, 1986; and D. K. Miller and T. E. Allen, *Fitness: a lifetime commitment,* 3rd ed., Edina, Minnesota: Burgess Publishing, 1986.

SHOULDER LIFT

The shoulder lift test is very similar to the shoulder-and-wrist elevation test, but it measures shoulder flexibility only. It measures absolute flexibility rather than relative flexibility.

Age Level. Six through college.

Equipment. Mat and two yardsticks, or one yardstick and a tape measure.

Validity. Face validity.

Reliability and Objectivity. Not reported.

Norms. Table 11-3 reports norms for college students.

Administration and Directions. The test performer lies prone on the mat with the chin to the mat, and the arms extended forward directly in front of the shoulders. A yardstick is held with the hands about shoulder-width. The wrists and elbows are kept straight as the yardstick is raised upward as far as possible, with the chin touching the mat. The distance in inches is measured from the bottom of the yardstick to the mat (Figure 11-4).

Scoring. The score is the best of three trials.

Figures 11-5 through 11-8 (Jensen and Hirst 1980) illustrate observation measures of flexibility. No score is recorded, but the measures may be used to identify individuals with inadequate flexibility.

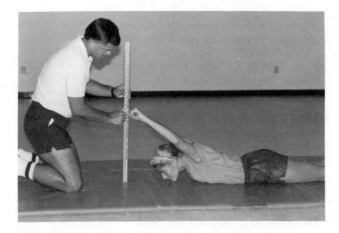

Figure 11-4. *Shoulder lift test.*

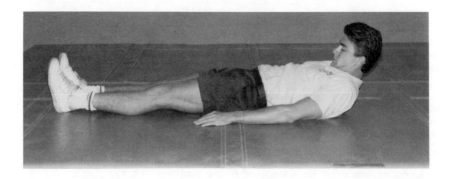

Figure 11-5. *Normal flexibility for the neck allows the chin to move closer to the upper chest.*

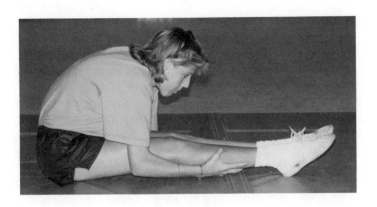

Figure 11-6. *Normal flexibility in the hips and lower back allows for flexion to about 135°.*

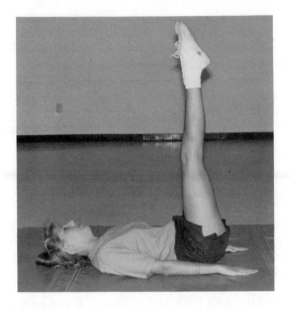

Figure 11-7. *Normal flexibility of the hamstring muscles allows straight-leg lifting to 90° from supine position.*

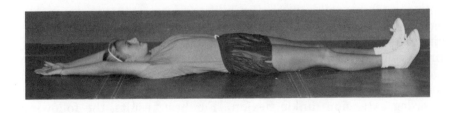

Figure 11-8. *Normal flexibility of chest muscles allows arms to be flexed to 180° of shoulders.*

EXERCISES TO DEVELOP FLEXIBILITY

As previously stated, individuals with poor flexibility are more susceptible to musculoskeletal problems as well as other ailments. Once these individuals have been identified, the appropriate flexibility exercises should be prescribed for them.

Three stretching techniques can be used to improve flexibility: static stretching, ballistic stretching and proprioceptive neuromuscular facilitation (PNF). Static stretching involves slowly moving to a position to stretch the designated muscle(s) and holding the position for a specified length of time. The recommended length of time for holding the stretch varies from 10 to 30 seconds, with the stretch for each muscle being repeated two to three times per stretching session.

Ballistic stretching makes use of repetitive bouncing motions. Though ballistic stretching can improve flexibility, it is not often recommended as a stretching technique. If the force produced by the effort to stretch is greater than the extensibility the muscle tissues can tolerate, injury to the muscle may occur. In addition, the use of a fast, forceful, bobbing type of stretching induces the stretch reflex (the reflex contraction of a muscle in response to being suddenly stretched beyond its normal length). The purpose of this reflex action is to prevent injury caused by overstretching. The amount and rate of the stretch reflex contraction vary directly in proportion to the amount and rate of the movement causing the stretch. The faster and more forceful the stretch, the faster and more forceful the reflex contraction of the stretched muscle. As the individual is attempting to stretch the muscle through a bouncing action, the stretch reflex responds to prevent the muscle from being stretched. This combination may result in muscle injury.

There are a number of different PNF techniques used for stretching, but all involve a combination of alternating contraction and relaxation of both agonist and antagonist muscles. The disadvantage of the PNF techniques is that they require the assistance of a partner to stretch.

Both static stretching and PNF techniques will improve flexibility, but there is lack of agreement regarding the superior technique. It is difficult to compare flexibility studies, as different designs for training programs, length of stretch time and number of PNF repetitions influence the results of the studies. Since it is accepted that static stretching will improve flexibility and no partner is required to perform the exercises, only descriptions of static stretching exercises will be provided. The exercises are designed to improve flexibility throughout the body, but the most important areas to consider are neck and shoulder flexion, back extension, trunk and hip flexion (including lower back and posterior upper-leg muscles) and posterior lower-leg extension (ankle flexion). For best results, the following guidelines should be observed when performing the exercises:

- Spend 20 to 30 seconds in gentle, static stretch with each exercise, and perform each exercise two to three times.
- Increase the extent of the stretch gradually and progressively, with full extension, flexion or both being placed on the joint.
- Breathe slowly, rhythmically and under control.
- Stretch beyond the normal length of the muscle, but stretch to the point that only a slight stretch pain is felt.
- Practice regularly; perform the exercises several times each day.

Flexibility is highly specific to each joint and activity; therefore, flexibility exercises should be performed for each joint in which increased flexibility is desired.

Neck
1. Place the hands behind the head and gradually press down; hold. The posterior neck muscles should feel stretched.
2. Bend the neck from side to side and then from front to back. Do not rotate the head.

Shoulder and Upper Chest
1. Stand in a doorway and grasp the door jamb above the head. Lean forward through the doorway until stretch is felt.
2. Stand with the feet shoulder-width apart and lock the hands behind the waist. Straighten the arms, raise and hold. Bending forward at the waist is a good variation.
3. Extend the arms overhead and interlace the fingers with the palms facing upward. Push upward and slightly backward.
4. Interlace the fingers in front of the chin with the palms turned out. Extend the arms forward.
5. Bring the right hand over the right shoulder to the upper back and reach down as far as possible. Bring the left under the left shoulder to the upper back. Grab fingers and hold. If you are unable to grasp the fingers together, hold a towel between them. Gradually move the left hand up the towel. Reverse hand positions and repeat.

Upper Back
1. Lie on the back with the knees bent and the feet flat on the floor. Interlace the fingers behind the head and gently pull forward until you feel a comfortable stretch. This stretch also may be performed while in standing position.

Lower Back
1. Lie on the back with knees bent and feet flat on the floor. Pull both knees to the chest with your hands, while simultaneously raising the head.
2. Sit on the floor with the legs crossed and arms at the sides. Tuck the chin and curl forward. Slide the hands forward on the floor, allowing the back to be rounded.

Trunk

1. Stand with the feet shoulder-width apart and toes pointed straight ahead. Extend both arms overhead; grasp the left hand with the right hand and bend slowly to the right. Pull the left arm over the head and down toward the ground with the right hand. Bend to the left, reversing the hand positions.
2. Stand and hold a towel overhead with the hands about 12 inches apart, the elbows straight and the feet 18 to 24 inches apart. Bend to one side as far as possible, keeping the elbows straight. Repeat to the other side.
3. Lie prone with the hands in the push-up position. Extend the arms fully to raise the shoulders and upper back. Keep the pelvis and legs on the floor.
4. Lie prone, bend the lower legs, and reach back and grasp the ankles. Pull slowly and hold the head up.

Posterior Hip and Upper Leg (also involves the lower back)

1. Sit on the floor with the legs straight and feet together. Bend forward at the waist (do not dip the head or round the back) and slide the hands down the lateral sides of the legs. Try to place the chest on the thighs and grasp the outer borders of the feet. Keep the toes pointed back to stretch the posterior lower leg muscles.
2. Sit on the floor. Extend one leg and place the sole of the other foot against the thigh of the extended leg. Lean forward at the waist and attempt to pull the toes of the extended leg back, to exert a stretch in the calf and hamstrings. Repeat with the other leg.
3. Lie flat on the back. Raise one leg straight up with the knee extended and ankle flexed to 90°. Grasp the leg around the calf and pull toward the head. Repeat with the opposite leg.

Anterior Hip and Thigh

1. In a standing position, draw one knee up to the chest and pull it tightly to the chest with the hands. Repeat with the other knee.
2. Stand on either leg. Bend the other knee and grasp the ankle behind you. Pull up on the leg as you lean forward slightly. Repeat with the opposite leg. It may be necessary to support yourself by leaning against a wall. This exercise may be performed by lying on the side, grasping the foot of the top leg and slowly pulling it back.
3. Squat with the bent knee of one leg forward and the other leg extended behind you. Push forward until the knee of the front leg is directly over the ankle. The knee of the backward extended leg should be resting on the floor. Without changing the position of the legs and feet, lower the front of your hips downward to create an easy stretch. Reverse the position of the legs and repeat.

Groin Area

1. Sit on the floor. Put the soles of the feet together and grasp the toes. Gently pull yourself forward, bending at the hips.

2. Sit against a wall, or anything that will give support. With the back straight and the soles of the feet together, gently push down on the inside of the thighs with the hands.

Posterior Lower Leg
1. Facing a wall, stand approximately three to four feet away. Lean forward and place the palms against the wall, with the arms straight and at shoulder height. Keep the feet flat and the body in a straight line. Allow the elbows to bend while leaning forward more. Do not allow the heels to rise off the floor.
2. Assume the same position as described in the previous exercise. Perform the same routine but also bend at the knees. Do not allow the heels to rise off the floor. You should feel the stretch in the area closer to the Achilles tendon.

Foot and Ankle
1. Kneel, with the toes and ankles stretched backward. Lean backward and put the body weight on the hands.
2. Stand with the feet apart. Reach back with one foot and touch the floor with the upper side of the toes. Press down until stretch is felt. Repeat with the other foot.

REVIEW PROBLEMS
1. Review additional flexibility tests found in other textbooks. Note the groups for whom the tests are intended and the validity, reliability and objectivity coefficients.
2. Administer one of the tests described in this chapter to several of your classmates. Ask them to provide constructive criticism of your test administration.
3. A physical education teacher administered the AAHPERD sit-and-reach test to 20 15-year-old students. After the students followed a 10-week flexibility program for the lower back and posterior thighs, the teacher again administered the test. Determine if the students significantly improved their flexibility scores.

Student	Pretest Scores	Posttest Scores
A	17.50	18.25
B	16.75	17.50
C	17.00	17.75
D	15.50	16.25
E	15.00	15.75
F	18.50	18.50
G	18.00	18.50
H	14.25	16.25
I	17.00	17.25

J	16.50	17.25
K	15.75	15.75
L	17.50	18.00
M	16.75	17.75
N	15.75	16.50
O	15.50	16.25
P	16.25	16.25
Q	15.75	16.00
R	15.25	15.25
S	16.00	16.50
T	17.00	17.75

12

Muscular Strength, Endurance and Power

Upon completion of this chapter, you should be able to:
1. Define and measure muscular strength, endurance and power;
2. State why muscular strength, endurance and power should be measured; and
3. Prescribe activities to improve muscular strength, endurance and power.

Muscular strength is the ability of a muscle or muscle group to exert maximum force. Dynamic strength is force exerted by a muscle group as a body part moves. Dynamic strength also may be referred to as isotonic strength. Static strength is the force exerted against an immovable object; that is, movement does not take place. This type of strength also is referred to as isometric strength. Both types of strengths are best measured by tests which require one maximum effort.

Muscular endurance is the ability of a muscle or muscle group to resist fatigue and to make repeated contractions against a defined submaximal resistance (dynamic endurance). It also may be the ability to maintain a certain degree of force over time (static endurance). Muscular strength and endurance are closely related, though weight-training methods for them are typically different. Generally, strength is best developed through a high-resistance, low-repetition program, while endurance is improved through a low-resistance, high repetition program. Strength and endurance can be improved through either program, however. Also, it is necessary to have some strength to develop endurance. For example, to develop abdominal muscular endurance through sit-ups, you must have the strength to perform at least one sit-up. The inability to perform one sit-up is due to lack of strength, not endurance.

169

Muscular power is the ability to generate maximum force in the fastest possible time. It also may be defined as the ability to release maximum muscular force in an explosive manner. Power is equal to the product of force times velocity. Force is generated by muscle strength (strength is a component of power), and velocity is the speed the force is used. Although power is not considered an essential component of physical fitness or good health, it is often the characteristic of a good athlete. Power usually is measured by some type of jump, throw or charge (the vertical jump, shot put or a charge at a blocking sled).

WHY MEASURE MUSCULAR STRENGTH, ENDURANCE AND POWER?

There are several reasons for measurement of muscular strength and endurance. Strength is essential for high level performance in many sports and, though not to the same degree, it also is essential for good health. Strong muscles help protect the joints, making them less susceptible to sprains, strains and other injuries. Strength is necessary for good posture. Such postural problems as sagging abdominal organs, round shoulders, and low back pain may be prevented if adequate strength is maintained. In addition, strength will enable you to perform routine tasks more efficiently, and to experience more satisfaction from leisure sport participation.

The need of muscular endurance is demonstrated in many of our daily activities. Have you ever experienced occasions when it was necessary to "keep going," though your arms, legs or entire body felt too tired to do so? Perhaps your arms felt this way when carrying the groceries from the car into the house. You had the strength to pick up the groceries, but they became heavier and heavier the farther you carried them. This can occur when pushing a stalled car, carrying a heavy suitcase or performing any task that involves sustained muscular contraction. Even if you do not lift and carry heavy loads, you probably lift light loads repeatedly or lift and move your body throughout the day. To avoid end-of-day fatigue, you need muscular endurance. Also, possessing adequate muscular endurance enables you to maintain good posture, thereby decreasing the likelihood that you will experience backaches and muscle injury while performing routine tasks.

As previously stated, muscular power is often a characteristic of a good athlete, but it is rarely necessary to have power when performing daily tasks. Because it is not considered to be an essential component of health and physical fitness, it is not usually emphasized in physical education and wellness programs. Occasionally, leisure sports participants feel that increasing their power will improve their sport performance.

Are you able to:
define muscular strength, endurance and power and state why
they should be measured?

TESTS OF MUSCULAR STRENGTH AND ENDURANCE

Though not required, dynamometers, cable tensiometers, electromechanical instruments, weight-training machines and free weights may be used for the testing of muscular strength and endurance. These equipment and instruments are expensive and are typically used in research studies when accuracy of measurement is essential. Two types of dynamometers are used to measure static strength, one for handgrip and one for back and leg strength. Cable tensiometers may be used to measure static strength of 38 different muscle groups. Electromechanical instruments measure static and dynamic strength, endurance and power. Through measurement of the intensity and frequency of muscle contractions, in terms of electrical activity, they are capable of determining the maximum contraction of a muscle group at a constant speed throughout the entire range of the movement. Many public schools and fitness centers have weight-training machines and free weights, but few have dynamometers, cable tensiometers and electromechanical instruments.

Tests with Weight-Training Equipment

If weight-training equipment is available, the measurement of dynamic muscular strength and endurance is a simple procedure. It is important, however, that hand grip, knee flexion, feet placement and all other considerations that may influence test performance be standardized and enforced. In addition, since motivational factors can influence the test results, the test administration must be standardized for motivation considerations. Test participants should warm up, but avoid overworking, and safety precautions should be observed, especially if free weights are used.

Dynamic strength is measured with one repetition maximum (1-RM). Since a direct relationship exists between body weight and weight lifted (heavier individuals generally can lift more), the maximum weight that can be lifted should be interpreted in relation to the individual's weight. The 1-RM is determined through trial and error. A weight the individual can lift comfortably is first selected. After performing the lift, the test participant is permitted to rest for two to three minutes. The weight is increased by five to 15 pounds, and another lift is attempted. With allowance for rest after each lift, this procedure is followed until the participant is unable to perform a successful lift. Although 1-RMs may be administered to measure most muscle groups, the body's major muscle groups may be tested with the bench press, standing press, arm curls and leg press. Table 12-1 reports the optimal strength values for these lifts for the various body weights.

Muscular endurance tests may be relative or absolute. In a relative endurance test, the performer works with a weight that is proportionate to the maximum strength of a particular muscle group, or to body weight. In an absolute endurance test, all performers work with the same amount of weight (the weight has no relationship to maximum strength or body weight of the test performer). When testing for muscular endurance, the weight should be lifted and returned without jerky movements. To encourage continuous, smooth movement, a three-second cadence may be used for each lift. The score is the number of repetitions completed, and the test is completed when a lift can no longer be properly executed or performed with the cadence. Pollock, Wilmore and Fox (1978) suggest that a fixed percentage of 70% of the maximum strength be used to test muscle endurance. This percentage would be the same for all muscle groups tested. No norms have been developed for this procedure, but on the basis of limited test data, the individual seeking health fitness should be able to perform 12 to 15 repetitions, and the competitive athlete should be able to perform 20 to 25 repetitions of each of the lifts tested.

Table 12-1. *Optimal Strength Values in Pounds for Various Body Weights (Based on 1-RM Test on Universal Gym Apparatus)**

BODY WEIGHT	BENCH PRESS	STANDING PRESS	ARM CURL	LEG PRESS
		MALES		
80	80	53	40	160
100	100	67	50	200
120	120	80	60	240
140	140	93	70	280
160	160	107	80	320
180	180	120	90	360
200	200	133	100	400
220	220	147	110	440
240	240	160	120	480
		FEMALES		
80	56	37	28	112
100	70	47	35	140
120	84	56	42	168
140	98	65	49	196
160	112	75	56	224
180	126	84	63	252
200	140	93	70	280

*Adapted from M. L. Pollock, J. H. Wilmore, and S. M. Fox, *Health and fitness through physical activity*, New York: John Wiley and Sons, 1978.

Tests Requiring Limited Equipment

The following tests for muscular strength, endurance and power are simple and practical, and they require little equipment for administration. However, reliability and objectivity coefficients are not reported for all the tests, and many of them are not appropriate for both sexes. If a test is designed primarily for one sex, that sex is indicated. Rest should be permitted when two or more test trials are administered.

SIT-UP TEST (STRENGTH) (Johnson and Nelson 1986)

Test Objective. To measure strength of abdominal and trunk flexion muscles.

Age Level. 12 through college.

Equipment. A mat, weight bar, dumbbell bar, weight plates and a 12-inch ruler.

Validity. Face validity.

Reliability. .91.

Objectivity. .98.

Norms. Johnson and Nelson provide norms (weight lifted divided by body weight) for college students.

Administration and Directions. The sit-up is performed with a weight plate, a dumbbell or a barbell behind the neck. If a dumbbell or barbell is used, the attached weight plates must not have a greater circumference than standard five-pound plates. The test performer (1) selects the amount of weight that is to be held during the sit-up; (2) assumes a supine position on a mat so the selected weight is behind the neck, flexes the knees and places the feet flat on the mat; (3) with a test partner holding a ruler under the knees, slides the feet toward the buttocks until the ruler can be held in place due to the flexion of the lower legs; (4) slowly slides the feet forward until the ruler falls — at that point the test administrator marks the heel line and the buttocks line, indicating the distance that should remain between the heels and the buttocks during the test; and (5) as the partner holds the performer's feet firmly to floor, attempts to sit-up while holding the weight behind the neck (Figure 12-1). The test administrator should be prepared to remove the weight at the completion of the sit-up.

Scoring. Two sit-ups are permitted and the greatest amount of weight lifted is recorded. The test score may be (1) the amount of weight lifted, or (2) the amount of weight lifted divided by body weight.

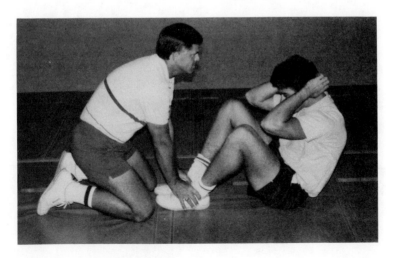

Figure 12-1. *Sit-up test for strength.*

SIT-UPS TEST (ENDURANCE) (AAHPERD 1980; Pollock, Wilmore and Fox 1978)

Test objective. To measure abdominal strength and endurance.

Age level. Five through adulthood.

Equipment. Mats and a stopwatch.

Validity. Logical validity.

Reliability. .68 to .94 for AAHPERD Modified Sit-ups Test.

Norms. Tables 12-2 and 12-3 include norms.

Administration and Directions. Two types of sit-up tests may be administered, but both are performed for 60 seconds. With the AAHPERD Modified Sit-ups Test, the test performer assumes a supine position on the mat with the knees flexed, feet flat on the mat, and the heels between 12 and 18 inches from the buttocks. The arms are crossed on the chest with the hands on opposite shoulders. A test partner holds the feet of the test performer to keep them in contact with the mat. On the signal, "Go," the test performer (1) curls to a sitting position and touches the thighs with the elbows, while maintaining arm contact with the chest and keeping the chin tucked on the chest (Figure 12-2); (2) curls back to the floor until the midback contacts the mat; and (3) continues

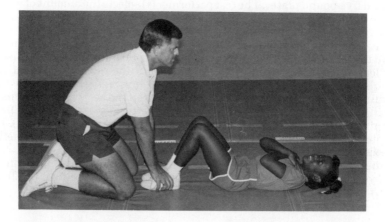

Figure 12-2. *AAHPERD modified sit-up test; (a) start position.*

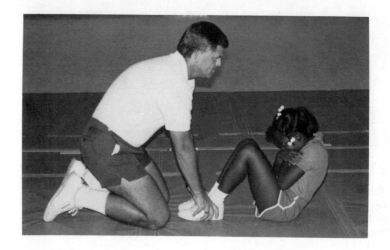

Figure 12-2b. *Up position.*

to perform as many sit-ups as possible in 60 seconds. The test administrator should use the signal, "Ready, Go," to begin the test, and the word "Stop," to conclude the test at the end of 60 seconds. Pausing between sit-ups is permitted. Table 12-2 includes norms for this sit-ups test for ages five through college.

A second type of sit-ups test is administered in a similar procedure, except the hands are interlocked behind the performer's neck, the elbows are touched to the knees, and the performer must return to the full lying position prior to starting the next sit-up (Figure 12-3). The performer should be cautioned not to use the arms to thrust the body into a sitting position. Table 12-3 includes norms for ages 20 through 69 for this sit-ups test.

Scoring. The score for both tests is the number of sit-ups correctly performed during the 60 seconds. Incorrect performance for the AAHPERD sit-ups test includes failure to curl up, failure to keep the arms against the chest, failure to touch the thighs with the elbows and failure to touch the midback to the mat. The distance between the heels and the buttocks should be monitored continuously. Incorrect performance for the second type of sit-ups test includes failure to keep the hands interlocked behind the neck, failure to touch the knees with the elbows and failure to return to the full lying position. If partners are permitted to count the number of sit-ups, the test administrator should observe to be sure the partners are counting only sit-ups that are performed correctly.

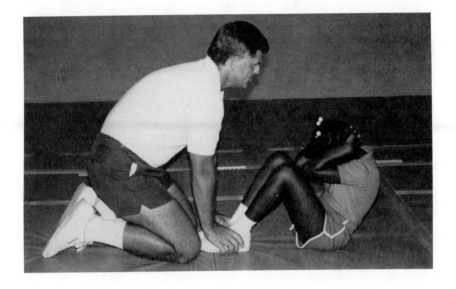

Figure 12-3. *Sit-up test (bent knee).*

PULL-UP TEST FOR MALES (STRENGTH) (Johnson and Nelson 1986)
Test Objective. To measure arm and shoulder girdle strength.
Age level. 12 through college.
Equipment. A horizontal bar; 2½-, 5-, 10- and 25-pound weight plates; a rope or strap to secure the weights to the waist of the test performer and a chair.
Validity. Face validity.
Reliability. .99.
Objectivity. .99.

Table 12-2. *Norms for AAHPERD Modified Sit-Ups Test for Ages Five through College**

| PERCENTILE | Age | | | | | | | | | | | | | |
	5	6	7	8	9	10	11	12	13	14	15	16	17+	College
MALES														
95	30	36	42	48	47	50	51	56	58	59	59	61	62	60
75	23	26	33	37	38	40	42	46	48	49	49	51	52	50
50	18	20	26	30	32	34	37	39	41	42	44	45	46	44
25	11	15	19	25	25	27	30	31	35	36	38	38	38	38
5	2	6	10	15	15	15	17	19	25	27	28	28	25	30
FEMALES														
95	28	35	40	44	44	47	50	52	51	51	56	54	54	53
75	24	28	31	35	35	39	40	41	41	42	43	42	44	42
50	19	22	25	29	29	32	34	36	35	35	37	33	37	35
25	12	14	20	22	23	25	28	30	29	30	30	29	31	30
5	2	6	10	12	14	15	19	19	18	20	20	20	19	21

*Adapted from *Health related physical fitness test manual*, Reston, Virginia: AAHPERD, 1980; and R. R. Pate, *Norms for college students: health related physical fitness test*, Reston, Virginia: AAHPERD, 1985.

Table 12-3. Norms for Sit-Ups Test (Muscular Endurance) for Ages 20 through
69*

	20–29	30–39	Age 40–49	50–59	60–69
PERFORMANCE LEVEL		**MALES**			
Above Average	43 and above	35 and above	30 and above	25 and above	20 and above
Average	37 to 42	29 to 34	24 to 29	19 to 24	14 to 19
Below Average	41 and below	33 and below	23 and below	18 and below	13 and below
		FEMALES			
Above Average	39 and above	31 and above	26 and above	21 and above	16 and above
Average	33 to 38	25 to 30	19 to 25	15 to 20	10 to 15
Below Average	32 and below	24 and below	18 and below	14 and below	9 and below

*Adapted from M. L. Pollock, J. H. Wilmore, and S. M. Fox, *Health and fitness through physical activity*, New York: John Wiley and Sons, 1978.

Norms. Johnson and Nelson provide norms for college males.
Administration and Directions. The horizontal bar is raised to a height so the test performer's feet will be off the floor. The test performer (1) secures the desired amount of weight to his waist and steps on the chair (test administrator should assist performer when he steps to and from the chair); (2) grasps the bar with the overhand grip (palms forward) and assumes a straight-arm hang (chair is removed); and (3) pulls upward until his chin is above the bar (chair is replaced under his feet). He may step down and readjust the weights before repeating the test.
Scoring. Two pull-ups are permitted and the greatest amount of weight lifted is recorded. The test score is the amount of weight lifted divided by body weight. The test performer who cannot lift more than his own body weight receives zero. No swinging action to move upward is permitted.

PULL-UPS TEST FOR MALES (ENDURANCE) (AAHPERD 1976)
Test Objective. To measure arm and shoulder girdle strength and endurance.
Age Level. Nine through college.
Equipment. Metal or wooden bar approximately 1½ inches in diameter (inclined ladder may be used).
Validity. Face validity.
Reliability. .87.
Norms. Table 12-4 includes norms for ages 9 through 17+.
Administration and Directions. The test performer hangs from the bar using the overhand grip (palms forward) with his legs and arms fully extended. His feet should not touch the floor. He pulls himself upward until his chin is over the bar and then lowers his body to a full hang position. He repeats the exercise as many times as possible.
Scoring. Only one trial is administered, unless it is obvious the performer can do better with a second attempt. The score is the number of completed pull-ups. The knees must not be flexed, and kicking motions, swinging and snap-up motions are not permitted. The test administrator may prevent these actions by holding an extended arm across the front of the performer's thighs.
  A test using the reverse grip (palms facing the body) is also administered

Table 12-4. *Norms for AAHPERD Pull-Ups Test for Males Ages Nine through 17+**

				Age				
	9-10	11	12	13	14	15	16	17+
PERCENTILE								
95	9	8	9	10	12	15	14	15
75	3	4	4	5	7	9	10	10
50	1	2	2	3	4	6	7	7
25	0	0	0	1	2	3	4	4
15	0	0	0	0	1	1	3	2

*Adapted from *AAHPERD youth fitness test manual*, Reston, Virginia: AAHPERD, 1976.

to measure arm and shoulder girdle strength and endurance. This is an acceptable grip, but since the test performers will be able to complete more repetitions with this grip, the AAHPERD norms should not be used for scoring.

MODIFIED PULL-UPS FOR FEMALES (ENDURANCE)
Test Objective. To measure arm and shoulder girdle endurance.
NOTE: Though designed for females, this test may be administered to males who are unable to perform the pull-ups previously described.
Age Level. 10 through college.
Equipment. Horizontal bar.
Validity. Face validity.
Norms. None.
Administration and Directions. The bar is adjusted to the height of the base of the performer's sternum when the performer is standing erect. The performer (1) grasps the bar with an overhand grip (palms forward) and slides the feet under the bar until the arms are straight and the angle between the arms and trunk is 90°; (2) keeps the body rigid and straight, and brings the chin over the bar; and (3) completes as many pull-ups as possible (Figure 12-4).
Scoring. Only one trial is permitted, and the score is the number of correct pull-ups completed.

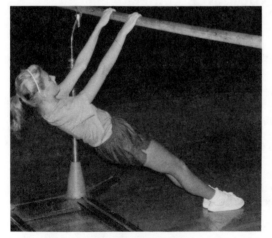
(a) Start position

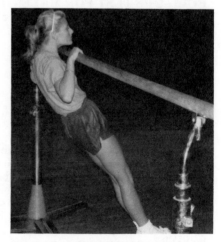
(b) Up position

Figure 12-4. *Modified pull-up for females.*

BAUMGARTNER MODIFIED PULL-UPS TEST (Baumgartner and Jackson 1982; Baumgartner et al. 1984)

Test Objective. To measure arm and shoulder girdle strength or endurance or both.

Age Level. Elementary school through college.

Equipment. The necessary equipment is sold commercially, or it may be constructed locally with inexpensive parts. The equipment consists of an inclined board with a rail system for a scooter board to slide on (Figure 12-5).

Validity. Face validity and construct validity since males performed significantly better than females.

Reliability. Reliability coefficients of .89 to .98 have been reported.

Norms. Table 12-5 reports norms for ages six through college.

Administration and Directions. The test performer lies prone on the scooter board and grasps the bar with an overhand grip, hands shoulder-width apart. The arms should be fully extended. The test is then performed like the regular pull-up test, chin over the bar and return to a straight-arm hanging position. The performer should pull evenly with both arms and not drag the toes.

Scoring. The score is the completed number of repetitions.

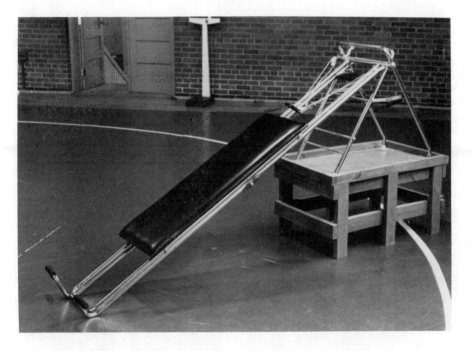

Figure 12-5. *Equipment for modified pull-up test.*
(Photograph provided by Ted Baumgartner, University of Georgia)

FLEXED-ARM HANG FOR FEMALES (AAHPERD 1978)

Test Objective. To measure arm and shoulder girdle endurance.

Age Level. 10 through college.

Equipment. A horizontal bar 1½ inches in diameter and a stopwatch.

Validity. Face validity.

Reliability. .90.

Objectivity. .99.

Table 12-5. *Norms for Baumgartner's Modified Pull-Ups Test**

MALES
Age

PERFORMANCE LEVEL	6	7	8	9-11	**	14	15	16	17-18	College
Above Average	18 and above	23 and above	26 and above	32 and above		30 and above	31 and above	35 and above	33 and above	34 and above
Average (40 to 60%)	13 to 17	18 to 22	19 to 25	25 to 31		25 to 29	27 to 30	30 to 34	29 to 32	28 to 33
Below Average	12 and below	17 and below	18 and below	24 and below		24 and below	26 and below	29 and below	28 and below	27 and below

FEMALES
Age

PERFORMANCE LEVEL	6	7	8	9-11	**	14-15	**	College
Above Average	18 and above	21 and above	19 and above	24 and above		14 and above		13 and above
Average (40 to 60%)	13 to 17	15 to 20	14 to 18	18 to 23		10 to 15		10 to 12
Below Average	12 and below	14 and below	13 and below	17 and below		9 and below		9 and below

*Adapted from A. Jackson et al., Baumgartner's modified pull-test for male and female elementary school aged children, *Research Quarterly for Exercise and Sport* 53: 163–164, 1982; and T. A. Baumgartner et al., Equipment improvements and additional norms for the modified pull-up test, *Research Quarterly for Exercise and Sport* 55: 64–68, 1984.

**Norms not reported for males ages 12 through 13, and females ages 12 through 13 and 16 through 18.

Norms. Table 12-6 includes norms for ages 9 through 17+.

Administration and Directions. The bar should be at a height that the test performer cannot touch the floor from the flexed-arm position. With the assistance of two spotters and using an overhand grip, the performer raises her body off the floor so that the chin is above the bar and the elbows are flexed. This position is held for as long as possible.

Scoring. The score is the number of seconds the proper position is maintained. The test administrator should begin the time as soon as the performer is in the flexed-arm position and should stop the time when the chin touches the bar, tilts backward or drops below the bar. Though developed for females, this test may be used for males who are unable to perform the pull-up test.

Table 12-6. *Norms in Seconds for AAHPERD Flexed-Arm Hang for Females Ages Nine through 17+**

	Age							
	9-10	11	12	13	14	15	16	17+
PERCENTILE								
95	42	39	33	34	35	36	31	34
75	18	20	18	16	21	18	15	17
50	9	10	9	8	9	9	7	8
25	3	3	3	3	3	4	3	3
15	1	2	1	1	2	2	1	2

*Adapted from *AAHPERD youth fitness test manual*, Reston, Virginia: AAHPERD, 1976.

DIP TEST FOR MALES (STRENGTH) (Johnson and Nelson 1986)

Test Objective. To measure arm and shoulder girdle strength.

Age Level. 12 through college.

Equipment. Parallel bars, weight plates, straps and a chair.

Validity. Face validity.

Reliability. .98.

Objectivity. .99.

Norms. Johnson and Nelson provide norms for college males.

Administration and Directions. The bars should be at a height that the test performer is freely above the floor while in the lowered bent-arm support position. After securing the desired amount of weight to the waist, the test performer (1) steps on the chair and takes a secure grip on the bars (should be assisted when he steps to and from the chair); (2) assumes a straight-arm support position (the chair is removed); (3) lowers himself until his elbows form a right angle; and (4) pushes to a straight-arm support position (chair is replaced). He may step down and readjust the weights before attempting the exercise again.

Scoring. Two dips are permitted. The greatest amount of weight lifted is recorded. The test score is the amount of weight lifted divided by body weight. The test performer is not permitted to swing or kick in returning to the straight-arm support position.

DIPS FOR MALES (ENDURANCE)

Test objective. To measure arm and shoulder girdle endurance.

Age level. 10 through college.

Equipment. Parallel bars.

Validity. Face validity.

Reliability. .90 (Johnson and Nelson 1986).

Objectivity. Not reported.

Norms. None reported.

Administration and Directions. The bars should be at a height that the test performer is freely above the floor while in the lowered bent-arm support position. The performer (1) jumps to a straight-arm support position between the bars; (2) lowers the body until the angle at the elbows is a right angle or less; and (3) completes the exercise as many times as possible.

Scoring. The score is the number of correct dips completed. Resting between dips, and kicking or swinging are not permitted.

PUSH-UPS FOR MALES (Johnson and Nelson 1986)

Test Objective. To measure arm and shoulder girdle endurance.

Age Level. 10 through adulthood.

Equipment. None required; mats may be used.

Validity. Face validity.

Objectivity. .99.

Norms. Table 12-7 reports norms for males and females (modified push-up) ages 20 through 69.

Administration and Directions. The test performer (1) lies face down on the floor with the body straight, arms bent and hands flat on the floor beneath the shoulders; (2) pushes upward to a straight-arm position; (3) lowers the body until the chest touches the floor; and (4) repeats the exercise as many times as possible, without rest. The body must stay rigid (not sag or pike upward) throughout the test. The counter may place his hand on the floor for the performer to touch with his chest.

Scoring. The score is the number of correct push-ups completed.

MODIFIED PUSH-UPS FOR FEMALES

Test Objective. To measure arm and shoulder girdle endurance.

Age Level. 10 through adulthood.

Equipment. None required; mats may be used.

Validity. Face validity.

Reliability. .93 (Johnson and Nelson 1986).

Objectivity. Not reported.

Norms. Table 12-7 provides norms for ages 20 through 69.

Administration and Directions. The test performer (1) lies face down on the floor with the body trunk straight, knees bent at right angles, arms bent

Table 12-7. Norms for Push-Ups Test (Muscular Endurance) for Ages 20 through 69*

			Age		
	20–29	30–39	40–49	50–59	60–69
PERFORMANCE LEVEL			**MALES**		
Above Average	45 and above	35 and above	30 and above	25 and above	20 and above
Average	35 to 44	25 to 34	20 to 29	15 to 24	10 to 19
Below Average	34 and below	24 and below	19 and below	14 and below	9 and below
			FEMALES (modified push-up)		
Above Average	34 and above	25 and above	20 and above	15 and above	5 and above
Average	17 to 33	12 to 24	8 to 19	6 to 14	3 to 4
Below Average	32 and below	11 and below	7 and below	5 and below	2 and below

*Adapted from M. L. Pollock, J. H. Wilmore and S. M. Fox, *Health and fitness through physical activity*, New York: John Wiley and Sons, 1978.

and hands flat on the floor beneath the shoulders; (2) pushes upward to a straight-arm position (Figure 12-6); (3) lowers the body until the chest touches the floor; and (4) repeats the exercise as many times as possible without rest. The body trunk must remain straight throughout the test. Modified push-ups also may be performed with a bench. The push-up is performed in the same manner as the push-ups for males except the hands are placed on a bench that is approximately 15 inches high and 15 inches long.

Scoring. The score is the number of correct push-ups completed.

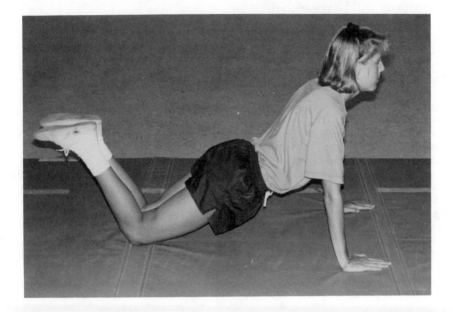

Figure 12-6. *Modified push-up.*

SQUAT THRUST

Test Objective. To measure general muscular endurance of the body.

Age Level. 10 through college.

Equipment. Stopwatch.

Validity. Face validity.

Reliability and Objectivity. Not reported.

Norms. None reported.

Administration and Directions. The test performer (1) from a standing position, squats and places the hands in front of the feet; (2) thrusts the legs backward and takes a front leaning rest position (push-up position); (3) returns to a squat position; (4) rises to a standing position; and (5) completes as many squat thrusts as possible. The sequence for this test is identical to the sequence for the agility squat thrust test described in Chapter 8. The test may be administered with a time limit; for example, the performer completes as many squat thrusts as possible in 30 seconds, 60 seconds, two minutes, or any reasonable time you select.

Scoring. The score is the number of correct squat thrusts completed.

MUSCULAR POWER

Two types of muscular power may be measured: athletic power and work power. The distance the body or an object can be propelled through space indicates athletic power (vertical jump and medicine ball put). If work power is to be measured, extraneous movements are controlled or eliminated, so that maximum effort must be put forth by the muscle groups being tested. For example, if the vertical jump is used to measure work power, the test performer is not permitted to swing the arms. Since power is rarely measured to determine the health or physical fitness status of an individual, only two athletic power tests will be presented.

VERTICAL JUMP (Sargent 1921)
Test Objective. To measure the explosive leg power.
Age Level. Nine through adulthood.
Equipment. A yardstick or measuring tape, chalk and a wall of sufficient height.
Validity. .78 using a criterion test of four power events in track and field.
Reliability. .93.
Objectivity. Coefficients >.90 have been reported.
Norms. Table 12-8 reports norms for ages 9 through 34.
Administration and Directions. A yardstick or tape measure is taped to the wall to measure the distance between two chalk marks. The test performer (1) stands with the dominant side toward the wall and feet flat on the floor; (2) holding a piece of chalk (one-inch in length) in the dominant hand, reaches as high as possible and makes a mark on the wall; and (3) jumps as high as possible and makes another mark at the height of the jump. Three trials are administered. (Rather than using a piece of chalk to make the mark, chalk can be placed on the fingertips.) All test performers should practice the jump until it can be executed correctly before attempting the test.
Scoring. For each jump the score is the distance between the two chalk marks, measured to the nearest half inch. The best jump score is the test score.

Table 12-8. *Norms in Inches for the Vertical Jump for Ages 10 through 17**

	Age							
	10	11	12	13	14	15	16	17
	MALES							
PERCENTILE								
95	15.5	16.5	17.5	19.0	20.5	21.5	22.5	24.0
75	12.5	13.5	14.5	16.0	17.5	18.5	19.5	21.0
50	11.0	12.0	13.0	14.5	16.0	17.0	18.0	19.5
25	9.0	10.0	11.0	12.5	14.0	15.0	16.0	17.5
5	6.0	7.0	7.0	8.5	10.0	11.0	12.0	13.5
	FEMALES							
95	14.0	14.5	15.0	15.5	16.0	17.0	17.0	17.0
75	11.5	12.0	12.5	13.0	13.5	14.5	14.5	14.5
50	10.0	10.5	11.0	11.5	12.0	13.0	13.0	13.0
25	8.5	9.0	9.5	10.0	10.5	11.5	11.5	11.5
5	6.0	6.5	7.0	7.5	8.0	9.0	9.0	9.0

*Adapted from *Physical fitness-motor ability test*, Austin, Texas: Texas Governor's Commission on Physical Fitness, 1973.

STANDING BROAD JUMP (AAHPERD 1976)
Test Objective. To measure explosive leg power.
Age Level. Six through college.
Equipment. A yardstick, tape and tape measure; mat is optional.

Validity. Face validity.

Reliability. Coefficients ranging from .83 to .99 have been reported.

Norms. Table 12-9 reports norms for ages 9 through 17+.

Administration and Directions. A tape measure should be taped to the floor or mat; the jump is performed close to, and parallel to it. The test performer (1) stands behind the restraining line with the feet parallel and several inches apart; (2) bends the knees and swings the arms forward; and (3) jumps forward as far as possible. The test administrator marks the landing point of the nearest heel to the restraining line with the yardstick (yardstick is placed perpendicular to tape measure). All test performers should be permitted to practice the jump until they are able to perform it correctly. Three trials are administered.

Scoring. The score is the number of inches between the restraining line and the nearest heel on landing. If the test performer falls backward on landing, the measurement is made from the restraining line to the nearest part of the body touching the floor or mat.

Table 12-9. *Norms in Feet and Inches for AAHPERD Standing Broad Jump for Ages Nine through 17+**

	Age							
	9-10	11	12	13	14	15	16	17+
	MALES							
PERCENTILE								
95	6' 0"	6' 2"	6' 6"	7'1"	7' 6"	8' 0"	8'2"	8' 5"
75	5' 4"	5' 7"	5' 9"	6'3"	6' 8"	7' 2"	7'6"	7' 9"
50	4'11"	5' 2"	5' 5"	5'9"	6' 2"	6' 8"	7'0"	7' 2"
25	4' 6"	4' 8"	5' 0"	5'2"	5' 6"	6' 1"	6'6"	6' 6"
5	3'10"	4' 0"	4' 2"	4'4"	4' 8"	5' 2"	5'5"	5' 3"
	FEMALES							
95	5'10"	6' 0"	6' 2"	6'5"	6' 8"	6' 7"	6'6"	6' 9"
75	5' 2"	5' 4"	5' 6"	5'9"	5'11"	5'10"	5'9"	6' 0"
50	4' 8"	4'11"	5' 0"	5'3"	5' 4"	5' 5"	5'3"	5' 5"
25	4' 1"	4' 4"	4' 6"	4'9"	4'10"	4'11"	4'9"	4'11"
5	3' 5"	3' 8"	3'10"	4'0"	4' 0"	4' 2"	4'0"	4' 1"

*Adapted from *AAHPERD youth fitness test manual*, Reston, Virginia: AAHPERD, 1976.

EXERCISES TO DEVELOP MUSCULAR STRENGTH AND ENDURANCE

Changes in muscular strength and endurance will take place within a few weeks if the correct exercises are done on a regular basis. Though weight-training programs typically involve the use of free weights, Universal Gym, or Nautilus equipment, muscular strength and endurance can be improved without the use of expensive equipment or a special room. To avoid extreme soreness or injury when the following, and similar, exercises are performed, certain guidelines should be observed:

1. Perform stretching and warm-up exercises before attempting muscular effort.
2. Since some exercises are more difficult than others, perform the ones that provide a mild overload, and gradually progress to the more difficult ones.
3. Unless otherwise indicated, begin with 10 repetitions and add

two or three repetitions each week, until the desired number is reached. If unable to perform 10 repetitions, begin with a lower number.

4. Perform the exercises three to five days per week.

Posterior Upper Arm, Shoulders, Chest and Upper Back
Chair push-up: (1) Place hands shoulder-width apart with fingertips forward on chair or bench, feet on the floor and weight supported on the toes; (2) straighten arms with chin up and chest forward; (3) bend arms and lower chest within one to two inches of chair; and (4) push back to starting position.

Modified push-up: Performed in same manner as modified push-up for females (endurance).

Push-up: Performed in same manner as push-up for males (endurance).

Advanced push-up: Performed in same manner as regular push-up, but feet are placed on a bench or chair.

Anterior Upper Arm, Shoulders, Chest and Upper Back
Modified chin-up: Performed in same manner as modified chin-up for females (endurance).

Chin-up: Performed in same manner as chin-up for males (endurance).

Chin-up with weight: (1) Fill two plastic milk or bleach bottles with equal amounts of water or sand, and tie a bottle to each end of a rope that is 24 to 36 inches long; (2) hang the bottles around the shoulders so they are in front of the body (may place padding between the rope and neck); and (3) perform the chin-ups.

Arm curls: (1) Fill two plastic milk or bleach bottles with equal amounts of water or sand, and tie a bottle to each end of a bar or heavy stick which is approximately 36 to 40 inches long; (2) stand erect with arms fully extended downward and grasp bar with palms up and shoulder-width apart; (3) raise bar to chest by bending arms (elbows should remain at sides and back should remain straight); and (4) perform two or three sets of six to 10 repetitions.

Abdomen
To perform these exercises, lie on the back with the knees bent and feet flat on the floor.

Trunk curl: (1) Clasp hands on top of head (placing the hands behind head may cause the head to jerk forward, straining the neck muscles); (2) roll head and shoulders forward and upward enough to feel tension; and (3) return to starting position.

Reverse Sit-up: (1) Place arms at sides and lift knees to chest, raising hips off the floor and (2) return to starting position.

Assisted flexed knee sit-up: Put hands under thighs to help pull the upper body up to position where no resistance is encountered. Perform the sit-up.

Flexed knee sit-up: Perform sit-up with arms at sides, folded across chest or hands clasped on top of head.

Sit-up with feet elevated: Same position as previous sit-ups but place feet on seat of chair, bed or bench; knees remain bent and arms may be placed in any position.

Lateral Trunk

Side bender: (1) Stand with feet shoulder-width apart and hands clasped behind head and (2) alternate bending to right and left while maintaining straight back and legs. Perform the same number of repetitions for each side. Exercise may be made more difficult by extending arms overhead or extending at sides, holding a weight in each hand.

Lower Back and Buttocks

Back tightener: (1) Lie face down with hands behind lower back and (2) raise head and chest, tense lower back and buttocks muscles. Do not overextend, and raise the head and chest slightly off floor.

Leg raise: (1) With body supported on hands and knees, extend and raise one leg behind the body and (2) perform the same number of repetitions with each leg. Wearing heavy shoes or adding weight to ankles will increase resistance.

Back leg raise: Lie face down, hands clasped behind head, and lift straight legs a few inches off floor. Hold head and chest down.

Back extension: (1) Lie on a bench face down and extend body from waist up over the edge of bench (will be necessary to strap feet down or have someone hold them) and (2) with hands clasped behind head, lift head and trunk. Do not overextend.

Lateral Hip and Thigh

Side leg raise: (1) Using the arms to maintain balance, lie on right side with legs straight; (2) lift left leg straight up from side as high as possible; (3) return to starting position; and (4) perform the same number of repetitions with each leg. Wearing heavy shoes or adding weight to ankles will increase resistance.

Leg Raise: (1) Lie on back with arms at sides and lift legs until they are perpendicular to floor; (2) open legs to a wide V-shape; and (3) close the V and return to starting position. May use heavy shoes or weights for added resistance.

Upper Legs

Two-leg squat: (1) Stand with feet 12 inches apart, with arms extended in front and parallel to floor; (2) squat until knees are bent at a 90° angle (do not go beyond this point); and (3) return to standing position.

Single leg knee dip (with assistance): (1) Stand facing a partner and hold right hands as if shaking hands (if necessary may use table or chair); (2) keeping left leg extended in front, squat down on right foot until knee is at a 90° angle (partner remains standing); (3) grab partner's hand with both hands to return to standing position; and (4) perform the same number of dips with each leg, though attempt no more than five to seven dips when first performing this exercise. Using partner's hand only for balance throughout exercise will increase difficulty.

Lower Legs

Heel raises: (1) Stand on a board, book, or something similar, with heels resting off the edge; (2) using arms for balance, rise up onto toes; and (3) return to starting position. Hanging weights around shoulders will increase resistance.

Jumps in place: With feet parallel, 12 inches apart, jump in place; maintain a steady pace. Do not attempt to jump too high and try to perform on a soft surface (mats, wood floor with carpet).

REVIEW PROBLEMS

1. Review additional muscular strength, endurance and power tests found in other textbooks. Note the groups for whom the tests are intended and the validity, reliability and objectivity coefficients.
2. Administer one of the muscular strength and one of the endurance tests described in this chapter to several of your classmates. Ask them to provide constructive criticism of your test administration.
3. Interview individuals responsible for weight-training programs at fitness or wellness centers. Inquire about tests that are used to measure muscular strength and endurance, interpretation of tests results and programs prescribed for development of muscular strength and endurance.
4. A physical education teacher administered the AAHPERD modified sit-ups test to students in the second grade. The scores listed below are for the 50 girls in the second grade. Determine the mode, median, mean and standard deviation for the scores. Refer to table 12-2, and compare the group with national norms.

15	34	20	31	22
29	16	39	27	31
23	33	24	30	32
21	35	15	38	20
37	18	21	33	22
29	37	40	22	6
19	18	24	30	22
20	29	18	28	14
36	22	18	29	28
25	18	38	17	31

13

Anthropometric Measurement and Body Composition

Upon completion of this chapter, you should be able to:
1. Define the terms somatotype, overweight, overfat, and lean body weight;
2. State why body structure and composition should be measured;
3. Correctly interpret height-weight tables;
4. Classify body frames; and
5. Perform skinfold measurements and estimate percent body fat.

Anthropometry, the measurement of the structure and proportions of the body, is one of the earliest forms of measurement in physical education. It may include measurement of height and weight, measurement of circumferences, diameters, and lengths of body segments and somatotyping (body typing).

Body composition refers to the component parts of the body. Though there are many component parts, for measurement purposes body composition is interpreted as referring to body fat weight and lean body weight. Because lean body weight is found by subtracting the weight of body fat from the total body weight, it is often interpreted as fat-free weight. Technically, however, it includes a small amount of essential lipid that is associated with a variety of tissues in the body, such as the nerve sheaths, the brain and the cell membranes. Depending on body size, about 1.5 to 3% of the weight of the lean body is essential lipids, while 40 to 50% is composed of muscle weight or mass. Organs and tissues, such as skin and bones, make up the remaining portion.

WHY MEASURE BODY STRUCTURE AND COMPOSITION?

Research involving somatotyping requires accurate body type classification, but understanding the concept of somatotyping and

189

being able to roughly determine body types can be of value to coaches, physical education teachers and fitness instructors. The values found in most weight tables are grouped into height and body type categories. Estimation of desirable weight through a height-weight table is not ideal, as no estimation of percent body fat can be made. If this method is used, however, individuals should realistically determine their body type. Additionally, body type classification may be useful when planning obtainable fitness goals. For example, individuals with thick abdomens, wide hips, heavy buttocks and short, heavy legs (endomorphic body type characteristics) usually do not perform as well on running tests as individuals with slender abdomens and hips and lean or muscular legs. This does not mean that certain individuals are to avoid running for health benefits, but it does mean that their running goals should be realistic in terms of their body type.

Height and weight measurements may be recorded for diagnostic purposes. Great differences exist in the physiological maturity of boys and girls, and not all individuals of the same age are expected to have identical heights and weights. The recording of these variables during the growing and developing years may serve to prevent the occurrence of long-term health problems. Young people who significantly deviate from either height or weight ranges, or both, for their ages probably should be observed to determine that no health problems exist. (This determination should be done in a way that is not embarrassing to the individuals.) Height and weight measurements also may be used for homogeneous grouping of youth for sports participation. Classification indexes based on height, weight and age were developed in the 1930s for this purpose; but, currently they are not extensively used.

The measurement of body composition is of importance to all physical educators. It has been estimated that more than 80 million Americans are overweight in that their percentage of body fat exceeds a desirable level. Possibly, as many as 40 million are obese, which means their body fat content exceeds 25% (men) or 30% (women) of the total body weight. This excess weight is not limited to the older population; 20 to 30% of teenagers are overweight. Indeed, overfatness is a national problem.

In an effort to combat overfatness, millions of Americans undertake weight-loss diets. They fail, however, to understand the difference between the loss of body fat and lean body weight, and the role of exercise in weight management. In addition, they mistakenly use weight as indicated on scales to determine the success or lack of success of their diet. Physical educators need to assume a leadership role in the counseling of individuals who are attempting to lose weight. We should be prepared to measure body composition and to advise individuals how to correctly lose body fat.

Furthermore, some people attempt to lose weight, though their percent body fat is acceptable. For example, some athletes have unrealistic images of what their weight should be, and they do not realize the implications of changes in their body composition. This is especially true of amateur wrestlers and gymnasts. Many distance runners also attempt to get their weight too low, with the belief that their running times will improve. This problem is not limited to athletes, however. There are other individuals creating health problems for themselves because they have an incorrect perception of a slender body. Many of these people have emotional problems and need professional counseling to overcome these problems, but possibly some would discontinue efforts to lose weight if they understood the relationship of body fat and good health.

> Are you able to:
> define somatotype, overweight, overfat and lean body weight?
> state why body structure and composition should be measured?

BODY TYPE CLASSIFICATION (SOMATOTYPING)

There are several methods of body type classification, but the classification described by Sheldon, Stevens and Tucker (1970) is the best known. Sheldon's morphological classification includes the ectomorph, the mesomorph and the endomorph. An ectomorph is a slender person with a light frame—the arms and legs are slender and long, the neck appears long and muscle tissue has little definition. A mesomorph is an athletic-looking individual—the shoulders are broad, the hips are narrow and muscle tissue is predominant. An endomorph is a thick individual—the arms and legs are short compared with the torso, the chest and waist are about the same size and the neck is thick.

Three numbers are used to designate the components of each of the three types, with 7 as the highest and 1 as the lowest rating for each. The first number refers to endomorphic, the second to mesomorphic, and the third to ectomorphic characteristics. The rating 7-1-1 designates a pure endomorph; 1-7-1, a pure mesomorph; and 1-1-7, a pure ectomorph. Such extreme ratings are rare, however; usually, at least two components of each type are present in an individual. A 2-5-4 designation indicates less than average endomorphic, more than average mesomorphic and an average number of ectomorphic characteristics. Simplified modifications of Sheldon's classification have been developed, but unless you are involved in research, rarely will it be necessary that you use a numbering system to designate body types.

By knowing the major characteristics of each body type, it is possible to estimate the two dominant body types of each individual and put the estimate to practical use. For example, a relationship exists between somatotypes and certain sports. A football lineman gains an advantage in blocking with a low center of gravity and wide hips and shoulders. Football linemen, therefore, usually rate high on the mesomorph and endomorph scales, and low on the ectomorph scale. On the other hand, individuals who play center on college or professional basketball teams, as well as long distance runners, rate high on the ectomorph scale. When advising individuals about the relationship of physical activity and body types, you should emphasize that training may result in improved performance, but it will not result in a change of body type.

HEIGHT-WEIGHT TABLES

Since 1959, many individuals have used the Metropolitan Life Insurance Company height-weight tables to determine their desirable weight. In 1983, the company released revised tables that were said to represent the weights associated with the lowest death rates among approximately 4,200,000 people observed for 22 years (Table 13-1).

Table 13-1. *1983 Metropolitan Height and Weight Tables for Men and Women of Ages 25 through 59*

Height (with shoes on; 1-in. heels)	Small Frame (lb)	Medium Frame (lb)	Large Frame (lb)
MEN (indoor clothing weighing 5 lb)			
5 ft 2 in.	128–134	131–141	138–150
5 ft 3 in.	130–136	133–143	140–153
5 ft 4 in.	132–138	135–145	142–156
5 ft 5 in.	134–140	137–148	144–160
5 ft 6 in.	136–142	139–151	146–164
5 ft 7 in.	138–145	142–154	149–168
5 ft 8 in.	140–148	145–157	152–172
5 ft 9 in.	142–151	148–160	155–176
5 ft 10 in.	144–154	151–163	158–180
5 ft 11 in.	146–157	154–166	161–184
6 ft 0 in.	149–160	157–170	164–188
6 ft 1 in.	152–164	160–174	168–192
6 ft 2 in.	155–168	164–178	172–197
6 ft 3 in.	158–172	167–182	176–202
6 ft 4 in.	162–176	171–187	181–207
WOMEN (indoor clothing weighing 3 lb)			
4 ft 10 in.	102–111	109–121	118–131
4 ft 11 in.	103–113	111–123	120–134
5 ft 0 in.	104–115	113–126	122–137
5 ft 1 in.	106–118	115–129	125–140
5 ft 2 in.	108–121	118–132	128–143
5 ft 3 in.	111–124	121–135	131–147
5 ft 4 in.	114–127	124–138	134–151
5 ft 5 in.	117–130	127–141	137–155
5 ft 6 in.	120–133	130–144	140–159
5 ft 7 in.	123–136	133–147	143–163
5 ft 8 in.	126–139	136–150	146–167
5 ft 9 in.	129–142	139–153	149–170
5 ft 10 in.	132–145	142–156	152–173
5 ft 11 in.	135–148	145–159	155–176
6 ft 0 in.	138–151	148–162	158–179

Source of basic data: *1979 Build Study*, Society of Actuaries and Association of Life Insurance Medical Directors of America, 1980. Courtesy of Metropolitan Life Insurance Company.

However, when the new tables were released, the American Heart Association (AHA) encouraged Americans to continue to use the 1959 recommendations (Table 13-2). The AHA took this position because the new tables list average weight range increases of 13 pounds for short men, and 10 pounds for short women; with little increases for medium-height men and women; and insignificant increases for tall men and women. The AHA noted that merely looking at death rates obscured health risks associated with the increased weights. The AHA also stated that few health problems are improved by gaining weight, pointing out that the incidence of heart disease, high blood pressure, and diabetes increases in relation to weight gained. Also, the new acceptable weights are most likely skewed upward by the fact that

Table 13-2. *1959 Metropolitan Life Insurance Company Table of Desirable Weights (in pounds) for Men and Women of Ages 25 and Over (indoor clothing)*

Height (with shoes on; 1-in. heels)	Small Frame (lb)	Medium Frame (lb)	Large Frame (lb)
MEN			
5 ft 2 in.	112–120	118–129	126–141
5 ft 3 in.	115–123	121–133	129–144
5 ft 4 in.	118–126	124–136	132–148
5 ft 5 in.	121–129	127–139	135–152
5 ft 6 in.	124–133	130–143	138–156
5 ft 7 in.	128–137	134–147	142–161
5 ft 8 in.	132–141	138–152	147–166
5 ft 9 in.	136–145	142–156	151–170
5 ft 10 in.	140–150	146–160	155–174
5 ft 11 in.	144–154	150–165	159–179
6 ft 0 in.	148–158	154–170	164–184
6 ft 1 in.	152–162	158–175	168–189
6 ft 2 in.	156–167	162–180	173–194
6 ft 3 in.	160–171	167–185	178–199
6 ft 4 in.	164–175	172–190	182–204
WOMEN			
4 ft 10 in.	92–98	96–107	104–119
4 ft 11 in.	94–101	98–110	106–122
5 ft 0 in.	96–104	101–113	109–125
5 ft 1 in.	99–107	104–116	112–128
5 ft 2 in.	102–110	107–119	115–131
5 ft 3 in.	105–113	110–122	118–134
5 ft 4 in.	108–116	113–126	121–138
5 ft 5 in.	111–119	116–130	125–142
5 ft 6 in.	114–123	120–135	129–146
5 ft 7 in.	118–127	124–139	133–150
5 ft 8 in.	122–131	128–143	137–154
5 ft 9 in.	126–135	132–147	141–158
5 ft 10 in.	130–140	136–151	145–163
5 ft 11 in.	134–144	140–155	149–168
6 ft 0 in.	138–148	144–159	153–173

NOTE: For those between 18 and 25, subtract one pound for each year under 25.
Source of data: Derived primarily from data of the *Build and Blood Pressure Study*, 1959, Society of Actuaries. Courtesy of Metropolitan Life Insurance Company.

cigarette smokers, who tend to be thinner than nonsmokers and who die at significantly younger ages, were not taken into account in calculating the new tables.

A major drawback to both the old and new tables is that some individuals do not correctly determine their frame size when selecting an appropriate weight range. Many small- or medium-framed, overfat individuals consider themselves large-framed and do not realistically examine their weight problem. On the other hand, some medium- or large-framed individuals with an acceptable percent of body fat view themselves as small-framed and mistakenly attempt to lose weight. Determination of body frame is best performed by trained personnel, but the following practical methods may be used.

Elbow Breadth

Extend the right arm and bend the forearm upward at a 90° angle. Keep the fingers straight and turn the palm away from the body. Place the thumb and index finger of the left hand on the two prominent bones on either side of the right elbow, and measure the space between the thumb and index finger of the left hand with a ruler or tape measure. Record the measurement, and compare with the standards in Table 13-3.

Ankle Girth

Pulling the tape as snug as possible, measure the girth of the right ankle at the smallest point, just above the bony prominences. Record the measurement and compare with the standards in Table 13-4.

Table 13-3. *Standards for Estimating Medium Frame Using Elbow Breadth and Height**

MALES		FEMALES	
Height (inches)	Elbow Breadth** (inches)	Height (inches)	Elbow Breadth** (inches)
61 to 62	2½ to 2⅞	57 to 58	2¼ to 2½
63 to 66	2⅝ to 2⅞	59 to 62	2¼ to 2½
67 to 70	2¾ to 3	63 to 66	2⅜ to 2⅝
71 to 74	2¾ to 3⅛	67 to 70	2⅜ to 2⅝
75 and above	2⅞ to 3¼	71 and above	2½ to 2¾

Adapted from the Metropolitan Life Insurance Company.
*Height without shoes
**Measurements lower than those listed indicate a small frame and higher measurements indicate a large frame.

Table 13-4. *Standards for Estimating Body Frame Size from Ankle Girth (inches)*

Sex	Small	Medium	Large
Male	Less than 8	8 to 9.25	More than 9.25
Female	Less than 7.5	7.5 to 8.75	More than 8.75

Source: P. B. Johnson et al. *Sport, exercise and you.* New York: Holt, Rinehart and Winston, 1975.

BODY COMPOSITION

Several methods are available for measurement of body composition. Using the computerized method of body impedance, electrodes are attached to the wrist and ankles and a tiny electrical current is sent through the body. The amount of water in the body affects the flow of the current. Since only fat-free tissue contains water, the readings can be converted into the percentage of body fat. An inaccurate reading may result if the individual has eaten recently, is dehydrated, bloated, or improperly positioned during the measurement.

One of the most valid methods of measurement of body composition is underwater weighing, as demonstrated in Figure 13-1. This method is based on the Archimedean principle of water displacement and the determination of body density. A body immersed in fluid is acted upon by a buoyancy force, which is equal to the weight of the water the body displaces. Thus, when an individual is weighed while totally submerged underwater, the total body volume is equal to the loss of weight in water. Specific gravity, which reflects body density, is obtained by dividing the body weight in air by the body weight displaced in water. The density of lean tissue (bone and muscle) is higher than water, while body fat is less dense than water. An individual with a small percentage of body fat and a high percentage of lean tissue will weigh heavier in water than the individual with a high percentage of fat tissue. Once body density and residual lung volume have been determined, equations are available for estimation of percent body fat. Unfortunately, because underwater weighing is costly and requires more time and trained personnel, it is rarely used for mass testing.

Skinfold Tests

The measurement of body composition may also be done through the measurement of subcutaneous body fat with skinfold calipers. The use of a skinfold caliper involves pinching a fold away from the underlying muscle and applying the caliper to the fold. All measurements are taken on the right side of the body, and they should not be taken immediately after exercise as the shift of body fluid to the skin will increase the skinfold size. The directions for skinfold testing are:

1. Grasp the skinfold firmly between the thumb and index finger about one-half inch from the site at which the caliper is to be applied. As the thickness of the fold reflects the percentage of body fat, it should be great enough to include two thicknesses of skin with intervening fat, but it should not include muscle or

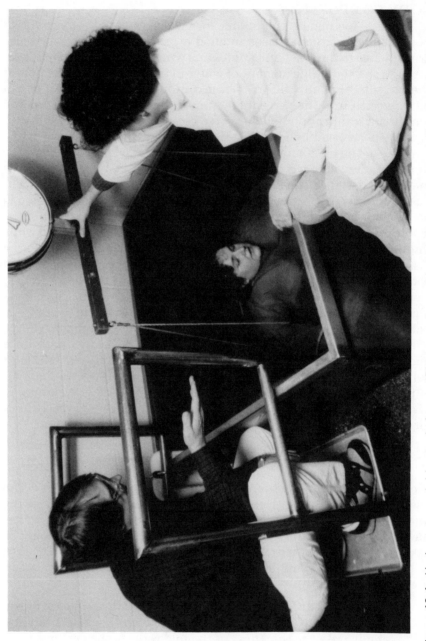

Figure 13-1. *Underwater weighing technique.* (*Photograph provided by Richard G. Israel, East Carolina University*)

fascia. The test administrator may ask the subject to tense the underlying muscles to determine if muscle tissue is included in the fold.

2. While continuing to hold the fold, apply the caliper perpendicular to the fold above or below the finger and slowly release the caliper grip so that full tension is exerted on the fold. The measurement is read to the nearest 0.5 millimeter about one to two seconds after the grip is released.

3. Take a minimum of two measurements at each site, and if they vary by more than one millimeter, take a third measurement. Specific test instructions sometimes differ in this step. For example, the AAHPERD Health Related Physical Fitness Test uses the median score of three measurements. Other tests require that two consecutive measurements agree within one-half millimeter. It is best to follow the instructions of the test being administered. Complete a measurement at one site before going to another site, but if consecutive measurements become smaller and smaller at the same site, complete the measurements at the other sites. Later, return to the trouble site. Consecutive measurements are sometimes smaller due to the compression of fat.

Skinfold measurements may be taken in several places, seven of which are described here. To ensure accuracy and consistency, the sites may be marked with a grease pencil. Figures 13-2 through 13-8 present the measurement sites.

1. Chest: a diagonal fold half of the distance between the anterior axillary line and nipple.

2. Axilla: a vertical fold on the midaxillary line at the level of the xiphoid process of the sternum.

3. Triceps: a vertical fold over the triceps muscle, halfway between the acromion and olecranon processes (arm should be extended and relaxed).

4. Subscapula: a diagonal fold parallel to the axillary border at the inferior angle of the scapula.

5. Abdominal: a vertical fold approximately one-half to one inch to the right of the navel.

6. Suprailium: a slightly diagonal fold on the crest of the ilium at the midaxillary line.

7. Thigh: a vertical fold on the anterior thigh midway between the hip and knee joints (weight should be on left foot).

Skinfold measurements rarely are performed outside the laboratory setting for two reasons: the expense of the skinfold calipers, and

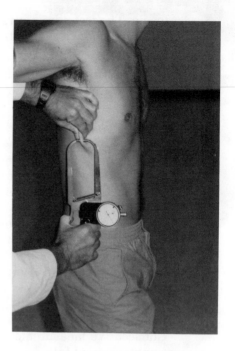

Figure 13-3. *Caliper placement for axilla skinfold.*

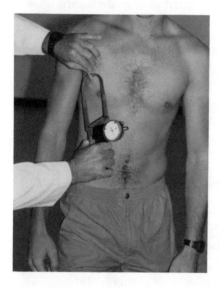

Figure 13-2. *Caliper placement for chest skinfold.*

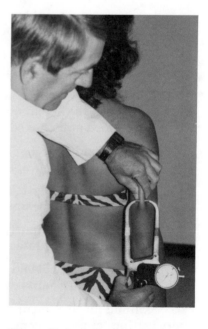

Figure 13-4. *Caliper placement for triceps skinfold.*

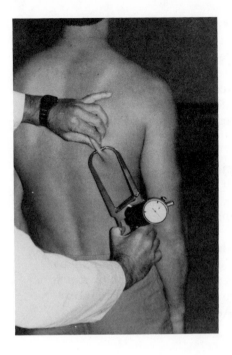

Figure 13-5. *Caliper placement for subscapular skinfold.*

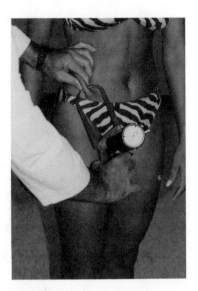

Figure 13-7. *Caliper placement for suprailium skinfold.*

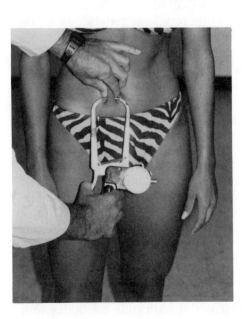

Figure 13-6. *Caliper placement for abdominal skinfold.*

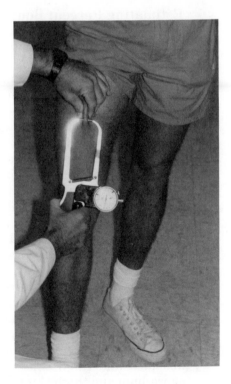

Figure 13-8. *Caliper placement for thigh skinfold.*

ANTHROPOMETRIC MEASUREMENT 199

the lack of confidence in the reliability of the measurements. A study by Lohman and Pollack (1981) concluded that the less expensive calipers may be suitable for a mass testing setting, if the test administrator is well trained. Differences between the scores of experienced and inexperienced testers occurred less often when an expensive metal caliper was used. However, Lohman and Pollack also found that when inexperienced testers were trained, similar scores were obtained when using a plastic caliper with a spring, and a caliper with a uniform tension independent of skinfold thickness. The major requirement for a skinfold caliper is that it exert a constant force of 10 gm/mm^2 at the skinfold site, regardless of the skinfold thickness. Inexpensive calipers are capable of exerting this force if the springs in them are not weakened.

Skinfold measurements can be reliable if testers are willing to practice performing the measurements. Consistency of measurement is obtained only through practice. Testers who are willing to measure many individuals can develop the skill to perform skinfold measurements with accuracy and consistency. As a physical educator, you should seek to develop this skill.

Estimating Percent Body Fat (Jackson and Pollock 1985)

Many regression equations with functions to predict hydrostatically measured body density from skinfold measurements have been published. These equations are termed population specific or generalized. Population specific equations were developed from homogeneous samples, meaning their application is limited to a similar sample (athletes, for instance). To eliminate this problem, generalized equations that can be used with samples varying in age and body fatness have been developed. The generalized equations were developed on large heterogeneous samples using regression models that account for age and the nonlinear relationship between skinfold fat and body density. The generalized approach makes it possible to use one equation rather than several, without a loss in prediction accuracy.

Computer and microcomputer programs are available, or may be developed, to determine body density and percent body fat after the skinfold measurements have been completed. However, computer-generated tables that provide percent body fat estimates have been developed, eliminating the need of calculations by the test administrator. Values published by Jackson and Pollock are presented in Tables 13-5 through 13-8. Jackson and Pollock (1985) found that two different sums of three skinfolds for males and females highly correlated with the sum of the seven skinfolds previously described. For males, chest, abdomen and thigh skinfolds were used, and for females, triceps, suprailium and thigh skinfolds were used. The researchers also found the sums of triceps, chest and subscapular skinfolds for males and triceps, abdomen and suprailium for females, to be similarly accurate. The test administrator has the option of using either combination, but the latter skinfolds may be more practical.

AAHPERD Health Related Physical Fitness Test (AAHPERD 1980)

The AAHPERD Health Related Physical Fitness Test includes a body composition component for ages six through 18. Though skinfolds are related to body fatness in children, the absolute amount of body fat cannot be accurately determined. The relation of skinfold fat to body fatness differs by sex, and also changes as children mature. Therefore, a given skinfold thickness does not correspond to the same body fat content for seven-year-olds as it does for 17-year-olds. Norms for the Health Related Physical Fitness Test are reported as percentile scores for the sums of triceps and subscapular skinfolds. Children scoring within the 50th to 90th percentile are considered to have an acceptable fat content. Skinfold measurements greater than the 90th percentile represent exceptional leanness, and weight reduction is not advised. When children score within the 25th to 50th percentile, it is recommended their weight not increase during the current year. Children who score below the 25th percentile need to be advised and motivated to reduce their body fat content until their skinfold scores are at a desirable level.

Percentile norms also have been published for college-age individuals. They are interpreted in the same way as the norms for younger ages.

The triceps and subscapula skinfold measurements are to be performed as previously described. Each measurement is to be taken three consecutive times, with the recorded score being the median of the three scores. Table 13-9 provides an adaptation of the norms for ages six through college.

DESIRABLE BODY WEIGHT

Though different optimal limits of percent body fat have been reported, to stay within good health standards adult males and females probably should not exceed 18% and 25%, respectively. Male endurance athletes may have a fat percentage as low as eight to 12%, and female endurance athletes may reach 10 to 15%. For the nonathlete, however, the percent body fat for males should be no lower than between five and 10%, and for the females it should be no lower than between 15 and 18%. Percentages lower than these may lead to health problems.

Once the percent body fat has been estimated, desirable weight can be determined. The desired weight is calculated from lean weight.

Table 13-5. *Percent Fat Estimate for Men: Sum of Chest, Abdomen and Thigh Skinfolds*

Sum of Skinfolds (mm)	Age to Last Year*								
	Under 22	23–27	28–32	33–37	38–42	43–47	48–52	53–57	Over 57
8–10	1.3	1.8	2.3	2.9	3.4	3.9	4.5	5.0	5.5
11–13	2.2	2.8	3.3	3.9	4.4	4.9	5.5	6.0	6.5
14–16	3.2	3.8	4.3	4.8	5.4	5.9	6.4	7.0	7.5
17–19	4.2	4.7	5.3	5.8	6.3	6.9	7.4	8.0	8.5
20–22	5.1	5.7	6.2	6.8	7.3	7.9	8.4	8.9	9.5
23–25	6.1	6.6	7.2	7.7	8.3	8.8	9.4	9.9	10.5
26–28	7.0	7.6	8.1	8.7	9.2	9.8	10.3	10.9	11.4
29–31	8.0	8.5	9.1	9.6	10.2	10.7	11.3	11.8	12.4
32–34	8.9	9.4	10.0	10.5	11.1	11.6	12.2	12.8	13.3
35–37	9.8	10.4	10.9	11.5	12.0	12.6	13.1	13.7	14.3
38–40	10.7	11.3	11.8	12.4	12.9	13.5	14.1	14.6	15.2
41–43	11.6	12.2	12.7	13.3	13.8	14.4	15.0	15.5	16.1
44–46	12.5	13.1	13.6	14.2	14.7	15.3	15.9	16.4	17.0
47–49	13.4	13.9	14.5	15.1	15.6	16.2	16.8	17.3	17.9
50–52	14.3	14.8	15.4	15.9	16.5	17.1	17.6	18.2	18.8
53–55	15.1	15.7	16.2	16.8	17.4	17.9	18.5	19.1	19.7
56–58	16.0	16.5	17.1	17.7	18.2	18.8	19.4	20.0	20.5
59–61	16.9	17.4	17.9	18.5	19.1	19.7	20.2	20.8	21.4
62–64	17.6	18.2	18.8	19.4	19.9	20.5	21.1	21.7	22.2

65–67	18.5	19.0	19.6	20.2	20.8	21.3	21.9	22.5	23.1
68–70	19.3	19.9	20.4	21.0	21.6	22.2	22.7	23.3	23.9
71–73	20.1	20.7	21.2	21.8	22.4	23.0	23.6	24.1	24.7
74–76	20.9	21.5	22.0	22.6	23.2	23.8	24.4	25.0	25.5
77–79	21.7	22.2	22.8	23.4	24.0	24.6	25.2	25.8	26.3
80–82	22.4	23.0	23.6	24.2	24.8	25.4	25.9	26.5	27.1
83–85	23.2	23.8	24.4	25.0	25.5	26.1	26.7	27.3	27.9
86–88	24.0	24.5	25.1	25.7	26.3	26.9	27.5	28.1	28.7
89–91	24.7	25.3	25.9	26.5	27.1	27.6	28.2	28.8	29.4
92–94	25.4	26.0	26.6	27.2	27.8	28.4	29.0	29.6	30.2
95–97	26.1	26.7	27.3	27.9	28.5	29.1	29.7	30.3	30.9
98–100	26.9	27.4	28.0	28.6	29.2	29.8	30.4	31.0	31.6
101–103	27.5	28.1	28.7	29.3	29.9	30.5	31.1	31.7	32.3
104–106	28.2	28.8	29.4	30.0	30.6	31.2	31.8	32.4	33.0
107–109	28.9	29.5	30.1	30.7	31.3	31.9	32.5	33.1	33.7
110–112	29.6	30.2	30.8	31.4	32.0	32.6	33.2	33.8	34.4
113–115	30.2	30.8	31.4	32.0	32.6	33.2	33.8	34.5	35.1
116–118	30.9	31.5	32.1	32.7	33.3	33.9	34.5	35.1	35.7
119–121	31.5	32.1	32.7	33.3	33.9	34.5	35.1	35.7	36.4
122–124	32.1	32.7	33.3	33.9	34.5	35.1	35.8	36.4	37.0
125–127	32.7	33.3	33.9	34.5	35.1	35.8	36.4	37.0	37.6

*Last calendar birthday

Source: A. S. Jackson and M. L. Pollock, Practical assessment of body composition, *The Physician and Sportsmedicine* 13(5): 76–90, 1985.

Table 13-6. *Percent Fat Estimate for Women: Sum of Triceps, Suprailium and Thigh Skinfolds*

Age to Last Year*

Sum of Skinfolds (mm)	Under 22	23–27	28–32	33–37	38–42	43–47	48–52	53–57	Over 57
23–25	9.7	9.9	10.2	10.4	10.7	10.9	11.2	11.4	11.7
26–28	11.0	11.2	11.5	11.7	12.0	12.3	12.5	12.7	13.0
29–31	12.3	12.5	12.8	13.0	13.3	13.5	13.8	14.0	14.3
32–34	13.6	13.8	14.0	14.3	14.5	14.8	15.0	15.3	15.5
35–37	14.8	15.0	15.3	15.5	15.8	16.0	16.3	16.5	16.8
38–40	16.0	16.3	16.5	16.7	17.0	17.2	17.5	17.7	18.0
41–43	17.2	17.4	17.7	17.9	18.2	18.4	18.7	18.9	19.2
44–46	18.3	18.6	18.8	19.1	19.3	19.6	19.8	20.1	20.3
47–49	19.5	19.7	20.0	20.2	20.5	20.7	21.0	21.2	21.5
50–52	20.6	20.8	21.1	21.3	21.6	21.8	22.1	22.3	22.6
53–55	21.7	21.9	22.1	22.4	22.6	22.9	23.1	23.4	23.6
56–58	22.7	23.0	23.2	23.4	23.7	23.9	24.2	24.4	24.7
59–61	23.7	24.0	24.2	24.5	24.7	25.0	25.2	25.5	25.7
62–64	24.7	25.0	25.2	25.5	25.7	26.0	26.7	26.4	26.7
65–67	25.7	25.9	26.2	26.4	26.7	26.9	27.2	27.4	27.7
68–70	26.6	26.9	27.1	27.4	27.6	27.9	28.1	28.4	28.6
71–73	27.5	27.8	28.0	28.3	28.5	28.8	29.0	29.3	29.5

*Last calendar birthday									
74–76	28.4	28.7	28.9	29.2	29.4	29.7	29.9	30.2	30.4
77–79	29.3	29.5	29.8	30.0	30.3	30.5	30.8	31.0	31.3
80–82	30.1	30.4	30.6	30.9	31.1	31.4	31.6	31.9	32.1
83–85	30.9	31.2	31.4	31.7	31.9	32.2	32.4	32.7	32.9
86–88	31.7	32.0	32.2	32.5	32.7	32.9	33.2	33.4	33.7
89–91	32.5	32.7	33.0	33.2	33.5	33.7	33.9	34.2	34.4
92–94	33.2	33.4	33.7	33.9	34.2	34.4	34.7	34.9	35.2
95–97	33.9	34.1	34.4	34.6	34.9	35.1	35.4	35.6	35.9
98–100	34.6	34.8	35.1	35.3	35.5	35.8	36.0	36.3	36.5
101–103	35.3	35.4	35.7	35.9	36.2	36.4	36.7	36.9	37.2
104–106	35.8	36.1	36.3	36.6	36.8	37.1	37.3	37.5	37.8
107–109	36.4	36.7	36.9	37.1	37.4	37.6	37.9	38.1	38.4
110–112	37.0	37.2	37.5	37.7	38.0	38.2	38.5	38.7	38.9
113–115	37.5	37.8	38.0	38.2	38.5	38.7	39.0	39.2	39.5
116–118	38.0	38.3	38.5	38.8	39.0	39.3	39.5	39.7	40.0
119–121	38.5	38.7	39.0	39.2	39.5	39.7	40.0	40.2	40.5
122–124	39.0	39.2	39.4	39.7	39.9	40.2	40.4	40.7	40.9
125–127	39.4	39.6	39.9	40.1	40.4	40.6	40.9	41.1	41.4
128–130	39.8	40.0	40.3	40.5	40.8	41.0	41.3	41.5	41.8

*Last calendar birthday

Source: A. S. Jackson and M. L. Pollock, Practical assessment of body composition, *The Physician and Sportsmedicine* 13(5): 76-90, 1985.

Table 13-7. Percent Fat Estimate for Men: Sum of Triceps, Chest and Subscapular Skinfolds

Sum of Skinfolds (mm)	Age to Last Year*								
	Under 22	23–27	28–32	33–37	38–42	43–47	48–52	53–57	Over 57
8–10	1.5	2.0	2.5	3.1	3.6	4.1	4.6	5.1	5.6
11–13	3.0	3.5	4.0	4.5	5.1	5.6	6.1	6.6	7.1
14–16	4.5	5.0	5.5	6.0	6.5	7.0	7.6	8.1	8.6
17–19	5.9	6.4	6.9	7.4	8.0	8.5	9.0	9.5	10.0
20–22	7.3	7.8	8.3	8.8	9.4	9.9	10.4	10.9	11.4
23–25	8.6	9.2	9.7	10.2	10.7	11.2	11.8	12.3	12.8
26–28	10.0	10.5	11.0	11.5	12.1	12.6	13.1	13.6	14.2
29–31	11.2	11.8	12.3	12.8	13.4	13.9	14.4	14.9	15.5
32–34	12.5	13.0	13.5	14.1	14.6	15.1	15.7	16.2	16.7
35–37	13.7	14.2	14.8	15.3	15.8	16.4	16.9	17.4	18.0
38–40	14.9	15.4	15.9	16.5	17.0	17.6	18.1	18.6	19.2
41–43	16.0	16.6	17.1	17.6	18.2	18.7	19.3	19.8	20.3
44–46	17.1	17.7	18.2	18.7	19.3	19.8	20.4	20.9	21.5
47–49	18.2	18.7	19.3	19.8	20.4	20.9	21.4	22.0	22.5
50–52	19.2	19.7	20.3	20.8	21.4	21.9	22.5	23.0	23.6
53–55	20.2	20.7	21.3	21.8	22.4	22.9	23.5	24.0	24.6
56–58	21.1	21.7	22.2	22.8	23.3	23.9	24.4	25.0	25.5
59–61	22.0	22.6	23.1	23.7	24.2	24.8	25.3	25.9	26.5

62–64	22.9	23.4	24.0	24.5	25.1	25.7	26.2	26.8	27.3
65–67	23.7	24.3	24.8	25.4	25.9	26.5	27.1	27.6	28.2
68–70	24.5	25.0	25.6	26.2	26.7	27.3	27.8	28.4	29.0
71–73	25.2	25.8	26.3	26.9	27.5	28.0	28.6	29.1	29.7
74–76	25.9	26.5	27.0	27.6	28.2	28.7	29.3	29.9	30.4
77–79	26.6	27.1	27.7	28.2	28.8	29.4	29.9	30.5	31.1
80–82	27.2	27.7	28.3	28.9	29.4	30.0	30.6	31.1	31.7
83–85	27.7	28.3	28.8	29.4	30.0	30.5	31.1	31.7	32.3
86–88	28.2	28.8	29.4	29.9	30.5	31.1	31.6	32.2	32.8
89–91	28.7	29.3	29.8	30.4	31.0	31.5	32.1	32.7	33.3
92–94	29.1	29.7	30.3	30.8	31.4	32.0	32.6	33.1	33.4
95–97	29.5	30.1	30.6	31.2	31.8	32.4	32.9	33.5	34.1
98–100	29.8	30.4	31.0	31.6	32.1	32.7	33.3	33.9	34.4
101–103	30.1	30.7	31.3	31.8	32.4	33.0	33.6	34.1	34.7
104–106	30.4	30.9	31.5	32.1	32.7	33.2	33.8	34.4	35.0
107–109	30.6	31.1	31.7	32.3	32.9	33.4	34.0	34.6	35.2
110–112	30.7	31.3	31.9	32.4	33.0	33.6	34.2	34.7	35.3
113–115	30.8	31.4	32.0	32.5	33.1	33.7	34.3	34.9	35.4
116–118	30.9	31.5	32.0	32.6	33.2	33.8	34.3	34.9	35.5

*Last calendar birthday

Source: A. S. Jackson and M. L. Pollock, Practical assessment of body composition, The Physician and Sportsmedicine 13(5): 76-90, 1985.

Table 13-8. *Percent Fat Estimate for Women: Sum of Triceps, Abdomen and Suprailium Skinfolds*

Sum of Skinfolds (mm)	Age to Last Year*								
	Under 22	23-27	28-32	33-37	38-42	43-47	48-52	53-57	Over 57
8-12	8.8	9.0	9.2	9.4	9.5	9.7	9.9	10.1	10.3
13-17	10.8	10.9	11.1	11.3	11.5	11.7	11.8	12.0	12.2
18-22	12.6	12.8	13.0	13.2	13.4	13.5	13.7	13.9	14.1
23-27	14.5	14.6	14.8	15.0	15.2	15.4	15.6	15.7	15.9
28-32	16.2	16.4	16.6	16.8	17.0	17.1	17.3	17.5	17.7
33-37	17.9	18.1	18.3	18.5	18.7	18.9	19.0	19.2	19.4
38-42	19.6	19.8	20.0	20.2	20.3	20.5	20.7	20.9	21.1
43-47	21.2	21.4	21.6	21.8	21.9	22.1	22.3	22.5	22.7
48-52	22.8	22.9	23.1	23.3	23.5	23.7	23.8	24.0	24.2
53-57	24.2	24.4	24.6	24.8	25.0	25.2	25.3	25.5	25.7
58-62	25.7	25.9	26.0	26.2	26.4	26.6	26.8	27.0	27.1
63-67	27.1	27.2	27.4	27.6	27.8	28.0	28.2	28.3	28.5
68-72	28.4	28.6	28.7	28.9	29.1	29.3	29.5	29.7	29.8
73-77	29.6	29.8	30.0	30.2	30.4	30.6	30.7	30.9	31.1
78-82	30.9	31.0	31.2	31.4	31.6	31.8	31.9	32.1	32.3
83-87	32.0	32.2	32.4	32.6	32.7	32.9	33.1	33.3	33.5
88-92	33.1	33.3	33.5	33.7	33.8	34.0	34.2	34.4	34.6

93–97	34.1	34.3	34.5	34.7	34.9	35.1	35.2	35.4	35.6
98–102	35.1	35.3	35.5	35.7	35.9	36.0	36.2	36.4	36.6
103–107	36.1	36.2	36.4	36.6	36.8	37.0	37.2	37.3	37.5
108–112	36.9	37.1	37.3	37.5	37.7	37.9	38.0	38.2	38.4
113–117	37.8	37.9	38.1	38.3	39.2	39.4	39.6	39.8	39.2
118–122	38.5	38.7	38.9	39.1	39.4	39.6	39.8	40.0	40.0
123–127	39.2	39.4	39.6	39.8	40.0	40.1	40.3	40.5	40.7
128–132	39.9	40.1	40.2	40.4	40.6	40.8	41.0	41.2	41.3
133–137	40.5	40.7	40.8	41.0	41.2	41.4	41.6	41.7	41.9
138–142	41.0	41.2	41.4	41.6	41.7	41.9	42.1	42.3	42.5
143–147	41.5	41.7	41.9	42.0	42.2	42.4	42.6	42.8	43.0
148–152	41.9	42.1	42.3	42.8	42.6	42.8	43.0	43.2	43.4
153–157	42.3	42.5	42.6	42.8	43.0	43.2	43.4	43.6	43.7
158–162	42.6	42.8	43.0	43.1	43.3	43.5	43.7	43.9	44.1
163–167	42.9	43.0	43.2	43.4	43.6	43.8	44.0	44.1	44.3
168–172	43.1	43.2	43.4	43.6	43.8	44.0	44.2	44.3	44.5
173–177	43.2	43.4	43.6	43.8	43.9	44.1	44.3	44.5	44.7
178–182	43.3	43.5	43.7	43.8	44.0	44.2	44.4	44.6	44.8

*Last calendar birthday

Source: A. S. Jackson and M. L. Pollock, Practical assessment of body composition, *The Physician and Sportsmedicine* 13(5): 76-90, 1985.

A sample calculation is provided.
Given: Body weight = 200 pounds; % fat = 24%

Calculation of fat weight (FW)

$$FW = \text{body weight} \times (\% \text{ fat} \div 100)$$
$$= 200 \times (24\% \div 100)$$
$$= 200 \times .24$$
$$FW = 48 \text{ pounds}$$

Calculation of lean body weight (LBW)

$$LBW = \text{body weight} - FW$$
$$= 200 - 48$$
$$LBW = 152 \text{ pounds}$$

Calculation of desirable body weight (DBW)

$$DBW = \frac{LBW}{1.00 - (\text{desired } \% \text{ fat} \div 100)}$$
$$= \frac{152}{1.00 - (19\% \div 100)}$$
$$= \frac{152}{1.00 - .19}$$
$$= \frac{152}{.81}$$
$$DBW = 187.7 \text{ pounds}$$

As measurement errors may occur, when estimating body density it is best to determine desirable body weight ranges. Generally, the upper limit of ideal weight for adult males should include no more than 15 to 18% fat, and for adult females, 22 to 25%. Values above these percentages indicate overfatness. Body fat content in excess of 25% and 30% indicates obesity for males and females, respectively.

Table 13-9. *Norms in Millimeters for Sum of Triceps and Subscapular Skinfolds for Ages Six through College**

PERCENTILE	6	7	8	9	10	11	12	13	14	15	16	17+	College
MALES													
95	8	9	9	9	9	9	9	9	9	9	9	9	12
75	11	11	11	11	12	12	11	12	11	12	12	12	16
50	12	12	13	14	14	16	15	15	14	14	14	15	21
25	14	15	17	18	19	22	21	22	20	20	20	21	26
5	20	24	28	34	33	38	44	46	37	40	37	38	40
FEMALES													
95	9	10	10	10	10	11	11	12	13	14	14	15	17
75	12	12	13	14	14	15	15	16	18	20	20	20	24
50	14	15	16	17	18	19	19	20	24	25	25	27	30
25	17	19	21	24	25	25	27	30	32	34	34	36	37
5	26	28	36	40	41	42	48	51	52	56	57	58	51

*Adapted from *Health related physical fitness test manual*, Reston, Virginia: AAHPERD, 1980; and R. R. Pate, *Norms for college students: health related physical fitness test*, Reston, Virginia: AAHPERD, 1985.

Cooper Method for Determining Ideal Weight (Cooper 1982)

When body fat cannot be estimated through skinfold measurements, the Cooper method may be used to calculate the ideal weight for men and women. Men multiply their height in inches by four, and then subtract 128. Women multiply their height in inches by 3.5, and then subtract 108. The resulting values will give men of medium bone structure a weight with roughly 15 to 19% body fat, and women of average build a weight with body fat of approximately 18 to 22%. Large-boned individuals should add 10% to the calculated figure to determine their ideal weight, and small-boned individuals should subtract 10%.

WEIGHT LOSS PROGRAMS

The best approach to reduction of body fat is through a program involving exercise and a modest decrease in caloric intake. With only a modest decrease in caloric intake, a permanent change in eating behavior is more easily made. By combining exercise and diet, 80 to 95% of the weight loss is through loss of fat tissue. If weight loss is accomplished strictly through dieting, 30 to 45% of the weight reduction is through loss of lean tissue. Unsound gimmicks or diets should be avoided, and weight reduction should be gradual, with a loss of no more than one to two pounds/week. For weight reduction purposes, exercise does not have to be intense. For example, walking a mile expends almost the same amount of calories as running a mile. If possible, percent body fat should be monitored during weight loss to be sure the body composition is not being altered in the wrong way.

REVIEW PROBLEMS

1. If skinfold calipers are available, perform skinfold measurements on several of your classmates. Use different types of calipers, if possible, on the same individuals and compare the results. Do you obtain similar measurements with different calipers?
2. Ask the directors of several local health or fitness clubs how they estimate percent body fat for their members.

14

Posture and Body Mechanics

Upon completion of this chapter, you should be able to:
1. Define proper posture and body mechanics;
2. State why posture and body mechanics should be measured;
3. Measure for proper posture while an individual is sitting, standing, walking, running for speed, running for distance, lifting heavy objects or walking with heavy objects; and
4. Prescribe activities and exercises for development of proper posture and movement mechanics.

Proper posture is the correct alignment of body parts, and a balance of forces that, with minimal effort, will provide: maximum support; the least amount of strain on the muscles, tendons, ligaments and joints; and the greatest mechanical efficiency. Good posture depends on good body mechanics. Body mechanics is the application of physical laws to the human body. The bones of the body act as levers (simple machines) while the muscles supply the force to move them. Therefore, through the application of mechanical laws, efficient movement can take place while avoiding strain or injury.

The postures that are maintained for various positions and movements are the result of conscious and unconscious practice, which usually lead to the formation of postural habits. As a person repeatedly assumes a given body alignment during work, play and relaxation, postural habits are developed. When in a position for extended periods of time, a response is established in the neuromuscular system. This response becomes habitual; it is produced when the person is unconscious of posture. The habitual postural response occurs regardless of good or bad habit, and many individuals mistakenly feel comfortable in a position that actually places a strain on the joints.

Posture is influenced by general health, emotions, body build, sex, adequate strength and endurance, visual and kinesthetic awareness, personal habits and the demands of work. The following examples illustrate how these factors influence posture: obese people often lean backward to shift the center of gravity backward over the feet (women in late pregnancy sometimes do the same thing); frail or tired individuals assume the "fatigue slouch," placing stress on the ligaments rather than the muscles; young, tall girls sometimes slouch to make themselves appear shorter (short men tend to stand in good posture to make themselves appear taller); and depressed and unhappy people usually slouch, while happy ones stand tall.

WHY MEASURE POSTURE AND BODY MECHANICS?

Poor posture can cause a number of health problems. Examples are:

1. Dysmenorrhea can occur, with greater severity among college women with a swayback posture.
2. A low but significant relationship exists between posture and trunk strength imbalance.
3. Dysmenorrhea, constipation and back pain are found with increased inclination of the pelvis.
4. Diseases and cardiac and pulmonary affectations occur more often among poor posture groups of elementary children.
5. Protruding abdomen and lumbar lordosis may contribute to painful menstruation, susceptibility to back injury and backache.
6. Rounded shoulders may impair respiratory capacity.
7. Hyperextended knees may lead to knee injury.
8. Unbalanced postural lines can cause tension in muscle groups, produce joint strain and stretch ligaments.
9. A forward lean of the head can cause headache and neck and shoulder pain.
10. Improper foot alignment and footwear cause most of the foot problems that occur.
11. Habitual misalignment of body parts can lead to structural changes in the skeletal system, and can restrict joint motion.

On the positive side, good posture contributes to a pleasing appearance, and can make a favorable first impression. It gives the appearance of alertness and confidence.

Undoubtedly, children in the elementary grades should be measured for postural deviations. The earlier the postural problems are identified, the less complicated the correction. Most individuals with incorrect posture and movement mechanics have minimal structure deviations. Their postural problems are primarily due to faults in body alignment. To correct their faulty posture, individuals must know (1) the mechanics of good posture, (2) their postural faults, and (3) activities and exercises to perform, in order to improve their posture and movement mechanics. Identification of postural faults occurs through measurement and evaluation of posture. However, knowledge alone is not always enough for individuals to work to improve their postural faults. Many must be motivated to correct their faults. Unfortunately, posture evaluation sometimes identifies individuals with serious structural deviation. These individuals need to be treated by medical specialists.

Finally, evaluation of posture may encourage all tested individuals to be more posture-conscious, thereby possibly preventing future problems.

> Are you able to:
> define posture and body mechanics and state why they should be measured?

MEASURES OF POSTURE

Numerous instruments and scales have been developed to measure posture. Though many of these instruments and scales have made positive contributions to posture evaluation, it is a mistake to expect all individuals to conform to the same postural standards. The variety of body types make it difficult to apply the same postural standards to everyone. Therefore, although certain body relationships are desirable and mechanical principles should be observed, there is probably no one best posture for all individuals. Use the standards provided here to diagnose possible postural problems, but do not insist that everyone conform to identical standards.

The only test with a numerical rating scale included in this group of tests, is the New York State Posture Rating Test. Since the primary purpose of postural screening is to identify postural deviations, you should not be concerned with the obtaining of scores for comparison purposes.

NEW YORK STATE POSTURE RATING TEST (New York State Education Department 1966)
Test Objective. To evaluate posture.
Age Level. Grades four through 12.
Equipment. Screen, rating chart and plumb line.
Validity. Logical validity.
Reliability. .93 to .98 for boys and girls at different grade levels.
Norms. Norms are provided by grade and sex in the reference.
Administration and Directions. The posture rating chart in Figure 14-1 is used to assess 13 areas of the body. The rating chart shows three profiles for each area: the correct position, a slight deviation and a pronounced deviation. The individual stands on a line that is three feet in front of a screen (parallel to the screen). A plumb line is suspended just in front of the line so the individual is standing between the plumb line and the screen. Another line is drawn at a right angle to the first line and extended 10 feet farther back from the screen. The total distance from the screen to the end of the line is 13 feet. The test administrator stands at this point.

The student is rated from two viewpoints, while standing comfortably and naturally. In one position, the student stands facing the screen with the plumb line bisecting the head and spine and passing down between the legs and feet. From this position, six areas of the body are rated.

The student then turns one quarter turn to the left (right side to the screen)

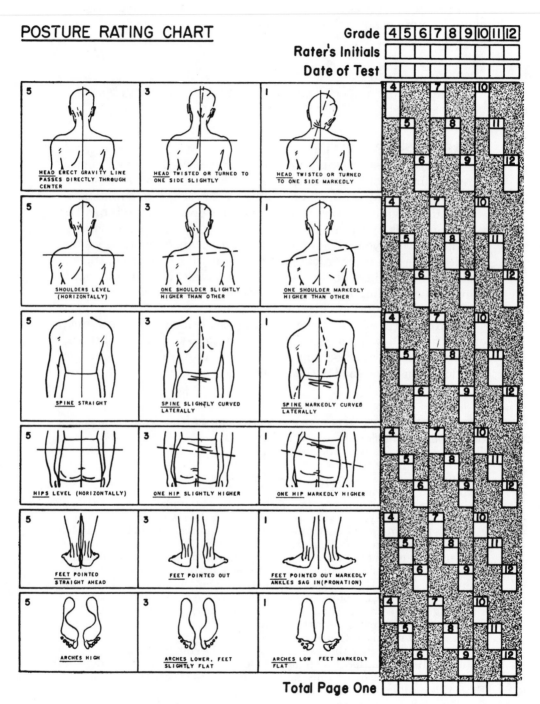

Figure 14-1. *New York State Posture Rating Chart.*
(Courtesy of the New York State Education Department)

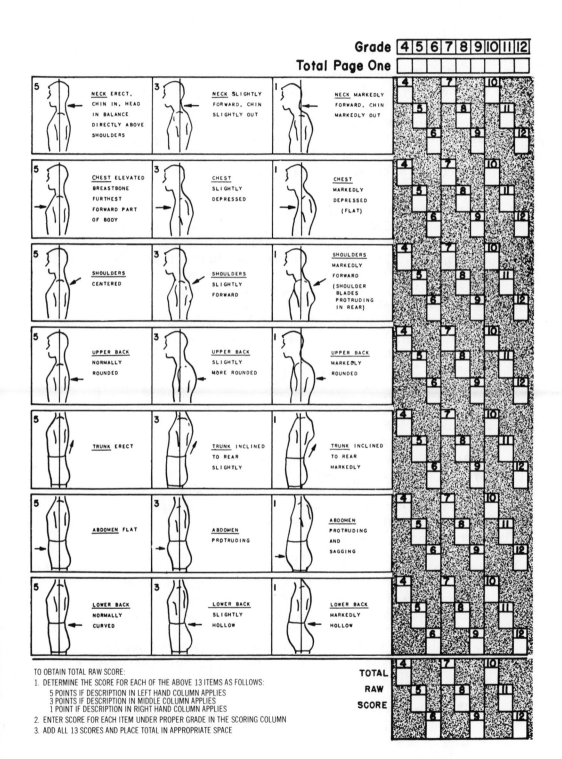

Grade 4 5 6 7 8 9 10 11 12

Total Page One

5 NECK ERECT, CHIN IN, HEAD IN BALANCE DIRECTLY ABOVE SHOULDERS
3 NECK SLIGHTLY FORWARD, CHIN SLIGHTLY OUT
1 NECK MARKEDLY FORWARD, CHIN MARKEDLY OUT

5 CHEST ELEVATED BREASTBONE FURTHEST FORWARD PART OF BODY
3 CHEST SLIGHTLY DEPRESSED
1 CHEST MARKEDLY DEPRESSED (FLAT)

5 SHOULDERS CENTERED
3 SHOULDERS SLIGHTLY FORWARD
1 SHOULDERS MARKEDLY FORWARD (SHOULDER BLADES PROTRUDING IN REAR)

5 UPPER BACK NORMALLY ROUNDED
3 UPPER BACK SLIGHTLY MORE ROUNDED
1 UPPER BACK MARKEDLY ROUNDED

5 TRUNK ERECT
3 TRUNK INCLINED TO REAR SLIGHTLY
1 TRUNK INCLINED TO REAR MARKEDLY

5 ABDOMEN FLAT
3 ABDOMEN PROTRUDING
1 ABDOMEN PROTRUDING AND SAGGING

5 LOWER BACK NORMALLY CURVED
3 LOWER BACK SLIGHTLY HOLLOW
1 LOWER BACK MARKEDLY HOLLOW

TO OBTAIN TOTAL RAW SCORE:
1. DETERMINE THE SCORE FOR EACH OF THE ABOVE 13 ITEMS AS FOLLOWS:
    5 POINTS IF DESCRIPTION IN LEFT HAND COLUMN APPLIES
    3 POINTS IF DESCRIPTION IN MIDDLE COLUMN APPLIES
    1 POINT IF DESCRIPTION IN RIGHT HAND COLUMN APPLIES
2. ENTER SCORE FOR EACH ITEM UNDER PROPER GRADE IN THE SCORING COLUMN
3. ADD ALL 13 SCORES AND PLACE TOTAL IN APPROPRIATE SPACE

TOTAL RAW SCORE

so the plumb line passes in a line through the ear, shoulder, hip, knee and ankle. Seven areas of the body are rated from this position.

Scoring. Each of the 13 areas is rated. For the correct position, five points are scored; for a slight deviation, three points are scored; and for a pronounced deviation, one point is scored. The total point value is the score, with a score of 65 being a perfect score.

Standing Posture Measurement

The subject backs up to a flat wall with the head, shoulders, hips, calves and heels touching the wall. The test administrator attempts to place a hand in the space between the wall and the small of the subject's back. The space should accommodate the fingers but not the palm. If the space is greater than the thickness of the hand, the subject probably has lordosis, with shortened lumbar and hip flexor muscles.

Foot Alignment Measurement

An estimated 80% of the adult population experiences some type of foot problem. The two major causes of foot problems are improper foot alignment and footwear. Improper foot alignment may be due to toeing in, toeing out, flat feet, foot pronation or congenital deformity. As with other postural deviations, it is important to initiate correction of improper foot alignment at an early age.

You can measure foot alignment by looking at the front of the body. A straight line should run from the knee cap, through the center of the ankle and to the second toe. From the rear, a straight line should pass through the center of the Achilles tendon.

DESCRIPTIONS OF PROPER POSTURE AND BODY MECHANICS

The following descriptions of the proper techniques for standing, walking, running for speed, running for distance, sitting, lifting heavy objects, carrying heavy objects and lying may be used to check posture and body mechanics. Remember, not everyone is expected to have identical posture, but if you discover postural deviations that may create health problems, you should attempt to correct them, or advise the individual to seek medical help.

Standing

1. The head and chin are centered over the trunk, and are held in a relaxed position at right angles to the front of the neck.
2. The shoulders are free and easy, and are not forward, back or elevated.
3. The shoulder blades are drawn down and flat on the back.
4. The chest is held up, not too high or leaning, and is not sagging.
5. The trunk is within normal limits of curves, not too straight and flat or too round and hollow.
6. The abdomen is up and in, and is not relaxed or protruding.
7. The hips are in line with the trunk and are not leading, or thrust back.

8. The arms hang naturally and relaxed at the sides, and are not held rigidly or too relaxed.
9. The knees are free and easy, and are not bent or thrust back.
10. The feet are parallel and slightly apart.
11. The weight falls ahead of the outer anklebone and is distributed toward the outside of each foot.

From the front view, the weight should be evenly distributed, about a vertical line through the midpoint of the body. From the side view, a vertical line should pass through the earlobe, through the middle of the shoulder and through the middle of the hip, slightly behind the kneecap and slightly in front of the outer anklebone. The center of gravity should be directly over the base of support.

Walking

1. The upper body (head, chin, shoulders and chest) is balanced on the trunk; it is not dragged forward by the pull of gravity.
2. The trunk is balanced in the pelvic basin. It does not come to an erect, rigid position between steps, but remains slightly forward to keep it in line with the extended rear leg, at the time of the push-off. The center of gravity remains within the base of support.
3. Motion originates in the hip joint, as the leading leg swings ahead of the body.
4. The leading leg is always parallel to or in advance of the trunk, so a new base of support is always ready to receive the body weight.
5. As a new base of support is established, the upper body remains in line with the axis of the rear leg.
6. The supporting and pushing leg applies its force directly through the center of gravity along the line of resistance of the trunk. This leg begins to push off before the front foot strikes the ground.
7. The heel strikes the ground first, directly in line with the direction of walk. The weight is transferred through the outer border of the foot to the ball of the foot.
8. The ankle joint is extended, as the final push, or thrust, is made with the big toe.
9. The weight shift of the alternate foot causes the pelvic girdle to oscillate back and forth. The arms and shoulders swing slightly to compensate for this oscillation, and to keep the body weight evenly distributed.
10. The leg muscles supply most of the energy for locomotion so the body makes as few extraneous motions as possible.

Running for Speed

1. At slower speeds runners are more erect, whereas at full speed the typical sprinter leans forward at about 15° from the perpendicular. Forward lean comes naturally with most sprinters, and conscious attempts to increase lean are not usually necessary.
2. Because a long lever develops more speed at the end than does a short lever, the lead leg is fully extended at the moment of the push from the rear leg. This action also enables the full force of the push to be converted into forward movement.

3. Any vertical movement is great enough to counteract the downward pull of gravity; but because the forward speed of the runner is decreasing, it is not great enough to produce an unnecessary bounce. The higher the center of gravity rises, the longer the body is off the ground.
4. As the foot leaves the ground after a vigorous push, the knee is bent. The faster the leg moves, the more the knee is bent, and the higher the foot is raised. By this action, the knee moves forward with greater angular velocity, due to the shorter radius of the arc through which the leg swings. The swing of the leg from the hip is in a straight forward and backward line.
5. The faster the runner moves, the higher the knee is raised in front. This movement delays the placing of the foot on the ground for its next thrust and permits the lead leg to reach full extension.
6. The runner lands on the ball of the foot. Landing on the heel of the foot causes the center of gravity to fall behind the contact foot, creating a retarding effect.
7. The faster the speed, the longer the stride. However, if the stride is too long, the foot contacts the ground ahead of the center of gravity, which produces a braking action.
8. The swing of the arms is coordinated with that of the legs, in order to balance the rotary effect of the leg swing on the trunk. The elbows are bent at right angles with the arms close to the sides.
9. Shoulder motion is kept to a minimum and the hands are relaxed.

Running for Distance
1. The head remains up, avoiding the tendency to watch the feet.
2. The back is straight but naturally comfortable. Do not throw the shoulders back or stick the chest out.
3. The buttocks are tucked in. In this position, a hypothetical line drawn through the shoulders and the hips is vertical, or nearly so.
4. The elbows are bent and held slightly away from the body. The arms are not placed out like wings, nor are they pressed to the chest. They are carried slightly above hip level.
5. The body is straight, as the legs move freely from the hips. The legs are lifted from the knees; the ankles are relaxed. Do not overstride; each foot falls just under the knee.
6. Using the heel-to-toe method for footstrike, land on the heel, then rock forward to take off from the ball of the foot. This method is the least tiring over long distances, and is the least wearing because the heel cushions the landing and the forward rocking distributes the pressure.
7. In the flat-foot method for footstrike, the foot falls under the knee in a quick, light action, with the entire foot landing on the ground at the same time. This type of landing provides a wide surface area to cushion the footstrike. The foot is not driven down but is allowed to pass beneath the body.

Sitting

1. The head, neck and shoulders are in the same position as standing.
2. The back of the buttocks touch the back of the chair.
3. Use one of the appropriate feet and leg positions. Put feet and knees close together with one foot slightly in the lead, or put feet together with both legs slanted to one side or crossed at the ankles. Regardless of feet and leg positions, the hips remain toward the back of the chair.
4. If writing or reading while sitting at a table, the chair is brought well under the table, so the edge of the table almost touches the front of the body. Sit all the way back in the chair and allow the trunk to slant forward slightly from the hip joint to bring the eyes in line with the work. Keep the head-neck-trunk line as straight as possible for maximum support of the head.

Lifting Heavy Objects

1. Stand close to the object being lifted.
2. The knees are bent; the back remains straight.
3. The feet are spread at about shoulder width.
4. The hands grasp the object with the fingers widely spaced under the object to provide the upward force.
5. The lifting is performed by straightening the legs.

Lifting an Object from a Height

1. Do not lift heavy objects down from a height without assistance.
2. Place one leg in front of the other in a stride position.
3. As the object is lifted down, shift the body weight to the rear leg.

Carrying Heavy Objects

1. The center of gravity is always above the base of support.
2. The body alignment is altered as little as possible.
3. The object is carried as close to the body's center of gravity, as possible and no higher than waist level.

Lying

1. If lying on the back, a pillow is placed under the knees to help prevent exaggerated curvature of the lower back. The head is elevated slightly.
2. If lying on the side, one or both knees are drawn up to relieve lower back strain.
3. If lying on the stomach, a pillow is placed under the stomach and hips to help keep the back straight.

EXERCISES TO CORRECT POSTURAL DEVIATIONS

(French and Jansma 1982)

Only a few exercises for several postural deviations will be described. You should refer to a source that describes the deviations in greater detail, and includes exercises for possible correction of the deviation. Textbooks dealing with physical education for special populations include this material.

Lumbar Lordosis

Lumbar lordosis is an increase in the lumbar curve. The exaggerated curve places a strain on the abdomen, causing it to weaken and become more prominent. The lower back muscles and hip flexors are shortened, the hamstrings and gluteal muscles may be weakened, the knees are hyperextended and the pelvis may be tilted forward and downward. Straight leg sit-ups and leg raises should not be performed by the lordotic individual. However, these individuals can:

1. Lie on the back with arms outstretched, press spine down until it is flat on the floor, tighten and hold stomach and seat muscles, and then relax.
2. Stand with feet apart, knees bent and hands on knees like a baseball player. Tighten seat and tuck in, drop head and round back, and relax. Repeat.
3. Stand erect against a wall with heels four inches from the wall, contract abdominal muscles, and push the lower back against the wall. Repeat.
4. Lie on the back with knees drawn to chest and arms wrapped around the lower legs to hold them close to the body. Rock forward and backward trying to come to a sitting position.
5. Lie on the back with arms at the sides, lift arms six to 10 inches, and roll the head and neck forward, then the shoulders. Roll as far forward as possible without lifting the lower back off the floor, hold the position and return to starting position. Repeat.
   As this exercise becomes easier, the individual may cross the arms with hands on the shoulders and roll up, touching the elbows to the knees. Do not anchor feet or place hands behind the head.

Kyphosis

Kyphosis involves an abnormal increase in the cervical curvature of the upper back. Round shoulders and forward head usually accompany this condition. The upper back extensors and the trapezius are weakened; the pectoral and intercostal muscles are shortened. Individuals with kyphosis should not perform push-ups. However, these individuals can:

1. Lie on stomach with hands behind the neck, pinch the shoulder blades together, and lift head and chest slightly above the floor. Lower the head and chest to the floor and repeat.
2. Stand tall and slowly swing both arms forward and upward reaching overhead to a full stretch. At the same time, rising high on the toes, turn the palms outward, and lower arms sideward and downward while forcefully pressing them back. Pull chin in, hold head high, and let heels drop to the floor. Avoid excessive arching of the back.

3. Lie on stomach with arms extended sideways. Lift arms while keeping the head, trunk and legs in contact with the floor. Slowly lower arms to floor and repeat.

Winged Scapula

Winged scapula is the postural deviation of one or both shoulder blades being farther than normal from the spinal column. This deviation may be caused by weakened rhomboids and trapezius, and tightened pectorals. Individuals with this deviation can:
1. Lie on back with knees bent and feet on the floor, holding a medicine ball in the hands. Raise the ball toward the ceiling, keeping feet together, body in correct alignment and back flat as possible. Repeat.
2. Lie on back with knees bent, feet on the floor, arms out to side and elbows bent. Pinch shoulder blades together while pressing arms, wrists, neck and lower back to floor. Repeat.

Scoliosis

Scoliosis is an abnormal lateral curvature of the vertebral column. There may be a single curve, known as a "c" curve, or a reverse "c" curve. This condition also may involve two or more curves in different directions. A double curve is usually shaped like the letter "s". Those afflicted with scoliosis can:
1. Hang by both arms, or the arm of the low shoulder, from a bar with the overhand grip.
2. Lie on back with legs extended and arms stretched overhead as far as possible.
3. Stand with the arm of the low shoulder raised directly overhead; slowly bend to the long side as far as possible for six seconds and return.
4. Facing a wall, stand erect, with feet approximately 18 inches apart. Reach up the wall with hand on the concave side of the scoliotic curve and down the wall with opposite hand. Repeat.

Knock Knees

Knock knees occurs when the knees are medially together (turned in), or even overlap. Usually, the medial ligaments of the knee are stretched, the external rotator muscles are weak, the tensor fasciae latae are tight and the feet are flat and everted. Correction of knock knees is possible if the condition is functional, and more effective if treated at a young age. Knock-kneed individuals can:
1. Stand with knees relaxed and feet parallel; bend the knees and turn both outward. Repeat.
2. Stand with knees relaxed and feet parallel; turn the knees out and pull the thighs and calves inward. Repeat.

Bowlegs

When the knees are laterally separated (turned out) while the feet are together, the individual has bowlegs. Faulty posture due to outer rotation of the legs is usually the cause of bowlegs in children. Those with bowlegs can:

1. Sit on the floor with back against a wall and legs extended. Roll the legs inward, and turn the feet outward. Repeat.
2. Lie on back with a pillow between the ankles. Spread straightened legs, and rapidly bring them together against the pillow. Repeat.

Toeing In and Toeing Out

When the feet are pointed inward while an individual is standing or moving, the condition is toeing in. Toeing out occurs when the feet are pointed outward while standing or moving. Usually exercise is only beneficial in very mild, functional cases of these conditions. Individuals afflicted with toeing in or toeing out can:

1. While sitting on the floor with the legs extended, slightly raise one leg (may use the hand to elevate the leg), fully extend the foot, and perform circles. Repeat with the foot flexed. Perform with other leg.
2. Sit in a chair, with a tennis ball between the feet. Roll it back and Rotate feet outward and inward without moving the heels.
3. Roller skate.

Flat Feet

Flat feet is a congenital or acquired condition in which the longitudinal arch is lower than normal. Acquired flat feet in children usually is caused by poor functional posture . Fallen arches occur in later life, as the muscle strength and elasticity decrease and the musculature is unable to support the bony arches. Having flat feet is not necessarily a serious problem, as only a few people experience pain with fallen arches. In cases of flat feet where no structural damage has occurred, exercise may be of remedial value. Individuals can try to:

1. Sit in a chair and attempt to pick up pencils or marbles with the toes and feet.
2. Sit in a chair, with a tennis ball between the feet. Roll it back and forth with the soles of the feet.
3. Sit on the floor with legs extended forward. Flex the toes while extending the feet as far away from the body as possible. Repeat.

Foot Pronation

Foot pronation occurs when the body weight is carried over the inner border of the foot. This act weakens the foot because downward force is exerted over the longitudinal arch, where there is not supporting contact with the floor. Symptoms of pronation include lowering of the arch height, protrusion of the inner ankle bones and deviation of the heel cords from a vertical line when viewed from the rear. Individuals with pronation can:

1. Sit barefoot with the soles of the feet on the floor. While holding the toes flat with the fingers, attempt to elevate the balls of the feet so the tendons stand out down the instep. The heels must remain on the floor, and the toes must not curl.

2. Sit in a chair and attempt to pick up pencils or marbles with the toes and feet.
3. Stand with the feet four inches apart and parallel. Curl the toes, and shift the weight to the outside of the feet; hold six seconds and relax. Repeat.

REVIEW PROBLEMS
1. Ask several friends to stand side by side. Compare their body types, limb lengths, weight, neck length, spinal curves and postures. Are their postures different? If so, what factors might contribute to the differences?
2. Observe the posture and body mechanics of students as they walk around the campus. Are there many individuals with poor posture and body mechanics?
3. Observe joggers for their posture and body mechanics. Are most mechanically sound in their jogging techniques?
4. Administer the New York State Posture Rating Test to one of your friends. Make note of any problems you experience in the test administration.

15

Physical Fitness

Upon completion of this chapter, you should be able to:
1. Define and measure health-related physical fitness and athletic performance-related physical fitness;
2. State why physical fitness should be measured; and
3. Prescribe activities and exercises for the development of physical fitness.

The terms fitness and physical fitness are often used interchangeably. Though both terms involve quality of life, they do not mean the same thing. Fitness includes emotional, mental, spiritual and social fitness, as well as physical fitness. Currently, a popular term for fitness is well-being. Everyone should be concerned with total fitness, but the responsibilities of physical educators are more related to physical fitness.

Different people and groups interpret fitness in different ways. It is sometimes defined as the capacity for sustained physical activity without excessive fatigue, or as the capacity to perform everyday activities with reserve energy for emergency situations. By these definitions many persons incorrectly classify themselves as physically fit. It is especially incorrect to accept these definitions when the relations between inactivity and health are considered. Some individuals consider physical fitness synonymous with cardiorespiratory fitness, while other groups limit their perception of physical fitness to muscular strength and endurance.

When defining physical fitness, it may be best to describe two types of physical fitness: health-related, and athletic performance-related. Both types require regular exercise, and both require proper nutrition and rest. However, health-related physical fitness includes cardiorespiratory fitness, muscular strength, muscular endurance, flexibility and body composition (leanness/fatness). Health-related physical fitness means the organic systems of the body are healthy and function efficiently, so you are able to engage in vigorous tasks and leisure activities. It exerts a positive influence on several risk factors associated with cardiovascular diseases, and it is effective in

227

reducing emotional stress. Health-related fitness enables you to look better, feel better and enjoy a healthy, happy and full life.

Athletic performance-related physical fitness may provide the same benefits as health-related physical fitness, but it also renders motor skills required in sports and specific types of jobs. For this reason, athletic performance-related fitness is sometimes referred to as skill-related physical fitness, or motor fitness. In addition to the five components — cardiorespiratory fitness, muscular strength and endurance, flexibility and body composition — athletic performance-related physical fitness includes agility, balance, coordination, power, reaction time and speed.

Exercise programs for the maintenance and development of health-related physical fitness are usually different than those programs for athletic performance-related physical fitness, particularly if the purpose of the program is to prepare the individual for athletic competition. Too often exercise programs for athletes place little emphasis on health-related components. In fact, because they have not made a commitment to health-related fitness, many athletes fail to continue an exercise program after they cease to participate in sports.

WHY MEASURE PHYSICAL FITNESS?

The relationship of good health and cardiorespiratory fitness, muscular strength and endurance, flexibility and body composition have been described in previous chapters. Because these components are developed and maintained through exercise, physical educators should be prepared to measure them, interpret the test results and prescribe the appropriate activities for the development of health-related physical fitness.

Though sports participation is not essential for a healthy lifestyle, many individuals enjoy taking part in sports. (The enjoyment is usually greater for individuals possessing athletic performance-related physical fitness.) The skills of agility, balance, coordination, power, reaction time and speed are important components of sports performance. These motor skills also are related to performance of many types of occupations and daily activities. Persons with adequate motor skills usually experience less job-related accidents, and are able to perform daily activities more efficiently. Diagnostic testing will enable the physical educator to prescribe the appropriate activities for individuals who do not possess adequate athletic performance-related physical fitness.

Are you able to:
define health-related and athletic performance-related physical fitness, and state why they should be measured?

TESTS OF HEALTH-RELATED PHYSICAL FITNESS

Establishing a single test battery that measures all components of health-related or athletic performance-related physical fitness is difficult. Since there is no one item that measures total body muscular strength, muscular endurance or flexibility, a decision must be made as to which parts of the body are to be measured for these components. Some tests include items that measure arm and shoulder girdle strength and endurance. Strength and endurance of the abdominal region and low back-posterior thigh flexibility are often included in tests because of their importance in prevention of low back disorders. Rather than selecting a single test battery, however, you may choose to measure either type of physical fitness through a combination of test items, presented in previous chapters. This approach is acceptable if you use items intended for the group (age and sex) you are testing.

Because most health-related physical fitness tests have similar components, only four are presented for your review. When reviewing these tests, note that only one test (the YMCA test) includes an item to measure arm-and-shoulder muscular strength and endurance.

AAHPERD HEALTH RELATED PHYSICAL FITNESS TEST (1980)
After years of study, the AAHPERD published the Health Related Physical Fitness Test in 1980. The specific criteria used for selection of the test items were:
1. a physical fitness test should measure a range that extends from severely limited dysfunction to high levels of functional capacity;
2. it should measure capacities that can be improved with appropriate physical activity; and
3. it should accurately reflect an individual's physical fitness status, as well as changes in functional capacity, by corresponding test scores and changes in these scores.

A test manual (1980) provides a description of the tests, tables of norms and criterion-referenced standards. A technical manual (1984) includes scientific evidence supporting the selection of the test items, and Pate (1985) provides norms for college students.
Age Level. Five through college.
Equipment. Flat running surface, stopwatch, skinfold caliper, mat, yard-sticks and bench, 12 inches high.
Test Components.
1. Cardiorespiratory function: The 1-mile run or 9-minute run is used for ages 5 through 18. The 1.5-mile or 12-minute run items are optional for ages 13 or older. These items are presented in Chapter 10.
2. Body composition (leanness/fatness): The sum of triceps and subscapular skinfolds; triceps skinfold is measured if only one site is used.
3. Abdominal and low back-hamstring musculoskeletal function: Modified, timed (one minute), bent-knee sit-ups (presented in Chapter 12), and sit-and-reach (presented in Chapter 11), are administered.

YMCA TEST (Golding, Meyers, and Sinning 1982)
The YMCA Test is for adult males and females and is administered as part of a health-related physical fitness program sponsored by the YMCA. (A medical examination is required before the test is administered.) Based on results of the test items, an exercise program is prescribed. The reference book includes standards for the test items.
Age Level. Adult.
Equipment. Skinfold caliper, yardstick, barbell and weights, mat and bicycle ergometer.
Test Components.
1. Body composition (percent body fat): The percent body fat is estimated

through skinfold measurements. For males, the sum of six skinfolds (chest, thigh, ilium, abdomen, triceps and scapula), or the sum of four (chest, ilium, abdomen and axilla) may be used. For females, the sum of five skinfolds (thigh, ilium, abdomen, triceps and scapula), or the sum of three (triceps, abdomen and ilium) may be used. Equations and tables based on age and sex are provided in the reference.

2. Flexibility: A form of the sit-and-reach test is used to measure flexibility of the low back and hamstring muscles. The test performer sits on the floor, with the heels 10-12 inches apart, and slowly reaches with both hands as far as possible. The near edge of the heel line is at the 15-inch mark of a yardstick. The score, in inches, is the most distant point reached on the yardstick. (If the test performer is unable to reach the 15-inch mark, the score is less than 15.)

3. Muscular strength and endurance: Three tests are used to measure these components.
   a. Two-arm curl. This test measures the number of times the test performer can repeatedly curl a barbell. Females curl 25 pounds, and males curl 40 pounds. The performer stands against a wall to standardize the movement, and a metronome, set at 44 beats/minute, regulates the rate of curls. On each click of the metronome there is an up or down movement. The score is the number of repetitions.
   b. Bench-press. This test measures the number of times the performer can repeatedly bench press a barbell. Females bench press 35 pounds, and males press 80 pounds. The press is performed at the same rate as the two-arm curl.
   c. One-minute sit-ups. The performer completes as many correct bent-knee sit-ups as possible, within a one-minute period.

4. Cardiorespiratory endurance: The bicycle ergometer is used to measure this component. Maximal oxygen uptake is predicted from the performer's response to a submaximal workload. The YMCA provides a graph to calculate VO_2 max.

SOUTH CAROLINA TEST (Pate 1978)
The South Carolina test includes both criterion and norm-referenced standards. Criterion-referenced standards for teachers are also included.
Age Level. Nine through adult.
Equipment. Flat running surface, skinfold caliper, mat, yardstick, bench and stopwatch.
Test Components.
1. Cardiorespiratory function: 1-mile run or 9-minute run for distance.
2. Body composition: The sum of triceps and abdominal skinfolds.
3. Abdominal and low-back musculoskeletal function: Timed (one minute) bent-knee sit-ups, and sit-and-reach.

MANITOBA PHYSICAL FITNESS PERFORMANCE TEST (Manitoba Department of Education 1977)
The Manitoba Physical Fitness Performance Test includes five health-related fitness components and one athletic performance-related fitness component. Tables of percentile norms for students, and criterion-referenced standards for students and teachers, are provided with the test.
Age Level. Five through 60+.
Equipment. Flat running surface, mat, horizontal bar, yardstick and skinfold caliper.
Test Components.
1. Abdominal muscular endurance: One-minute bent-knee sit-ups.
2. Flexibility: Sit-and-reach test.
3. Upper body muscular endurance: Flexed-arm hang.

4. Agility: Shuttle run is administered similarily to AAHPERD shuttle run, except to begin, performer lies face down with hands at the sides of chest and the forehead on the starting line.
5. Cardiovascular endurance: Distance run. 800-meter for ages five through nine; 1600-meter for ages 10 through 12; and 2400-meter for ages 13 through 60.
6. Body composition: Percent body fat estimated from biceps, triceps, subscapula and suprailium skinfolds measurements.

TESTS OF ATHLETIC PERFORMANCE-RELATED PHYSICAL FITNESS

Rarely does a single test battery include all components of athletic performance-related physical fitness. If you prefer a certain test, but would like to measure additional components, add the components to the test. However, remember to administer components that are appropriate for the group. Due to the similarity of many athletic performance-related tests, only three tests are described in this chapter.

AAHPERD YOUTH FITNESS TEST (AAHPERD 1976)
The AAHPERD Youth Fitness Test was developed by a group of physical educators who logically selected the test items. It was published in 1958 and revised in 1975 and 1976.
Age Level. Nine through 17+.
Test Components.
1. Arm and shoulder girdle strength and endurance: Pull-up test for males and flexed-arm hang test for females described in Chapter 12.
2. Abdominal strength and endurance: One-minute bent-knee sit-ups test.
   Equipment. Mat and stopwatch.
   Administration and Directions. The test performer lies on the back with the knees bent, feet flat on the floor and heels not more than 12 inches from the buttocks. The angle at the knees should be less than 90°. The hands are put behind the neck with the fingers clasped, and the elbows are placed squarely on the mat. A partner holds the feet to keep them from leaving the mat. On the start signal, the performer curls up, touching the elbows to the knees, and returns to the starting position (elbows on the mat). This action is repeated as many times as possible in 60 seconds. No rest is permitted between sit-ups, and only one trial is given, unless the test administrator believes the individual did not have a fair opportunity to perform. The performer should be cautioned against using the arms to thrust the body into the sitting position.
   Scoring. The item score is the number of correctly executed sit-ups performed in 60 seconds. Table 15-1 reports percentile norms.
3. Agility in running and changing direction: Shuttle run, described in Chapter 8.
4. Leg power: Standing long jump, described in Chapter 12.
5. Speed: The 50-yard dash.
   Equipment. A flat running area and a stopwatch accurate to one-tenth second per runner (may use one stopwatch accurate to one-tenth second with a split timer).
   Administration and Directions. Permit all performers to take one or two warm-up trials. Two performers should run at the same time (for competition) and all runners should be instructed not to slow down before crossing

Table 15-1. Norms for AAHPERD Youth Fitness Sit-Ups Test for Ages Nine through 17+*

	9–10	11	12	13	14	15	16	17+
					Age			
MALES								
PERCENTILE								
95	47	48	50	53	55	57	55	54
75	38	40	42	45	47	48	47	46
50	31	34	35	38	41	42	41	41
25	25	26	30	30	34	37	35	35
5	13	15	18	20	24	28	28	26
FEMALES								
95	45	43	44	45	45	45	43	45
75	34	35	36	36	37	36	35	35
50	27	29	29	30	30	31	30	30
25	21	22	24	23	24	25	24	25
5	10	9	13	15	16	15	15	14

*Adapted from *AAHPERD youth fitness test manual*, Reston, Virginia: AAHPERD, 1976.

the finish line. The test performers take a position behind the starting line. The starter uses the commands "Are you ready?" and "Go!" On the signal, "Go," the starter makes a downward sweep of the arm, as a signal to the timer. The timer stands at the finish line and stops the watch when the runner crosses the line.

Scoring. Scores are recorded to the nearest one-tenth of a second. Table 15-2 reports percentile norms.

6. Cardiorespiratory function: 600-yard run.

Equipment. A flat, running course and a stopwatch.

Administration and Directions. On the signal, "Ready, Go!" the test performers start running the 600-yard distance as fast as possible. Walking is permitted, but it is not encouraged. Pairing the test performers permits one partner to record the time of the performer. The test also may be administered with a scorer recording the times, as a timer calls out the times

Table 15-2. Norms in Seconds and Tenths of Second for AAHPERD 50-Yard Dash for Ages Nine through 17+*

	9–10	11	12	13	14	15	16	17+
					Age			
MALES								
PERCENTILE								
95	7.3	7.1	6.8	6.5	6.2	6.0	6.0	5.9
75	7.8	7.6	7.4	7.0	6.8	6.5	6.5	6.3
50	8.2	8.0	7.8	7.5	7.2	6.9	6.7	6.6
25	8.9	8.6	8.3	8.0	7.7	7.3	7.0	7.0
5	9.9	9.5	9.5	9.0	8.8	8.0	7.7	7.9
FEMALES								
95	7.4	7.3	7.0	6.9	6.8	6.9	7.0	6.8
75	8.0	7.9	7.6	7.4	7.3	7.4	7.5	7.4
50	8.6	8.3	8.1	8.0	7.8	7.8	7.9	7.9
25	9.1	9.0	8.7	8.5	8.3	8.2	8.3	8.4
5	10.3	10.0	10.0	10.0	9.6	9.2	9.3	9.5

*Adapted from *AAHPERD youth fitness test manual*, Reston, Virginia: AAHPERD, 1976.

when the runners cross the finish line. As with other running tests, the runners should warm-up prior to the test, and they should practice proper pacing.

Scoring. The time is recorded in minutes and seconds. Table 15-3 provides percentile norms.

Comments. Optional long distance runs include the 1-mile or 9-minute run for ages 10 through 12 years, and the 1.5 mile or 12-minute run for ages 13 years or older. Descriptions and norms for these runs are provided in Chapter 10.

Table 15-3. *Norms in Minutes and Seconds for AAHPERD 600-Yard Run Test for Ages Nine through 17+**

	Age							
	9–10	11	12	13	14	15	16	17+
MALES								
PERCENTILE								
95	2:05	2:02	1:52	1:45	1:39	1:36	1:34	1:32
75	2:17	2:15	2:06	1:59	1:52	1:46	1:44	1:43
50	2:33	2:27	2:19	2:10	2:03	1:56	1:52	1:52
25	2:53	2:47	2:37	2:27	2:16	2:08	2:01	2:02
5	3:22	3:29	3:06	3:00	2:51	2:30	2:31	2:38
FEMALES								
95	2:20	2:14	2:06	2:04	2:02	2:00	2:08	2:02
75	2:39	2:35	2:26	2:23	2:19	2:22	2:26	2:24
50	2:56	2:53	2:47	2:41	2:40	2:37	2:43	2:41
25	3:15	3:16	3:13	3:06	3:01	3:00	3:03	3:02
5	4:00	4:15	3:59	3:49	3:49	3:28	3:49	3:45

*Adapted from *AAHPERD youth fitness test manual*, Reston, Virginia: AAHPERD, 1976.

THE PRESIDENT'S CHALLENGE (President's Council on Physical Fitness and Sports 1986)

The President's Challenge can be used to qualify students for the Presidential Physical Fitness Award Program. (Previously, the AAHPERD Youth Fitness Test was used for this purpose.) All items are the same for males and females. To receive the award, students must score at, or above, the 85 percentiles on all five items of the test. The award standards are presented in Table 15-4.

Age Level. Six through 17.

Test Components.

1. Arm and shoulder girdle strength and endurance: Pull-up test, described in Chapter 12.
2. Cardiorespiratory endurance: One-mile run/walk, described in Chapter 10.
3. Leg muscle strength and endurance: Shuttle run, described in Chapter 8.
4. Abdominal muscle strength and endurance. Abdominal curl-ups (sit-ups).

    Administration and Directions. Administration and scoring of this item are the same as the AAHPERD Youth Fitness sit-ups test previously described, with the following exceptions: the test performer crosses the arms and places the fingers on the opposite shoulder; the arms are held in contact with the chest at all times; the elbows touch the thighs when the performer curls up; and the performer lowers the back to the surface so the scapula touches, before starting another curl-up.
5. Low back and hamstring flexibility: V-sit reach (the AAHPERD sit-and-reach test described in Chapter 11 also may be used to measure this component).

Table 15-4. *Performance Standards to Qualify for the Presidential Youth Fitness Award (85th Percentile)**

TEST ITEM	Age											
	6	7	8	9	10	11	12	13	14	15	16	17+
MALES												
Pull-ups (number)	2	4	5	5	6	6	7	7	10	11	11	13
One-mile run (minutes and seconds)	10:15	9:22	8:48	8:31	7:57	7:32	7:11	6:50	6:26	6:20	6:08	6:06
Shuttle run (seconds)	12.1	11.5	11.1	10.9	10.3	10.0	9.8	9.5	9.1	9.0	8.7	8.7
Curl-up (number)	33	36	40	41	45	47	50	53	56	57	56	55
V-sit reach (inches)	3.5	3.5	3.0	3.0	4.0	4.0	4.0	3.5	4.5	5.0	6.0	7.0
FEMALES												
Pull-ups (number)	2	2	2	2	3	3	2	2	2	2	1	1
One-mile run (minutes and seconds)	11:20	10:36	10:02	9:30	9:19	9:02	8:23	8:13	7:59	8:08	8:23	8:15
Shuttle run (seconds)	12.4	12.1	11.8	11.1	10.8	10.5	10.4	10.2	10.1	10.0	10.1	10.0
Curl-up (number)	32	34	38	39	40	42	45	46	47	48	45	44
V-sit reach (inches)	5.5	5.0	4.5	5.5	6.0	6.5	7.0	7.0	8.0	8.0	9.0	8.0

*Adapted from *The presidential physical fitness award program*, The Presidential Council on Physical Fitness and Sports, 1986.

Equipment. Yardstick and floor marking tape.

Administration and Directions. A straight line (baseline) two feet long is marked on the floor. At the midpoint of the baseline, a line of four feet (two feet on each side) is marked perpendicular to the baseline. This line serves as the measuring line. One inch and one-half inch marks are placed on the measuring line on each side of the base line. The baseline intersect is the "0" point. After removing shoes, the test performer sits on the floor, so the legs are eight to 12 inches apart, the measuring line is between the legs and the soles of the feet are just behind the baseline. The performer then clasps thumbs so the hands are together, with the palms turned down. With the soles of the feet perpendicular to the floor and a partner holding the legs down, the performer reaches forward along the measuring line as far as possible, keeping the fingers in contact with the floor. Three practice reaches are given. On the fourth extension, the test performer holds the farthest point for a count of three seconds, while the distance is recorded.

Scoring. The farthest point reached and held for three seconds is recorded as the score. A plus score is given when the ends of the fingers go beyond the baseline, and a minus score is given when the reach is short of the baseline. If the reach is exactly to the baseline, the score is 0. All scores are recorded to the nearest half-inch.

AAU PHYSICAL FITNESS TEST (AAU 1986)

The Amateur Athletic Union Physical Fitness Test is for males and females. It includes four required items and six optional items. Each participant must complete one of the optional items. An Outstanding Achievement award is earned by students who score in the top 20% of their age group for each of the four required events and one optional event. Students scoring above the 45th percentile, but not above the 80th percentile, receive the Attainment certificate. Individuals scoring at or below the 45th percentile on the four required events and one optional event, receive the Participation certificate.

The AAU provides a test brochure and a test record sheet which may be copied. The cost of award certificates is limited to postage and handling.

Age Level. Six through 17.

Equipment. Flat running surface, stopwatch, mat, yardstick, horizontal bar, tape measure and 2" x 2" x 4" blocks or erasers.

Test Components.
1. Cardiorespiratory endurance: Distance run. One-quarter mile for ages six through seven; one-half mile for ages eight through nine; three-quarter mile for ages 10 through 11; and one-mile for ages 12 through 17.
2. Trunk strength and endurance: One-minute bent-knee sit-ups.
3. Flexibility of the hamstrings and lower back: Sit-and-reach test. Yardstick or tape measure is placed on the floor and heels of test performer are even with 15-inch mark.
4. Upper body strength and endurance: Pull-ups (palms toward body) for males, and flexed-arm hang (palms toward body) for females.

Optional components and test items are:
1. Leg strength and efficiency of control of body mass in space: Standing broad jump.
2. Upper body static endurance (males): Isometric push-up. The test performer takes a push-up position. On the command to begin, the body is pushed up until the elbows are bent at a 90° angle. The score is the time this position can be held.
3. Upper body strength and endurance (females): Modified push-ups with 30 second time limit.
4. Static leg endurance: Isometric leg squat. With back flat against wall, the test performer slides down the wall until the knees form a 90° angle. The feet

should point directly forward and must be flat on the floor, and the arms should hang at the sides. The score is the length of time this position can be held.

5. Agility and quickness: Shuttle run. This item is similar to the AAHPERD Shuttle Run, except three blocks are used. After placing two blocks individually on the starting line, the test performer picks up the third block and runs across the starting line with it.

6. Speed, quickness and anaerobic capacity: Sprint. 50 yards for ages nine through 12; 100 yards for ages 13 through 17.

PRESIDENT'S COUNCIL ON PHYSICAL FITNESS AND SPORTS

The President's Council on Physical Fitness and Sports is an organization based in Washington, D. C. Its primary purpose is to promote physical fitness and sports. The Council offers the Presidential Physical Fitness Award to any student who scores at or above the 85th percentile on all items on the President's Challenge (for his or her appropriate age). Information on the awards is available by writing to the PCPFS, Washington, D. C. 20001. Program materials may be ordered from the American Alliance for Health, Physical Education, Recreation and Dance.

FITNESSGRAM

Developed by the Institute for Aerobic Research in Dallas, Texas, the FITNESSGRAM is a national program sponsored the AAHPERD, Campbell Soup Company, the President's Council on Physical Fitness and Sport and the Institute for Aerobic Research. The program, designed to measure and contribute to the improvement of youth fitness, can be used with both the Health-Related Physical Fitness and the Youth Fitness Test. The FITNESSGRAM program is a computerized system for reporting raw scores on the test items, the percentile rank against a national norm for each item and an overall fitness score and percentile rank. Based on the results of the test, an exercise prescription is provided for the student and a message to the parents.

The Institute for Aerobic Research will produce the fitness reports for a school district, and assist in the development of microcomputer software that will enable a school district to produce FITNESSGRAM locally. For information write to: Youth Fitness, Institute for Aerobic Research, 12200 Preston Road, Dallas, Texas 75230.

DEVELOPMENT OF HEALTH-RELATED AND ATHLETIC PERFORMANCE-RELATED PHYSICAL FITNESS

If either type of physical fitness is to be developed, a program must consist of different activities and exercises. One particular type of activity or exercise usually will not develop all components. For example, though running is an excellent activity for the development of cardiorespiratory fitness, other activities must be performed for the development of arm and shoulder strength and flexibility. The same is true of many cardiorespiratory fitness programs. Also, weight-lifting programs are excellent for muscular strength and endurance, but other types of programs are better for cardiorespiratory fitness. Activities and exercises that may be used to develop the components of health-related and athletic performance-related physical fitness have been described in previous chapters. Through selection of the appropriate activities for different ages, you should be able to design sound programs.

REVIEW PROBLEMS

1. Review additional health-related and athletic performance-related physical fitness tests in other sources. Do the tests include any components not reported in this textbook? If so, do you consider them as components of health-related or athletic performance-related physical fitness?
2. Interview several teachers in the local school system about their use of health-related and athletic performance-related physical fitness tests. Ask which tests they prefer, and why.
3. Administer the AAHPERD Health Related Test or the AAHPERD Youth Fitness Test to several of your fellow students. Ask them to provide constructive criticism of your test administration.
4. Design a program to develop health-related physical fitness for the age group 16 through 18.

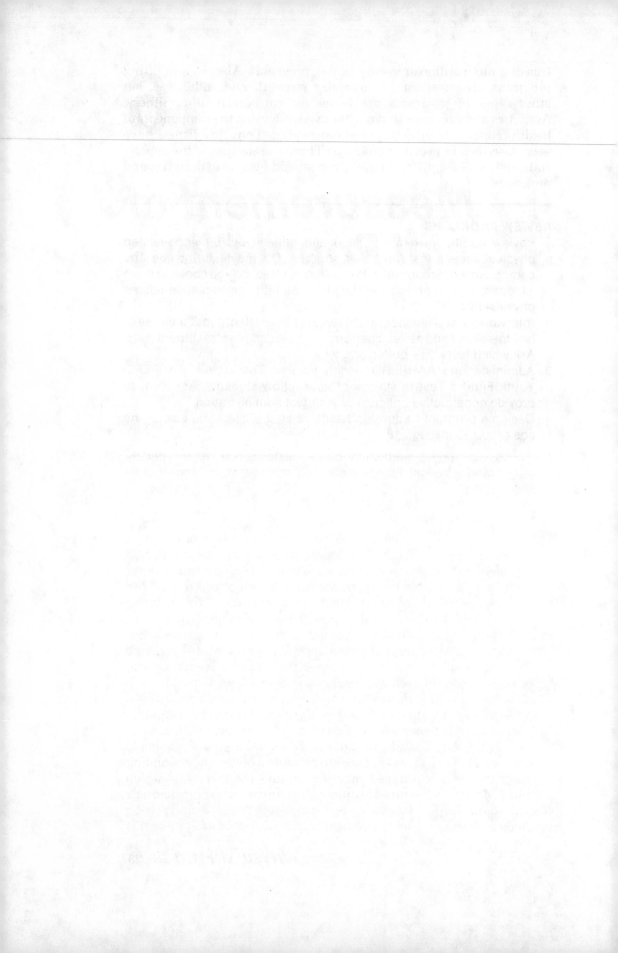

16

Measurement of Special Populations

Upon completion of this chapter, you should be able to:
1. Define the term special populations, and state what must be done in public physical education programs to meet the needs of special populations;
2. Describe the role of physical performance measurement in special physical education programs;
3. Justify the use of norm-referenced and criterion-referenced tests with special populations; and
4. Select appropriate perceptual-motor performance, motor performance and physical fitness tests, and administer them to special populations.

The term "special populations" is used when referring to handicapped, impaired or disabled individuals. Federal laws require all public agencies to ensure a continuum of alternate placements to meet handicapped children's needs for special education and related services; the children are to be educated in the least restrictive environment in which their educational needs can be provided. Therefore, when handicapped individuals cannot benefit from placement in a regular physical education program, federal laws dictate the program must be adapted or modified to meet their needs. As a physical educator you should seek approaches to these adaptations that will emphasize what the individuals can do; accentuate the positive. However, the adaptations will not be the same for everyone. Special needs vary for persons with different handicaps, and with similar degrees of the same handicap. Your professional preparation should include one or two courses that seek to promote a better understanding of the needs of handicapped individuals, and the means by which physical educators can provide appropriate and worthwhile programs for all handicapped students. The purpose of this chapter is to emphasize the place of measurement in physical education programs for special populations, and to provide examples of perceptual-motor performance, motor performance and physical fitness tests that may be used for screening and diagnostic purposes. Many tests are available. Though a few tests are described in this chapter, you should review other available tests, and select the one that best meets your needs.

No activities for development of perceptual-motor abilities, motor abilities and physical fitness will be described at the conclusion of this chapter. However, many activities, or modifications of them, described in previous chapters may be used for such purposes. Additionally, there are many types and degrees of handicaps, and the activities for development of perceptual-motor abilities, motor abilities and physical fitness may vary with the types of handicap.

WHY MEASURE SPECIAL POPULATIONS?

The Education for All Handicapped Children Act of 1975, P. L. 94-142, emphasizes the importance of evaluation in the education of handicapped children. Through the law a framework has been established, in which evaluation is the key to the type of program provided. All aspects of the law pertaining to evaluation will not be described here, but the major points are:

1. Every state is required to develop a plan for identifying, locating and evaluating all handicapped students.

2. All handicapped children and their parents are guaranteed procedural safeguards. Known as due process, this requirement means that parents and their children must be informed of their rights, and they may challenge educational decisions they feel are unfair. This requirement also means: the parents must give written permission for their child to be evaluated, the results of the evaluation must be explained to the parents, the parents may request that an independent evaluation be conducted outside the school, and if the parents and the school cannot agree on the evaluation findings, a special hearing must be held. All evaluation results must be kept confidential.

3. Standards for evaluation must be followed. Tests must be used that measure achievement level rather than impaired sensory, manual or speaking skills, and more than one test procedure must be utilized to determine the student's educational status. Since many handicapped students have communication problems, tests must be administered to test ability rather than communication skills. Finally, a multidisciplinary team of qualified professionals must administer the test and interpret the results.

If you assume a professional position that includes responsibilities with special populations, you should be familiar with all aspects of P. L. 94-142.

Regardless of federal laws, if the best possible physical education program is to be provided for handicapped students, evaluation must be included. Fait and Dunn (1984) state that a strong evaluation component serves to:

1. Identify individuals who have physical and motor deficiencies.
2. Establish eligibility for special physical education service. Individuals identified through the initial screening process are referred for further evaluation to confirm results of the initial screening (definitive diagnosis should not be based on one assessment). Further testing also helps pinpoint specific strengths and weaknesses, and the individual's particular needs.
3. Aid in the development of individualized physical education programs.
4. Help teachers and students recognize progress, which in turn permits effective exchange of communication between school and home. As a result of an evaluation that includes objective test scores, the teacher should feel more comfortable discussing the student's achievement.
5. Enable teachers to use results of student progress to analyze their own effectiveness, methods of instructions and curricular materials. Lack of progress may lead to changes in the program.

NORM-REFERENCED OR CRITERION-REFERENCED TESTS?

Should norm-referenced or criterion-referenced tests be used with special populations? Really, it is not a choice of using only one or the other, for there is need of both norm-referenced and criterion-referenced tests when working with handicapped students. Norm-referenced tests serve the same purposes as they do for other populations; standardized norms are useful in screening for motor problems, in comparing students with similar handicaps, in program evaluation and in the placement of students. Criterion-referenced tests are especially useful in measuring student progress, and for making instructional decisions about individual students. These tests also may be used for screening purposes when students are asked to perform certain basic skills.

> Are you able to:
> define the term special populations, and state what must be done in public physical education programs to meet the needs of special populations?
> describe the role of physical performance measurement in special physical education programs?
> state why norm-referenced and criterion-referenced measurement should be used in physical education programs for special populations?

PERCEPTUAL-MOTOR PERFORMANCE TESTS

Perceptual-motor performance tests sample the ability of children to integrate sensory information with past experience, with making decisions about movement. Since there is little doubt that perception is an important aspect of successful movement, perceptual-motor performance tests can be valuable educational tools. However, they should not be interpreted as providing an overall measurement of motor ability. Rather, each item of the test battery should be used to measure a separate, specific factor. Components of perceptual-motor efficiency include balance, postural and locomotor awareness, visual perception, auditory perception, kinesthetic perception, tactile perception, body awareness and laterality and directionality. Perceptual-motor programs for the handicapped are important, but they should not be used in place of physical education programs. A strong physical education program is essential to every child's motor development. Some handicapped children may need both programs.

Prior to any formal testing of the handicapped, you should try to be familiar with their basic motor behavior patterns. You may obtain much information through the informal techniques of observation, self-testing, discussion with others and rating scales and checklists. The preferred hand and foot should be determined, as well as any movement patterns that can be used in a positive way. Preliminary measurement of such skills as running, skipping, balancing, catching, throwing, striking an object and kicking, may be conducted with a rating scale by asking the students to perform these skills while you observe. This type of preliminary testing may prevent problems during the formal testing.

Many perceptual-motor tests are available, but only three are presented, as examples to illustrate the types of test components that may be included in perceptual-motor tests. You should refer to other sources prior to selecting a test. The test you choose to administer will depend on your needs, and the age group you wish to test.

PURDUE PERCEPTUAL MOTOR SURVEY (Roach and Kephart 1966)
Though referred to as a test, the Purdue Perceptual Motor Survey is a survey. The survey manual includes clear and precise instructions for scoring and administering each item, as well as illustrations clarifying exactly what the child is expected to do. Forms for recording each child's performance are provided. The survey may be purchased from Charles E. Merrill Publishing Co. in Columbus, Ohio.
Age Level. Six through 10.
Equipment. Visual achievement forms, chalkboard, chalk, yardstick and penlight.
Test Components.
1. Balance and posture: Walking forward, backward and sideward on a walking board and performing a series of jumping, hopping, and skipping tasks while maintaining balance.
2. Body image and differentiation: Identification of body parts, imitation of movement, and participation in various obstacle-course activities.
3. Perceptual-motor match: Drawing circles and lines on a chalkboard and performing eight rhythmic writing tasks.

4. Ocular control: Ocular-pursuit tasks involving individual eye movement and simultaneous eye movement.

5. Form-perception: Drawing various geometric shapes on a sheet of paper.

AYRES SOUTHERN CALIFORNIA PERCEPTUAL-MOTOR TESTS
(Miller and Sullivan 1982)

To perform this test, it is important the child understands simple verbal directions. In addition, as five of the six items call for adequate motor responses, caution must be taken in testing children with neuromuscular impairment. The test battery can be administered in approximately 20 minutes. The test may be purchased from Western Psychological Services, Los Angeles, California.

Age Level. Four through eight.

Equipment. Watch, table and chairs.

Test Components.

1. Imitation of postures: Imitate 12 postures demonstrated by the instructor.
2. Crossing mid-line of body: Point at, or touch, the designated ear or eye, using the left or right hand.
3. Bilateral motor coordination: Use the palms of the hands to gently slap or touch the thighs, with a rhythmical motion.
4. Right-left discrimination: Identify own left and right sides, those of another pupil, or of various objects.
5. Standing balance, eyes open: Maintain balance while standing on one foot, then change to the other foot. Each foot-balance is timed.
6. Standing balance, eyes closed: Same as component 5, except the eyes are kept closed throughout.

ANDOVER PERCEPTUAL-MOTOR TEST (Nichols, Arsenault, and Giuffre 1980)

The Andover Perceptual-Motor Test measures the basic perceptual-motor areas necessary for normal development and motor learning. The test should be used as a quick screening device, and not as a diagnostic tool. It can be administered to a group of 25 in two, 30-minute class sessions.

Age Level. Four through seven.

Equipment. Primary balance beam, two eight-inch balls, marking tape and dowel or stick.

Test Components.

1. Balance: The ability to maintain static and dynamic balance.
2. Eye-hand coordination: The ability to coordinate the eyes and hands to accomplish a task.
3. Locomotion: The ability to ambulate the body through space; a combination of strength, coordination and balance is needed to perform this item.
4. Spatial awareness: The ability to make spatial judgments, and perceive the body in relation to other objects in space.
5. Rhythm: The ability to hear, interpret the sounds heard and respond to what is interpreted.

MOTOR PERFORMANCE TESTS

For many years, educators have been interested in the relationship of age and motor performance. As a result of this interest, many tests have been established for measurement of motor skills, and to compare an individual's motor performance to that of other individuals of similar age. (Many of these tests have been described in previous chapters.) Motor performance tests also have been established to serve as screening instruments, to help identify individuals with motor deficiencies, and those in need of special education.

However, these tests often are incorrectly used to measure individual growth and progress over a period of time. Some teachers mistakenly believe that improvement in test scores will occur if students participate in a variety of movement experiences. But, you should not expect changes in test scores, unless the students practice items or skills that are very similar to the test items. Since many motor performance skills are highly specific, transfer of learning does not always occur as a result of participation in general movement experiences. On the other hand, assuming that no improvement in motor performance has taken place if test scores do not change, is incorrect. The students may have improved in skills that are not measured by the test. In addition, a general background in motor performance serves as a foundation for the development of specific motor skills. There are many motor performance tests, but only three will be presented as examples.

THE BRUININKS-OSERETSKY TEST OF MOTOR PROFICIENCY
(Arnheim and Sinclair 1985, and Safrit 1986)
The Bruininks-Oseretsky Test of Motor Proficiency can be administered in two forms: as a complete form, or as a short form. The complete form consists of eight subtests comprised of 46 separate items. Four subtests measure gross motor skills, three measure fine motor skills, and one measures both fine and gross motor skills. The complete test requires 45 to 60 minutes to administer. The short form also consists of eight subtests, but only 14 items. The short form can be administered in 15 to 20 minutes. The division of the test into eight basic areas permits the teacher to be specific in determining where to place the emphasis in remedying the children's movement problems. No special training is required of test administrators. The test kit may be purchased from the American Guidance Service in Circle Pines, Minnesota.
Age Level. 4½ through 14½.
Equipment. Balance beam, ball, mazes, scissors, balance rod, matchbook, coins, small boxes, thread, playing cards, matchsticks, ballpoint pen and paper.
Test Components.
LONG FORM
Subtest 1: Running speed and agility (one item).
Subtest 2: Balance (eight items).
Subtest 3: Bilateral coordination (eight items).
Subtest 4: Strength (three items).
Subtest 5: Upper-limb coordination (nine items).
Subtest 6: Response speed (one item).
Subtest 7: Visual-motor control (eight items).
Subtest 8: Upper limb speed and dexterity (eight items).
SHORT FORM
Subtest 1: Running speed and agility.
Subtest 2: Standing on preferred leg while making circles with fingers. Walking forward heel-to-toe on balance beam.
Subtest 3: Tapping feet alternately while making circles with feet. Jumping up and clapping hands.
Subtest 4: Standing broad jump.
Subtest 5: Catching a ball with both hands. Throwing a ball at a target with preferred hand.
Subtest 6: Response speed.

Subtest 7: Drawing a line through a straight path with preferred hand.
Copying a circle on paper with preferred hand.
Copying overlapping pencils with preferred hand.
Subtest 8: Sorting shape cards with preferred hand.
Drawing dots in circles with preferred hand.

THE BASIC MOTOR ABILITY TESTS (Arnheim and Sinclair 1979)
The Basic Motor Ability Tests (BMAT) are a battery of nine tests designed to evaluate the selected motor responses of small- and large-muscle control, static and dynamic balance, eye-hand coordination and flexibility. Each of the nine subtests requires little training to administer. One child can be tested in approximately 12 to 15 minutes, while a group of five children can be tested in about 25 minutes, by one test administrator.

Age Level. Four through 12.

Equipment. One-half-inch beads; 18-inch round shoe lace with three-quarter-inch plastic tip; 4″ x 5″ bean bags; wastepaper basket, 14 inches high; table; chair; transfer board consisting of two eight-ounce margarine containers, four inches in diameter, attached to and positioned on the board 12 inches apart; 30 regular size marbles; yardstick; 4′ x 6′ mat; blindfold; stopwatch; balance board with width of one and three-quarter inches; basketball; 50-foot tape measure; two Nerf balls (three-inch diameter ball, and 10-inch diameter ball); target consisting of four vertical lines, one inch wide and eight feet high which are connected at the top by a horizontal line one-inch wide (vertical lines are two feet apart); playground ball, 10 inches in diameter; and four cones.

Test Components.
Subtest 1: Bilateral eye-hand coordination and dexterity — bead stringing with 40-second time limit.
Subtest 2: Eye-hand coordination — target throwing with bean bags and wastepaper basket.
Subtest 3: Speed of hand movement, crossing from one side of the body to the other — transfer of marbles from one container to another; both hands are tested with 20-second time limit for each hand.
Subtest 4: Flexibility of back and hamstring muscles — sit-and-reach.
Subtest 5: Strength and power in the thigh and lower leg muscles — standing long jump.
Subtest 6: Speed and agility in changing from a prone to a standing position — move from face down to standing position and touch mark on wall; repeat cycle as many times as possible in 20 seconds.
Subtest 7: Static balance — static balance on one and three-quarter inch balance board; performed with eyes open and blindfolded on preferred foot and other foot; maximum of 10 seconds per trial.
Subtest 8: Arm and shoulder girdle explosive strength — two hand chest past with basketball; three trials.
Subtest 9: Coordination associated with striking — ability to strike Nerf ball with hand, and hit target drawn on wall; five swings with each arm.
Subtest 10: Eye-foot coordination — ability to kick ball at target; five kicks with each foot.
Subtest 11: Agility — rapidly move the body, and alter direction; zigzag pattern around cones.

THE STOTT, MOYES AND HENDERSON TEST OF MOTOR IMPAIRMENT (Miller and Sullivan 1982)
The objective of the Stott, Moyes and Henderson Test of Motor Impairment is to ascertain and assess motor impairment of functional or presumed neurological origin. The test was derived from the original Oseretsky test and the

revised Lincoln-Oseretsky test. The revised form contains sets of five test items each, one set for each year, ages 4 to 14. It can be administered to most pupils in approximately 20 minutes. Test procedures are available from Brook Educational Publishing Ltd., P. O. Box 1171, Guelph, Ontario N1H6N3.

Age Level. Five through 14.

Equipment. See test items (equipment varies for each age).

Test Components.
1. Control and balance of the body while immobile.
2. Control and coordination of the upper limbs.
3. Control and coordination of the body while in motion.
4. Manual dexterity with emphasis on speed.
5. Tasks that emphasize simultaneous movement and precision.

Age Five
1. Balancing on tiptoes; feet together, eyes open.
2. Bouncing a ball and catching it in two hands.
3. Jumping over a cord at knee height.
4. Posting coins into a bank box.
5. Placing counters simultaneously into a box.

Age Six
1. Balancing on one leg; eyes open.
2. Bouncing a ball and catching it in one hand.
3. Hopping forward for five yards, between two lines.
4. Threading beads onto a lace.
5. Tracing a circular track with a pencil.

Age Seven
1. Balancing on one foot with arms raised; eyes open.
2. Following a track of holes in a wooden board with a pencil.
3. Walking heel-to-toe along a line.
4. Placing pegs on a board, one by one.
5. Touching tips of the fingers in order.

Age Eight
1. Balancing on one foot with other placed on the knee; eyes open.
2. Throwing a ball at a wall and catching the rebound.
3. Jumping sideward, three jumps, with feet together.
4. Threading a lace through a series of holes in a wooden board.
5. Walking while balancing a bead on a board.

Age Nine
1. Balancing on a wide board; eyes open.
2. Catching a ball in one hand.
3. Jumping and clapping twice before landing.
4. Placing a wooden pin through a series of holes.
5. Placing pegs simultaneously into a board.

Age 10
1. Balancing on a narrow board; eyes open.
2. Guiding a ball round an obstacle course on a table.
3. Jumping over a knee-height cord; taking off with two feet together and landing on one foot.
4. Placing matchsticks in four small boxes.
5. Placing holed-squares simultaneously on two rods.

Ages 11-12
1. Balancing heel-to-toe on two narrow boards; eyes open.
2. Hitting a target with a ball.
3. Hopping sidewards into two squares.
4. Piercing holes in paper track.
5. Placing pegs on a board and squares on pins, simultaneously.

Ages 13-14
1. Balancing on the toes of one foot.
2. Moving a ring along a rod.

3. Jumping backward and forward inside large circles.
4. Moving a pen round a track.
5. Piercing holes simultaneously with two styluses.

PHYSICAL FITNESS TESTS

The development of physical fitness is important for special populations for the same reasons it is important for other individuals. All children should be instructed in the why and how of a healthy lifestyle, and they should be provided the opportunity for development of health-related and athletic performance-related physical fitness.

There is another important reason why special populations need to develop and maintain physical fitness: poor physical fitness can limit a child's performance and slow the rate of improvement in motor performance. For example, scores on balance and agility tests may be influenced by a child's poor muscular endurance and cardiorespiratory fitness. Any individual whose fitness limitations restrict progress in motor development should be involved in a program to strengthen those weaknesses.

The health-related and athletic performance-related physical fitness of many handicapped individuals may be measured with the same tests or test items presented in Chapter 15. Adjustments in the items may be necessary, depending on the type and degree of handicap. For example, the distance run on the AAHPERD Health-Related Fitness Test may be reduced in distance. If it is necessary to reduce the distance to the point that it is no longer a valid measure of cardiorespiratory fitness, the run may be used as a motivational item. (When it is necessary to adjust a test item for an individual, it is important you do not compare the resulting score with scores achieved by individuals who are able to perform the item without adjustments.)

AAHPERD MOTOR FITNESS TEST FOR THE MODERATELY MENTALLY RETARDED (Johnson and Londeree 1976)
The AAHPERD Motor Fitness Test for the Moderately Mentally Retarded is a modification of the AAHPERD Youth Test. It is intended to be used when testing mentally retarded children who are capable of learning (IQs ranging from 50 to 70). The test may include 13 items, but six items are recommended as sufficient for testing the motor fitness of the moderately retarded. The remaining items of height, weight, sitting bob-and-reach, hopping, skipping, tumbling progression and target throw may be used in local situations.
Age Level. Norms are published for boys and girls, ages six through 20.
Equipment. Metal or wooden bar one and one-half inches in diameter, tumbling mat, stopwatch, tape measure, softballs and flat running surface.
Test Components.
1. Arm-and-shoulder strength and endurance — flexed-arm hang.
2. Abdominal strength and endurance — 30-seconds sit-ups.
3. Explosive leg power — standing long jump.
4. Coordination — softball throw for distance.
5. Speed — 50-yard dash.
6. Cardiorespiratory fitness — 300-yard run-walk.

SPECIAL FITNESS TEST FOR MILDLY MENTALLY RETARDED PERSONS (AAHPERD 1976)
This test battery is a modification of the AAHPERD Youth Fitness Test. The

norms are different, but the components are similar to those of the Motor Fitness Test for the Moderately Mentally Retarded.

Age Level. Eight through 18.

Equipment. Metal or wooden bar one and one-half inches in diameter, tumbling mat, stopwatch, tape measure, softballs and flat running surface.

Test Components.
1. Arm-and-shoulder strength and endurance — flexed-arm hang.
2. Abdominal strength and endurance — one- minute straight-leg sit-ups.
3. Agility — shuttle run.
4. Explosive leg power — standing long jump.
5. Speed — 50-yard dash.
6. Coordination — softball throw for distance.
7. Cardiorespiratory fitness — 300-yard run.

FAIT PHYSICAL FITNESS TEST FOR MILDLY AND MODERATELY MENTALLY RETARDED STUDENTS (Fait and Dunn 1984)

This test is suitable for use with the educable and a majority of the medium and high trainables, if they do not have other handicaps which prevent safe performance of the test.

Age Level. Nine through 20.

Equipment. Horizontal bar or doorway bar, mat and flat running surface.

Test Components.
1. Speed — 25-yard run.
2. Static muscular endurance of the arm and shoulder girdle — bent arm hang.
3. Dynamic muscular endurance of the flexor muscles of the leg and of the abdominal muscles — leg lift.
4. Static balance — balance on one leg with eyes closed.
5. Agility — 20-second squat thrust.
6. Cardiorespiratory endurance — 300-yard run-walk.

BUELL AAHPERD YOUTH FITNESS ADAPTATION FOR THE BLIND (Buell 1982)

This test is an adaptation from the AAHPERD Youth Fitness Test.

Age Level. 10 through 17.

Equipment. Horizontal bar or doorway bar, mat, stopwatch, tape measure, basketball and flat running surface.

Test Components.
1. Arm and shoulder girdle strength and endurance — pull-ups (boys), and flexed-arm hang (females).
2. Abdominal strength and endurance — one-minute bent-knee sit-ups.
3. Leg power — standing long jump.
4. Speed — 50-yard dash.
5. Cardiorespiratory function — 600-yard run-walk.
6. Upper body power — basketball throw.

The norms for pull-ups (boys), flexed-arm hang (girls), sit-ups and standing long jump are the same as in the revised AAHPERD Youth Fitness Test (1975). Separate norms were developed for the 50-yard dash and for the 600-yard run-walk. The shuttle run test was eliminated, and a basketball throw was added to measure upper body power.

REVIEW PROBLEMS

1. Ask physical education teachers in the local schools to describe the tests they are using to screen special populations.
2. Review in other sources additional perceptual-motor performance, motor performance and physical fitness tests for special populations.

17

Sports Skills

Upon completion of this chapter, you should be able to:
1. Measure sports skills;
2. State how sports skills tests may be used in physical education; and
3. Locate and select individual and dual sports skills tests.

Many sports skills tests are described in the professional literature you will read. Some of these tests are valid and reliable, while others are not. No attempt is made in this chapter to describe all good sports skills tests, but a very adequate sampling is provided. Unless indicated otherwise, the described tests may be administered to males and females. Collins and Hodges (1978) is an excellent source for skills tests, as the authors describe 103 tests for 26 sports.

Selection of any sports skills test should be based on the criteria described in Chapter 3. In addition to selecting a good test, you should recognize that some tests measure only one aspect of a sport. When such a test is administered, no generalization should be made about an individual's overall skill in a particular sport.

Norms are available for many sports skills tests, but unless you wish to make national comparisons, it may be more appropriate to develop local norms. Often local norms are more meaningful, due to differences in movement experiences, and the socioeconomic environment of the group being tested and the group used to develop the test norms.

WHY MEASURE SPORTS SKILLS?

Perhaps the most popular purpose of sports skills measurement is to determine an individual's progress or level of achievement in a particular sport. Other important purposes for the measurement of sports skills are described below.

Classification: A skills test can be administered early in the instructional process of a sport to classify all participants. This eliminates the need of observing the individuals for several group meetings before attempting to classify them.

Diagnosis: Determining the strengths and weaknesses of the students can aid in the planning of unit objectives and can help identify students who may need special attention.

Motivation: Used correctly, a skills test can motivate individuals to improve their abilities in a sport. The challenge of competing against one's own scores often motivates more than the challenge of competing against others.

Practice: While performing the test items, the students are actually practicing the skills of the sport.

Program Accountability: Test scores, as well as other information, can be used to demonstrate to administration, parents and public, the objectives and values of physical education. When no such information is available, many individuals' perception of physical education as a play period is reaffirmed.

INDIVIDUAL AND DUAL SPORTS

Archery
AAHPERD Archery Test (AAHPERD 1967)
Test Objective. To measure archery skill.
Age Level. 12 through 18.
Equipment. Standard 48-inch target faces, bows ranging from 15 to 40 pounds in pull, matched arrows (eight to 10 per person) 24 to 28 inches in length, archery accessories (arm guards, finger tabs).
Validity. Face validity.
Reliability. No reliability estimate is provided, but test manual states that no test item in the battery has a reliability less than .70.
Administration and Directions. No more than four archers should shoot at one target. Two ends of six arrows (total of 12) are shot at distances of 10, 20, and 30 yards for boys, and 10 and 20 yards for girls. All archers begin at the 10-yard distance and move to the 20-yard line when the two ends have been completed. This process is repeated for each line. However, individuals who do not score at least 10 points at one distance may not advance to the next distance. Each archer is given four practice shots at each distance.
Scoring. Standard target scoring is used, with the point values 9, 7, 5, 3, and 1 for the respective circles from the center outward. Arrows falling outside the outer circle or missing the target are scored 0. Arrows passing completely through or rebounding off the target are awarded 7 points.

Badminton
FRENCH SHORT SERVE TEST (Scott 1941)
Test Objective. To measure the ability to serve accurately, with a low and short placement (degree of serving skill should be developed before the test is administered).
Age Level. Junior high through college.
Equipment. Badminton racket, shuttles, rope to stretch above net and floor marking tape.
Validity. Using tournament rankings as a criterion, a coefficient of .66 was reported.
Reliability. Using college women as subjects, coefficients of .51 to .89 were reported.
Administration and Directions. A rope is stretched 20 inches directly above and parallel to the net. A series of two-inch lines in the form of arcs are placed at distances of 22, 30, 38 and 46 inches from the midpoint of the

intersection of the center line and the short-service line of the right service court. Each measurement includes the width of the two-inch lines. The test performer may stand anywhere in the right service area, diagonally opposite the target. Twenty legal serves (may be two groups of ten) are attempted at the target (Figure 17-1). To earn points, the serve must pass between the rope and net and land somewhere in the proper service court area for doubles play.

Scoring. The scorer stands in a position (center of left service court, facing the target) to determine if the shuttle passes between the rope and net, and to determine the point value of each serve. A score is awarded to any legal serve that passes between the rope and net and lands in the proper service court for doubles play. A score of 0 is recorded for any shuttle that does not pass between the rope and net. The awarded points (5, 4, 3, 2, and 1) are based on the placement of the shuttle. Shuttles that land on a target line are awarded the point value of the higher area. If a shuttle hits the rope, the trial is not counted. Illegal serves may be repeated. The test score is the sum of the 20 serves.

Comment. The test performers should have the opportunity to practice this skill before attempting the test, as the reliability of the test is not as high for unskilled players. Drawing the target on the corner of a sheet or canvas for placement on the court will prevent the need of placing tape on the floor each time the test is administered.

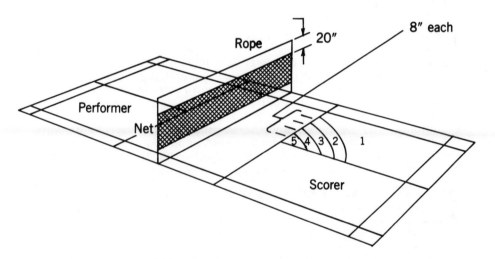

Figure 17-1. *French short serve test.*

SCOTT AND FOX LONG SERVE TEST (Scott and French 1959)
Test Objective. To measure the accuracy of the long serve.
Age Level. High school through college.
Equipment. Badminton racket, shuttles and floor marking tape.
Validity. A coefficient of .54 was found by correlating the scores of college women, with the subjective rating of judges.
Reliability. The internal-consistency of reliability estimates with college women were .77 and .68.
Administration and Directions. With the use of additional standards, a rope is stretched across the court 14 feet from and parallel to the net at a height of eight feet. Floor markings are identical to those described for the French Short Serve Test, except for their location. The intersection of the long service line and the left side boundary line for singles is utilized for placement of the target (Figure 17-2). Standing anywhere in the service court diagonally across

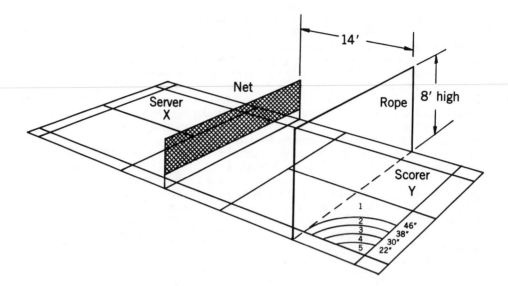

Figure 17-2. *Scott and Fox long serve test.*

from the target, the performer attempts 20 legal serves over the net and rope, to the target area.

Scoring. A score (5, 4, 3, 2 or 1) is awarded to any legal serve that passes over the net and rope, and lands in the target area. Serves that hit the rope are taken over, and shuttles that land on a target line are awarded the point value of the higher target. Illegal serves may be repeated. The test score is the sum of the 20 serves.

Comments. Any serve that lands beyond the back line receives 0 points. Because most opponents play serves that would land close to the back line, the test administrator may choose to develop a point system that includes an area two to three inches beyond the back line.

POOLE FOREHAND CLEAR TEST (Poole and Nelson 1970)

Test Objective. To measure ability to hit the forehand clear from the back court, high and deep into the opponent's court.

Age Level. High school through college.

Equipment. Badminton rackets, shuttles and floor marking tape.

Validity. Using tournament play as a criterion measure, a coefficient of .70 was found.

Reliability. With the test-retest method, a coefficient of .90 was found.

Administration and Directions. The scoring zones are marked as shown in Figure 17-3. A 15″ x 15″ square is drawn 11 feet from the net astride the center line (0 in Figure 17-3). Another square of equal size is drawn on the other side of the court at the intersection of the doubles long-service line and the center line (X in Figure 17-3). If right-handed, the test performer stands with the right foot on the X square (left-handed, left foot), and a player stands at point O with a racket extended overhead. The performer places a shuttle, with the feather end down, on the forehand side of the racket, tosses the shuttle into the air and hits it with an overhead forehand clear over the player's extended racket. The player calls out, "low," if the shuttle fails to pass over the racket.

Scoring. The point value of the zone in which the shuttle lands is recorded, and the best 10 of 12 shots are totaled for the test score. Shuttles landing on a target line are given the higher point value, and one point is deducted for any shuttle that fails to clear the extended racket of the player. The maximum score is 40.

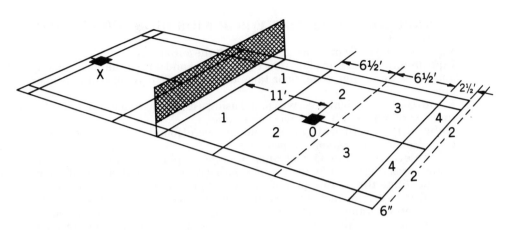

Figure 17-3. *Poole forehand clear test.*

Comments. The test performer should practice the tossing of the shuttle. The test also can be used to measure the backhand clear: The right-handed performer stands with the left foot in the X square, places the shuttle on the forehand side of the racket, tosses it into the air, and executes a backhand clear deep into the opponent's court.

Golf

Outdoor golf tests are preferable, and many such tests are available. In addition, it would not be difficult for you to devise accuracy tests for various clubs. Because of time and space limitations, however, it is sometimes necessary to administer indoor tests.

CLEVETTS'S PUTTING TEST (Clevett 1931)
Test Objective. To measure general golf putting ability.
Age Level. Junior high through college.
Equipment. Putters, golf balls and smooth carpet, 20 feet long and 27 inches wide (marked as shown in Figure 17-4).
Validity and Reliability. Not reported.
Administration and Directions. The carpet is placed on a level, smooth surface. It is divided into three equal nine-inch sections running the full length of the putting surface. Beginning eight feet from the starting point, 48 scoring areas, each nine inches square, are marked off. The square 10, or the imaginary hole, is located 15 feet from the starting line. Ten putts are attempted.
Scoring. Each putt receives a numerical score based on the square on which the ball stops. The final score is the total points for the 10 putts. Balls that stop on a line are given the higher point value. The test performer should be advised to putt too long rather than too short.
Comments. Cutting a hole in the 10 square makes the test more realistic. Also, with additional carpet, the distances can be varied.

Start		1	1	1	1	2	2	2	2	6	7	7	5	5	3	3	3
		1	1	1	1	2	2	2	6	6	10	8	8	8	4	4	4
		1	1	1	1	2	2	2	2	6	7	7	5	5	3	3	3

◄——— 8' ———►

Figure 17-4. *Clevett's putting test.*

INDOOR GOLF SKILL TEST FOR JUNIOR HIGH SCHOOL BOYS

(Shick and Berg 1983)

Test Objective. To measure golf skill with the 5-iron.

Equipment. Two 5-iron clubs (one right-handed and one left-handed), plastic golf balls, an orange cone, floor tape, tape measure, driving mat and floor mat.

Validity. A coefficient of .84 was found using a criterion measure of the best of three scores on a par-3, nine-hole golf course.

Reliability. Coefficients of .97 and .91 were found for single test and test-retest administrations, respectively.

Administration and Directions. A target is placed on the floor of the testing area (Figure 17-5). Identifying the scoring areas with different colors will facilitate the scoring process. A mat is placed at the front edge of the target, and a driving mat is placed on the mat one foot from the target line. The test performer stands on the mat and hits the plastic ball as far as possible off the driving mat with a 5-iron, aiming for the orange cone. After two practice trials, 20 test trials are completed.

Scoring. Each trial score is the landing point of the ball on the target. Balls landing beyond the target but in line with the 4, 6, 4 target areas are given the point value of the closest target area. A topped ball that rolls through the scoring area is given one point. A ball landing on a target line is given the value of the highest adjacent target area. The test score is the sum of the 20 trial scores.

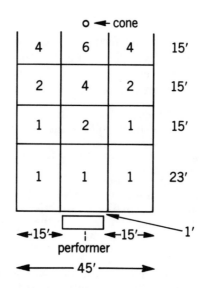

Figure 17-5. *Indoor golf skill test.*

Handball

TYSON HANDBALL TEST (Tyson 1970)

Test Objective. To measure essential handball skills.

Age Level. College men.

Equipment. Handballs, gloves and stopwatch.

Validity. The coefficient of .92 was found for the three-item battery. Coefficients of .87, .84 and .76 were found for the thirty-second volley, front wall kill with the dominant hand and back wall kill with the dominant hand, respectively.

Reliability. Coefficients of .82, .82 and .81 were found for the items in their order of previous presentation.

THIRTY-SECOND VOLLEY

Administration and Directions. Standing behind the short line holding a handball, the test performer puts the ball into play with a toss to the front wall. He then volleys the ball against the front wall as many times as possible within the 30-second time period. Each return must be hit from behind the short line. Returns do not count when the short line is violated, or the ball has bounced more than once. If the performer loses control of the ball, the test administrator quickly tosses him another ball. Either hand may be used.

Scoring. The item score is the total number of legal hits made in 30 seconds.

FRONT WALL KILL WITH DOMINANT HAND

Administration and Directions. If right-handed, the test performer assumes a position in the doubles service box against the left side wall, or if left-handed, the right side wall. The test administrator stands in the middle of the service zone and begins the trial by tossing the ball against the front wall so it rebounds to the right of the right-handed performer, or to the left of the left-handed performer. As soon as the test administrator releases the ball, the performer is free to move, being sure to cross behind the test administrator to get into a better position for hitting the ball. Five trials to place the ball in the target area on the front wall and floor are attempted (Figure 17-6).

Scoring. The item score is the total number of points accumulated on the five trials, with 25 points being the maximum.

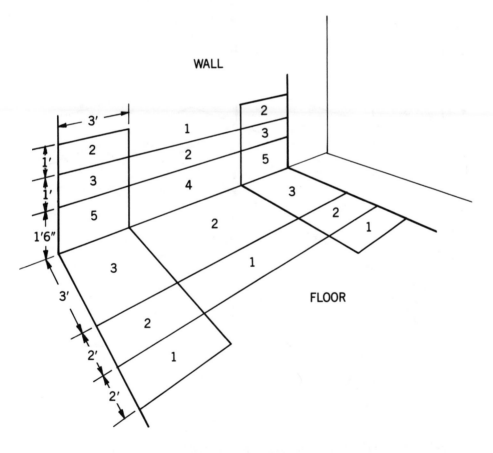

Figure 17-6. *Front wall kill with dominant hand test.*

BACK WALL KILL WITH DOMINANT HAND

Administration and Directions. The initial position of the test performer is the same as that for the front wall kill item. The test administrator, however, is now positioned in the center of the court, six feet behind the short line. The test administrator tosses the ball to the front wall so it rebounds and bounces eight to 12 feet behind the short line and approximately 10 feet from the right side wall for a right-handed performer, or 10 feet from the left side wall for a left-handed person. For best results, the toss should be aimed for a spot between 15 and 18 feet high on the front wall. (A bad toss does not have to be played.) As the toss is made, the test performer may leave his starting position and move into a position that allows him to hit the ball with his dominant hand, as the ball rebounds off the back wall. Five trials to place the ball in the target area on the front wall and floor are attempted (Figure 17-7).

Scoring. The item score is the points accumulated on the five trials, with 25 being the maximum.

Comments. The test administrator should practice the different tosses before administering the test items. Test performers should be aware that they do not have to return bad tosses.

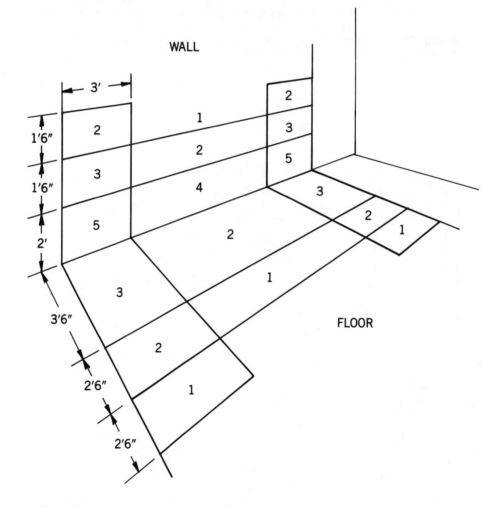

Figure 17-7. *Back wall kill with dominant hand test.*

Racquetball

RACQUETBALL SKILLS TEST (Hensley, East, and Stillwell 1979)
Test Objective. To measure basic racquetball skills.
Age Level. High school through college.
Equipment. Racquets, four new racquetballs, colored floor marking tape and stopwatch.
Validity. Using instructor ratings as the criterion, concurrent coefficients of .79 and .86 were found for the short wall volley and the long wall volley, respectively.
Reliability. Test-retest coefficients ranging from .76 to .86 for the short wall volley and long wall volley for college men and women were found.

SHORT WALL VOLLEY TEST
Administration and Directions. The test consists of two 30-second trials, preceded by a 30-second practice period. Holding two racquetballs, the test performer stands behind the short line, drops a ball, and volleys it against the front wall for 30 seconds. All strokes must be made from behind the short line. The ball may be hit in the air or after bouncing one or more times, and any stroke may be used to keep the ball in play. If the ball does not return past the short line or if the performer misses it, the ball may be retrieved or a new ball may be put into play. The test administrator should be standing near the back wall with two additional racquetballs in the event they are needed. Each time a new volley is started, the ball must be put into play by being bounced behind the short line. The stopwatch is started when the performer drops the ball to begin the volley.
Scoring. The item score is the sum of the legal hits against the front wall for the two trials.

LONG WALL VOLLEY TEST
Administration and Directions. The testing procedures for this item are the same as for the short wall volley test item, except the ball must be volleyed from behind a restraining line drawn 12 feet behind the short line. Two extra balls are placed in the crease of the back wall, as the test administrator should not be in the court during this test.
Scoring. The scoring is the same as for the short wall test.

Tennis

HEWITT'S REVISION OF THE DYER BACKBOARD TENNIS TEST (Hewitt 1965)
Test Objective. To classify beginning and advanced tennis players, by measuring rallying ability.
Age Level. High school through college.
Equipment. A smooth wall 20 feet high and 20 feet wide, tennis racket, at least one dozen new tennis balls, a basket, tape measure, stopwatch and floor and wall marking tape.
Validity. Coefficients ranging from .68 to .73 for beginner classes, and from .84 to .89 for advanced classes were found.
Reliability. Using the test-retest method, coefficients of .82 and .93 were found for beginner and advanced classes, respectively.
Administration and Directions. A line one-inch wide, 20 feet long, and at a height of three feet is placed on the wall. A restraining line one-inch wide, 20 feet long, and 20 feet from the wall is placed on the floor. A basket of tennis balls is placed at one end of the restraining line. The test performer, standing behind the restraining line with two tennis balls and a racket, serves the ball against the wall. (Any type of serve is allowed.) The stopwatch is started when the ball hits above the net line on the wall. On the rebound, the performer begins a rally from behind the restraining line and attempts to hit the ball

continuously against the wall so it hits on or above the line on the wall. If the ball gets away, the test performer may take another ball from the basket. Each time a new rally is started, the ball must be served. Three trials of 30 seconds each are given.

Scoring. One point is scored each time the ball hits on or above the wall line. If the test performer steps on or in front of the restraining line to hit a ball, the rally is continued but no point is scored. No points are scored on the serve. The test score is the average of the three trials.

HEWITT TENNIS ACHIEVEMENT TEST (Hewitt 1966)

Test Objective. To measure the basic tennis skills of the service, forehand drive and backhand drive.

Age Level. High school through college.

Equipment. Tennis rackets, 36 new tennis balls, court markings, poles or standards and rope, longer than width of court.

Validity. Coefficients ranging from .52 to .93 were found.

Reliability. Coefficients ranging from .75 to .94 were found.

SERVICE PLACEMENT

Administration and Directions. A rope is placed seven feet above the ground, and parallel to the net. The right service court is marked as shown in Figure 17-8. A 10-minute warm-up is permitted. The test performer stands to the right of the center line behind the base line and serves 10 balls into the marked service court. The ball must be served between the rope and net. Net balls and balls that hit the rope are repeated.

Scoring. The point value for the zone in which each ball lands is totaled for the 10 trials. Balls going over the rope are given a score of 0.

SPEED OF SERVICE

Administration and Directions. The court is divided into zones as shown in Figure 17-8. The distance the ball bounces after it hits in the service area gives an indication of the speed the ball travels. The score is based on the zone in which the second bounce lands. Ten trials are given. This test can be conducted at the same time as the service placement test.

Scoring. The point value for the zone in which each ball bounces is totaled for the 10 trials.

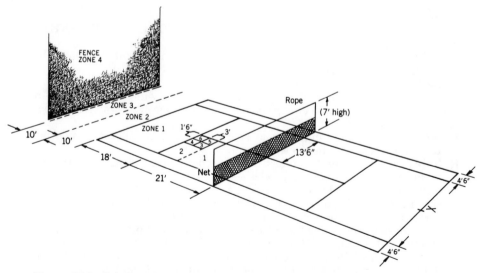

Figure 17-8. *Service placement and speed of service test.*

FOREHAND AND BACKHAND DRIVE TESTS

Administration and Directions. A rope is placed seven feet above the ground, and parallel to the net. The court is marked as shown in Figure 17-9. The test performer stands at the center of the baseline. The test administrator is positioned, with a basket of balls, on the other side of the net at the intersection of the center line and the service line. The administrator hits five practice balls to the performer, who uses either the forehand or backhand to return the balls. The balls hit by the administrator should land just beyond the service line. Twenty test trials are then administered the same way, the performer choosing which 10 balls to hit with the forehand and which 10 balls to hit with the backhand. If the drive goes between the net and rope, points are scored, as indicated in Figure 17-9. Balls hit over the rope and landing in the scoring zones score one-half the regular value. All net balls and those that hit the rope are repeated.

Scoring. The point value for the zone in which each ball lands is totaled for the 20 trials. Balls hit over the rope and landing in the scoring zones score one-half the regular value.

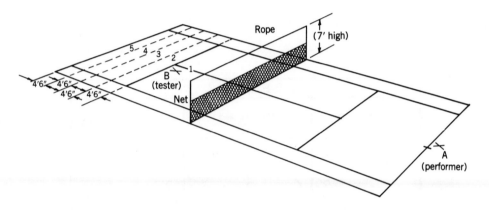

Figure 17-9. *Forehand and backhand drive test.*

TEAM SPORTS

Basketball

AAHPERD BASKETBALL SKILLS TEST (Hopkins, Shick, and Plack 1984)

Age Level. 10 through college.

Equipment. Basketballs, stopwatch, floor and wall marking tape, tape measure and six cones.

Validity. Coefficients ranging from .37 to .91 for all ages and both sexes on individual test items, and from .65 to .95 for test battery as a whole were found.

Reliability. Using the test-retest method, coefficients ranging from .82 to .97 for all ages and both sexes on individual test items were found.

SPEED SPOT SHOOTING

Test Objective. To measure skill in rapidly shooting from different positions, and to a limited extent, also measure agility and ball handling.

Administration and Directions. Floor markers are placed on the floor as shown in Figure 17-10. The distances for spots B, C, and D are measured from the center of the backboard, while those for spots A and E are measured from the center of the basket. For fifth and sixth graders, the shooting distance is nine feet; for grades seven, eight and nine, it is 12 feet; and for grades 10 through college, it is 15 feet. Holding a basketball, the test performer begins the test with one foot behind any one of the five markers. On the signal, "Ready, go," the performer shoots, retrieves the ball, and dribbles to and shoots from another spot. At least one shot must be taken from each of the five markers. A maximum of four lay-up shots may be attempted, but no two may be taken in succession. Three 60-second trials are administered, with the first being a practice trial.

Scoring. Two points are given for each shot made, and one point is given for each unsuccessful shot that hits the rim (from above). The item score is the sum of scores for the two trials. The test administrator must record the number of lay-ups attempted, the point value of the attempted shots, and if the performer attempts at least one shot from each of the five markers. No score is given for shots that follow ball-handling infractions such as traveling and double dribbling, or for more than four lay-up attempts. If the performer fails to shoot from each of the five markers, the trial is repeated.

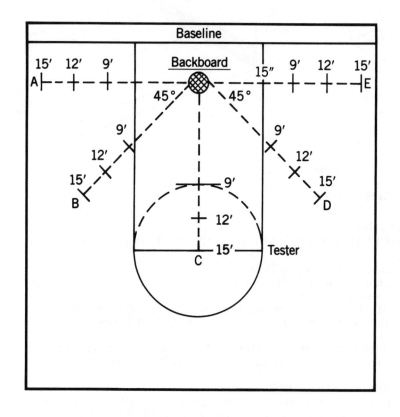

Figure 17-10. *Speed spot shooting test.*

PASSING

Test Objective. To measure skill in chest passing and recovering the ball while moving.

Administration and Directions. A restraining line is drawn on the floor eight feet from the wall and parallel to it, and squares are marked on the wall (as shown in Figure 17-11). Only chest passes are permitted. Holding a basketball, the test performer stands behind the restraining line facing target A. On the signal, "Ready, go," the ball is passed to target A. The rebound is recovered while moving to be in line with target B. The ball is then passed to target B. This sequence is continued until target F is reached, where two passes are attempted. The performer then moves back toward target A. Three 30-second trials are taken, with the first being a practice trial.

Scoring. Each pass that lands in the target or on the target line earns two points. Passes hitting the wall between the targets earns one point. The item score is the sum of the two trials. No points are given if: the performer's foot is on or over the line, a second pass is made at targets B, C, D, or E, and a pass other than a chest pass is used.

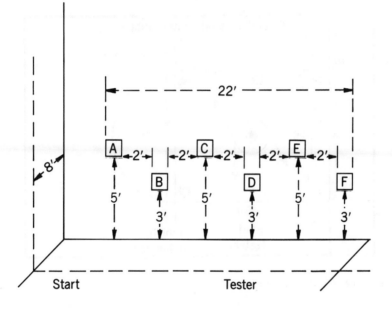

Figure 17-11. *Basketball passing test.*

CONTROL DRIBBLE

Test Objective. To measure ball-handling skill (dribbling) while moving.

Administration and Directions. Six cones are placed as shown in Figure 17-12. On the signal, "Ready, go," the test performer begins dribbling with the nondominant hand from the nondominant side of cone A to the nondominant side of cone B. For the remainder of the course the performer may use the dominant hand, and hands may be changed when appropriate. Three timed trials are given, with the first being a practice trial.

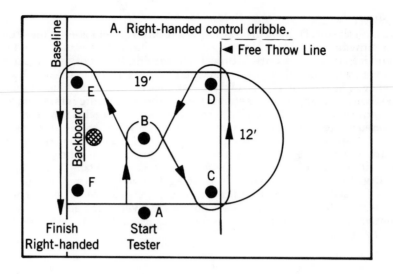

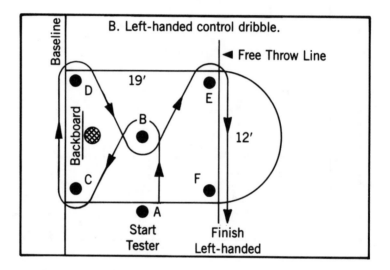

Figure 17-12. *Control dribble test.*

Scoring. The trial score is recorded to the nearest one-tenth of a second. The item score is the sum of the two trials. The trial is retaken for ball-handling infractions, failure of the performer or ball to remain outside any cone, and failure to continue the test from the spot where loss of ball control occurred.

DEFENSIVE MOVEMENT
Test Objective. To measure basic defensive movement skills.
Administrative and Directions. The court is marked as shown in Figure 17-13. The boundaries are the free-throw line, the end line behind the basket, and the free-throw lane lines. The middle lines on the free-throw lane serve as markers for C and F. Marks A, B, D, and E must be made with floor tape. The test performer stands at point A, facing away from the basket. On the signal, "Ready, go," the performer slides to the left, without crossing the feet, to point B and touches the floor outside the lane, with the left hand. Then, executing a

dropstep (changing defensive direction by moving the trailing foot in a sliding motion, in the direction of the next move), the performer slides to point C and touches the floor outside the lane, with the right hand. The test is continued (as shown in Figure 17-13) until both feet cross the finish line. Three timed trials are given, with the first being a practice trial.

Scoring. The trial score is recorded to the nearest one-tenth of a second. The item score is the sum of the two trials. The trial is repeated for crossing the feet during the slide or turn, running, failure to touch the hand to the floor outside the lane, and performing the dropstep before the hand touches the floor.

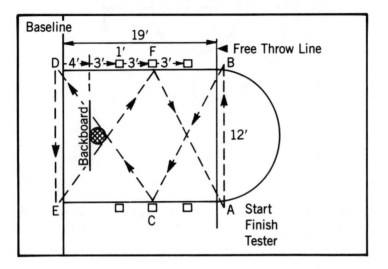

Figure 17-13. *Defensive movement test.*

Field Hockey
CHAPMAN BALL CONTROL TEST
Test Objective. To measure the ability to combine quickness in stick movement with ability to control the force that is necessary to move the ball.

Age Level. High school through college.

Equipment. Hockey sticks, hockey balls, floor marking tape and stopwatch.

Validity. Logical validity and, using a criterion measure of ratings of stickwork skills, concurrent validity coefficients of .63 and .64 were found.

Reliability. With single test administration, the coefficient of .89 was found.

Administration and Directions. A pattern is placed on the gymnasium floor (as shown in Figure 17-14). The lines that divide the outer circle into three equal segments are one-eight of an inch wide. (It is recommended that these segments be of a color that contrasts with both the hockey ball and the gymnasium floor.) The ball is placed just outside the outer circle, and on the signal, "Ready, go," the performer taps the ball through or in and out of the center circle with a hockey stick. Each time the ball is tapped through or out of the center circle, it must roll outside the outer circle. Three 15-second trials are given. It is recommended the test administrator be assisted by a separate time keeper who can start and stop the trials at the end of 15 seconds. An alternate administration method is to tape record the "go" and "stop" commands at 15 second intervals, so the test administrator does not have to observe the stopwatch and the test performer simultaneously. Test administration should

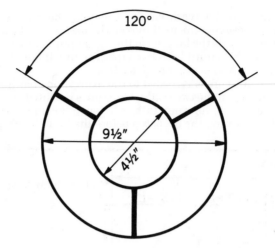

Figure 17-14. *Chapman ball control test.*

include a demonstration of the scoring techniques, a brief practice period and rest between all test trials. Providing two practice targets enables two performers to practice while a third is tested.

Scoring. One point is scored each time the ball is tapped (not pushed) through or into the center circle. A point also may be scored when the ball is tapped from the center circle to outside of the outer circle, and if it passes through a different segment from the one it entered. Points can only be scored when the ball is tapped outside of the outer circle or from within the center circle. No points are scored when the ball is tapped while inside the outer circle, or when it is tapped with the rounded side of the stick.

Football
AAHPER FOOTBALL SKILLS TEST (AAHPER 1965)
This test includes 10 items that measure different football skills. Eight items, which measure skills also used in touch or flag football, are described in this chapter. No validity or reliability coefficients were reported.

Test Objective. Each item measures a single basic skill.

Age Level. 10 through 18; although designed for males, some of the items may be administered to females.

Equipment. Footballs, 8′ X 11′ canvas, five chairs, kicking tee and tape measure.

FORWARD PASS FOR DISTANCE

Administration and Directions. The pass is made from within a six-foot restraining area. The contact point of the performer's first pass is marked with a metal or wooden stake. Three trials are given, with the stake being moved when the second or third pass is longer. If the test item is administered on a football field, the restraining area should be placed parallel to the yard lines. (Administration of the test on a football field facilitates the measurement process, as it is necessary to measure only the distance from the stake to the yard line immediately behind the stake.) The distance is measured to the last foot passed, and at a right angle to the throwing line.

Scoring. The item score is the best pass of the three trials.

50-YARD DASH WITH FOOTBALL

Administration and Directions. While carrying football, the performer runs as fast as possible for 50 yards. The starter shouts, "go," and simultaneously swings a white cloth down. The timer starts the watch with the downward arm movement of the starter, and stops it when the runner crosses the finish line. Two trials are administered, with a rest period between.

Scoring. The score is the better time of the two trials to the nearest one-tenth second.

FORWARD PASS FOR ACCURACY

Administration and Directions. A target is painted on an 8' X 11' canvas. The diameter of the center circle is two feet; four feet for the middle circle; and six feet for the outer circle. The bottom of the outer circle is three feet from the ground. The target is hung from the cross bar of the goal posts, and tied to the goal posts so it remains taut. A restraining line is placed 15 yards from the target. The test performer runs two or three small steps along the line in the direction of the dominant arm, turns, and throws the football at the target. The pass should be made with good speed. Ten trials are administered.

Scoring. The target values are three (inner circle), two (middle circle), and one (outer circle). Passes striking a line are given the higher value. The score is the point total for the 10 trials.

PUNT FOR DISTANCE

Administration and Directions. The performer takes one or two steps within a six-foot kicking zone, and punts the ball as far as possible. The test is administered the same as the forward pass for distance.

Scoring. Same as forward pass for distance.

BALL-CHANGING ZIGZAG RUN

Administration and Directions. Five chairs are placed in a line, with the first chair 10 yards from the starting line and the others 10 yards apart. The test performer stands behind the starting line, holding a football under the right arm. On the signal, "go," the performer runs to the right of the first chair, shifts the ball to the left arm and runs to the left of the second chair. The run is continued in and out of the chairs (as shown in Figure 17-15). The ball must be under the outside arm and the inside arm must be extended (as in stiff arming an opponent) each time a chair is passed. The runner is not permitted to touch the chairs. Two trials are administered.

Scoring. Each trial is timed to the nearest one-tenth of a second from the signal, "go," until the performer passes back over the starting line. The score is the better time of the two trials.

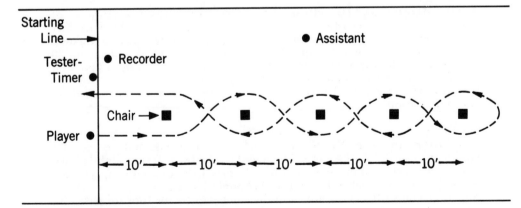

Figure 17-15. *Ball-changing zigzag test.*

CATCHING THE FORWARD PASS

Administration and Directions. Two end marks, located nine feet to the right and left of the center, are placed on the scrimmage line. Turning points are placed 30 feet in front of the end marks (Figure 17-16). The test performer stands on the right end mark and faces straight ahead. On the signal, "go," the performer runs toward the turning point directly in front of him, makes a 90° right turn behind the turning point, and while continuing to run parallel to the scrimmage line, prepares to receive a pass at the passing point. On the "go" signal the center snaps the ball to the passer. The passer then takes one backward step to be in position to pass the ball directly over the passing point, slightly above the head of the receiver. The same pattern is run from the left end mark, except the performer makes a left turn at the turning point. Ten trials are run around each turning point. Poorly thrown passes are repeated.
Scoring. One point is awarded for each pass caught. The score is the sum of the passes caught from both sides.

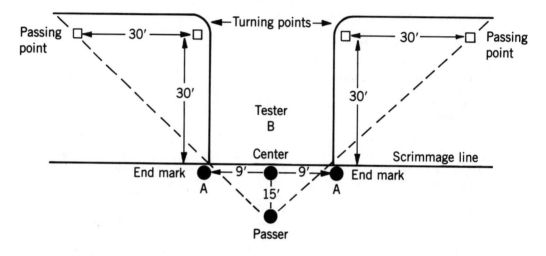

Figure 17-16. *Catching forward pass.*

PULLOUT

Administration and Directions. The test performer assumes a three-point stance midway between two goal posts. On the signal "go," the performer turns to the right and runs parallel to the imaginary scrimmage line, makes a 90° turn around the goal post, and races straight ahead across a finish line 30 feet away. Two time trials are administered, with the time starting on "go" and stopping when the performer crosses the finish line.
Scoring. The score is the better time of the two trials, measured to the nearest one-tenth second.

KICKOFF

Administration and Directions. A kicking tee is placed in the center of a yard line on the field. The football is placed on the tee so it tilts slightly back toward the kicker. Taking as long a run as he needs, the kicker attempts to kick the ball as far as possible. Three trials are administered.
Scoring. The score is determined in the same way as the forward pass and punt for distance tests.

Soccer

MCDONALD SOCCER TEST (McDonald 1951)

Test Objective. To measure general soccer ability.

Age Level. High school through college.

Equipment. Three soccer balls and stopwatch.

Validity. A coefficient of .85 was found by correlating the test scores of 53 college soccer players from three varsity levels, with the subjective ratings of three coaches.

Reliability. Not reported.

Administration and Directions. A restraining line is marked nine feet from a wall, 30 feet wide and 11½ feet high. A soccer ball is placed on the restraining line. On the signal, "go," the test performer kicks the ball against the wall as many times as possible in 30 seconds. Two soccer balls are placed nine feet behind the restraining line in the center of the test area. In the event of a wild kick, the test performer may retrieve the original ball or use one of the two additional balls. The hands may be used to retrieve a ball. Any type of kick may be used, but all kicks must be kicked from the ground behind the restraining line. Four trials are administered.

Scoring. The number of legal kicks in each 30-second period is recorded. The test score is the highest total of any three trials.

MITCHELL SOCCER TEST (Mitchell 1963)

Test Objective. To measure general soccer ability.

Age Level. Originally designed for fifth and sixth grade boys, but may be administered to girls and boys in grades five through junior high.

Equipment. Soccer balls and stopwatch.

Validity. With fifth and sixth grade boys serving as subjects, coefficients of .84 and .76 were found.

Reliability. Using the test-retest method, correlations of .93 and .89 were found.

Administration and Directions. A target four feet high from the base of the wall and eight feet long, is marked on a smooth, unobstructed wall. The total width of the kicking area on the wall should be at least 14 feet (three feet on each side of the target). A restraining line is marked six feet from the wall, and a boundary line is marked 12 feet from the wall (six feet behind the restraining line). A soccer ball is placed on the restraining line, and individuals who serve as ball retrievers are positioned around and behind the boundary line. On the signal, "go," the test performer kicks the ball against the wall target as many times as possible in 20 seconds. Any kicking technique may be used with either foot or leg, but the hands or arms may not be used. If the test performer miskicks or fails to block a kick, the retrievers stop the ball and place it back on the boundary line at the point where it rolled out. The performer retrieves the ball from that point (may not use hands), repositions it, and continues the test. The trial is given again for any action by the retrievers that causes an unnecessary time delay. The performer may go anywhere to retrieve the ball, but all legal kicks must be made from behind the restraining line. Three consecutive trials are administered.

Scoring. The test score is the total number of legal kicks made in the three trials. Use of the hands or arms at any time results in a one point reduction.

Softball

FIELDING GROUNDERS-AGILITY, SPEED AND ACCURACY TEST (Fringer 1961)

Test Objective. To measure the ability to field grounders, to run to a base, and to throw quickly and accurately to a target.

Age Level. Originally designed for high school girls, but also may be administered to high school boys.

Equipment. Softball glove, several quality softballs, floor marking tape and stopwatch.

Validity. Utilizing high school girls, a coefficient of .70 was found.

Reliability. A test-retest coefficient of .72 was found.

Administration and Directions. A floor space of 30' x 40' with a 20' x 20' wall is needed. A target is placed on the wall, and markings are placed on the floor (as indicated in Figure 17-17). Dimensions for the base markings are the same as for a softball base. The test performer stands with a foot on the start mark with a softball and glove. On the signal "go," the performer runs to either base, throws the ball at the target, rushes to field the ball, and quickly runs to the other base to make another throw at the target. The bases must be alternated for the throws and a foot must be in contact with the base on each throw. Two 45-second trials are administered with rest permitted between trials.

Scoring. Balls hitting on or in the target circle count. The test score is the sum of the target hits made in the two trials.

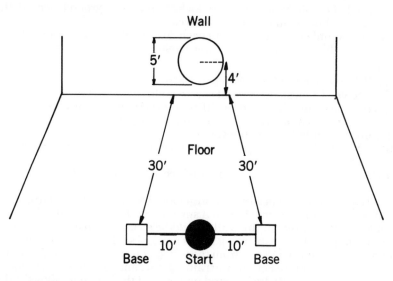

Figure 17-17. *Fielding grounders-agility-speed and accuracy test.*

SHICK SOFTBALL TEST BATTERY (Shick 1970)

Test Objective. To measure defensive softball skills.

Age Level. Originally designed for college women, but the test also may be administered to males and females in high school through college.

Equipment. Several softballs and stopwatch.

Validity. Utilizing two general softball classes of 59 college females, a coefficient of .75 was found by correlating expert ratings with the test battery.

Reliability. A coefficient of .88 was found for the test battery.

REPEATED THROWS

Administration and Directions. A line is drawn on the wall 10 feet from and parallel to the floor. A restraining line is drawn on the floor 23 feet from and parallel to the wall. The test performer stands behind the restraining line, holding a softball. On the signal "go," the student throws the ball against the wall above the 10-foot line (overhand or sidearm throw is required), and attempts to catch the rebound in the air or field it from the floor. This action is repeated as many times as possible in 30 seconds. If fielding errors occur, the performer must recover the ball. However, there is no penalty other than the loss of time. The test consists of four 30-second trials, and the performer is given one practice throw before each trial.

Scoring. A ball thrown with the test performer stepping on or across the restraining line, or one hitting below the wall line does not count. The test score is the sum of the legal hits for the four trials.

FIELDING TEST

Administration and Directions. A line is drawn on the wall four feet from and parallel to the floor. A line also is drawn on the floor 15 feet from and parallel to the wall. The procedures are the same as those for the repeated throws test, except any type throw may be used, and all throws are to hit below the wall line.

Scoring. The scoring method is identical to the repeated throws scoring, except no ball that hits above the wall line is counted.

TARGET TEST

Administration and Directions. The dimensions of the wall and floor targets are shown in Figure 17-18. The wall target is 66 inches square, and its center is 36 inches from the floor. The target value areas are color coded as follows: five = red, four = medium blue, three = bright yellow, two = pale aqua and one = black. A restraining line is marked on the floor 40 feet from and parallel to the wall. The test performer stands behind the restraining line for all throws. Two trials of 10 throws each are administered. Two practice throws are permitted.

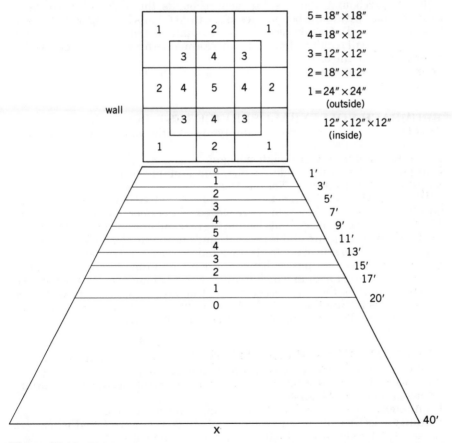

Figure 17-18. *Shick target test.*

Scoring. Each throw is given two scores: one for the wall hit and one for the hit of the first bounce on the floor. Any hit outside the scoring areas of the wall and floor is recorded as 0. The test score is the sum of the two trials. The highest possible test score is 200 (50 per trial for the wall, and 50 per trial for the floor).

Volleyball

BRADY VOLLEY TEST (Brady 1945)
Test Objective. To measure general volleyball playing ability.
Age Level. College, but may also be appropriate for some high school groups. If administered to younger groups, it is suggested the height of the target be lowered.
Equipment. Volleyballs, wall tape, tape measure and stopwatch.
Validity. Utilizing college males, a coefficient of .86 was found for the correlation between test scores and the subjective ratings of four qualified judges.
Reliability. A test-retest coefficient of .93 was found.
Administration and Directions. A target consisting of a horizontal line five feet in length and 11½ feet from the floor is marked on a smooth wall. Vertical lines at the end of the horizontal line are extended toward the ceiling. The wall should be at least 15 feet high and 15 feet wide. No restraining line is used. The test performer begins the test by throwing the volleyball against the wall. On the rebound, and all subsequent rebounds, the performer attempts to volley the ball within the boundaries of the target (balls landing on the target lines are counted). One 60-second trial is administered. Catching or losing control of the ball requires that the test performer re-throw the ball against the wall to continue the test.
Scoring. The test score is the number of legal hits in 60 seconds. Thrown balls do not count.

BRUMBACH VOLLEYBALL SERVICE TEST (Brumbach 1967)
Test Objective. To measure the ability to serve the volleyball low and deep into the opponent's court.
Age Level. Junior high through college.
Equipment. Rope, tall standards, floor tape and tape measure.
Validity and Reliability. Not reported.
Administration and Directions. A rope is placed four feet above and parallel to the net, and markings are placed on the floor (as shown in Figure 17-19). The test performer stands behind the rear end line and attempts to serve the ball between the net and rope, so it lands deep into the backcourt on the opposite side. Two sets of six trials are administered (total of 12).
Scoring. A serve that passes between the net and rope receives the higher value for the target area in which it lands. Serves going over the rope receive the lesser value for the target areas. Serves that hit the rope are repeated. Foot faults, serves hitting the net and serves landing outside the target area are given a 0 score. The test score is the sum of the 10 best trials.

RUSSELL-LANGE VOLLEYBALL TEST (Russell and Lange 1940)
Test Objective. To measure volleyball playing ability.
Age Level. Junior and senior high girls, but the serve item is also appropriate for junior and senior high boys.
Equipment. Volleyballs, floor and wall tape and stopwatch.
Validity. Coefficients of .51 (volley) and .79 (serve) were found when test scores were correlated with ability ratings of seven judges.
Reliability. Coefficients of .89 (volley) and .84 (serve) were found.

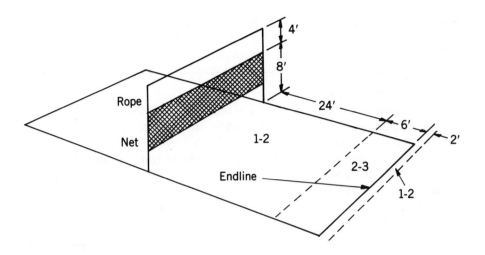

Figure 17-19. *Brumbach volleyball service test.*

VOLLEY

Administration and Directions. A line, two inches wide and 12 feet long, is placed with the lower edge seven and one-half feet above the floor. A restraining line is placed six feet from and parallel to the wall. Standing behind the restraining line, the test performer uses an underhand movement to toss the ball against the wall. She then repeatedly volleys the ball on or above the wall line, while remaining behind the restraining line. Three 30-second trials are administered.

Scoring. The legal volleys hit from behind the restraining line that hit on or above the wall line are recorded. The test score is the best score of three trials.

SERVE

Administration and Directions. The court is marked as shown in Figure 17-20. Standing behind the rear boundary line, the test performer attempts to serve the ball deep into the opponent's court. Two trials of 10 legal serves are administered. Serves touching the net but landing in the opponent's court are repeated.

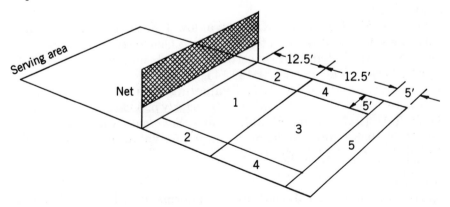

Figure 17-20. *Russell-Lange volleyball serve test.*

Scoring. Serves landing on a target line are given the higher target value, and serves in which foot faults occur are given a 0 score. The test score is total points of the best trial.

REVIEW PROBLEMS

1. Administer one individual and one team sports skills test to several of your classmates. Ask them to provide constructive criticism of your test administration.
2. Additional sports skills tests are presented at the conclusion of this chapter. Review at least one test for each sport, noting the validity and practicability of the test.
3. Ask several physical education instructors of activity classes what sports skills tests they use and why?

SOURCES OF ADDITIONAL SPORTS SKILLS TESTS

Archery

Hyde, E. I. 1937. An achievement scale in archery. *Research Quarterly* 8:109-116.

Shifflett, B., and Schuman, B. 1982. A criterion-referenced test for archery. *Research Quarterly for Exercise and Sport* 53:330-335.

Zabik, R. M., and Jackson, A. S. 1969. Reliability of archery achievement. *Research Quarterly* 40:254-255.

Badminton

French, E., and Statler, E. 1949. Study of skill tests in badminton for college women. *Research Quarterly* 20: 257-272.

Lockhart, A., and McPherson, F. A. 1949. The development of a test of badminton playing ability. *Research Quarterly* 20: 402-405.

Miller, F. A. 1951. A badminton wall volley test. *Research Quarterly* 22: 208-213.

Thorpe, J., and West, C. 1969. A test of game sense in badminton. *Perceptual and Motor Skills* 28: 159-169.

Basketball

Boyd, C. A., MacCachren, J. R., and Waglow, I. F. 1955. Predictive ability of a selected basketball test. *Research Quarterly* 26: 364-365.

Broer, M. R. 1958. Reliability of certain skill tests for junior high school girls. *Research Quarterly* 29: 139-145.

Elbel, E. R., and Allen, F. C. 1941. Evaluating team and individual performance in basketball. *Research Quarterly* 5: 538-555.

Knox, R. D. 1947. Basketball ability tests. *Scholastic Coach* 17(3): 45.

Stroup, F. 1955. Game results as a criterion for validating a basketball skill test. *Research Quarterly* 26: 353-357.

Bowling

Martin, J., and Keogh, J. 1964. Bowling norms for college students in elective physical education classes. *Research Quarterly* 35: 325-327.

Olson, J., and Liba, M. R. 1967. A device for evaluating spot bowling ability. *Research Quarterly* 38: 193-201.

Philips, M., and Summers, D. 1950. Bowling norms and learning curves for college women. *Research Quarterly* 21: 377-385.

Field Hockey

Schmithals, M., and French, E. 1940. Achievement tests in field hockey for college women. *Research Quarterly* 11: 84-92.

Football

Borleske, S. E. 1936. Borleske touch football test. In Barrow, H. M., and McGee, R. 1979. *A practical approach to measurement in physical education.* 3rd ed. Philadelphia: Lea & Febiger.

Golf

Cotten, D. J., Thomas, J. R., and Plaster, T. 1972. A plastic ball test for golf iron skill. In Johnson, B. L., and Nelson, J. K. 1986. *Practical measurements for evaluation in physical education.* 4th ed. Edina, Minn.: Burgess Publishing.

Rowlands, D. J. 1974. Rowlands golf skills test battery. In Barrow H. M., and McGee, R. 1979. *A practical approach to measurement in physical education.* 3d ed. Philadelphia: Lea & Febiger.

West, C., and Thorpe, J. 1968. Construction and validation of an eight-iron approach test. *Research Quarterly* 49: 1115-1120.

Handball

Cornish, C. 1949. A study of measurement of ability in handball. *Research Quarterly* 20: 215-222.

Montoye, H. J., and Brotzman, J. 1951. An investigation of the validity of using the results of a doubles tournament as a measurement of handball ability. *Research Quarterly* 22: 214-218.

Pennington, G. G. et al. 1967. A measure of handball ability. *Research Quarterly* 38: 247-253.

Racquetball

Karpman, M., and Isaacs, L. 1979. An improved racquetball skills test. *Research Quarterly* 50: 526-527.

Soccer

Heath, M. L., and Rogers, E. G. 1932. A study in the use of knowledge and skill tests in soccer. *Research Quarterly* 3: 33-53.

Johnson, J. R. 1963. Johnson soccer test. In Johnson, B. L., and Nelson, J. K. 1986. *Practical measurements for evaluation in physical education.* 4th ed. Edina, Minn.: Burgess Publishing.

Smith, G. 1947. Smith kick-up test. In Barrow, H. M., and McGee, R. 1979. *A practical approach to measurement in physical education.* 3d ed. Philadelphia: Lea & Febiger.

Vanderhoff, M. 1932. Soccer skills tests. *Journal of Health and Physical Education* 3: 42.

Warner, G. F. 1950. Warner soccer test. *Newsletter of the National Soccer Coaches Association of America* 6: 13-22.

Softball

Broer, M. R. 1958. Reliability of certain skill tests for junior high school girls. *Research Quarterly* 29: 139-143.

Fox, M. G., and Young, O. G. 1954. A test of softball batting ability. *Research Quarterly* 25: 26-27.

O'Donnell, D. J. 1950. O'Donnell Softball Skill Test. In Collins, D. R., and Hodges, P. B. 1978. *A comprehensive guide to sports skills tests and measurement.* Springfield, Illinois: Charles C. Thomas.

Underkofler, A. 1942. Underkofler softball skills test. In Collins, D. R., and Hodges, P. B. 1978. *A comprehensive guide to sports skills tests and measurement.* Springfield, Illinois: Charles C. Thomas.

Swimming

Fox, M. G. 1957. Swimming power test. *Research Quarterly* 28: 233-237.

Hewitt, J. E. 1948. Swimming achievement scales for college men. *Research Quarterly* 19: 282-289.

Hewitt, J. E. 1949. Achievement scale scores for high school swimming. *Research Quarterly* 20: 170-179.

Resentswieg, J. 1968. A revision of the power swimming test. *Research Quarterly* 39: 818-819.

Wilson, C. T. 1934. Coordination tests in swimming. *Research Quarterly* 5: 81-88.

Tennis

Avery, C., Richardson, P., and Jackson, A. 1979. A practical tennis serve test: measurement of skill under simulated game conditions. *Research Quarterly* 50: 554-564.

Broer, M. R., and Miller, D. M. 1950. Achievement tests for beginning and intermediate tennis. *Research Quarterly* 21: 303-313.

DiGennaro, J. 1969. Construction of forehand drive, backhand drive, and service tennis tests. *Research Quarterly* 40: 496-501.

Dyer, J. T. 1938. Revision of the backboard test of tennis ability. *Research Quarterly* 9: 25-31.

Edwards, J. 1965. Wisconsin wall test for serve. In Barrow, H. M., and McGee, R. 1979. *A practical approach to measurement in physical education.* 3d ed. Philadelphia: Lea & Febiger.

Fox, K. 1953. A study of the validity of the Dyer backboard test and the Miller forehand-backhand test for beginning tennis players. *Research Quarterly* 24: 1-7.

Hewitt, J. E. 1968. Classification tests in tennis. *Research Quarterly* 39: 552-555.

Johnson, J. 1957. Tennis serve of advanced women players. *Research Quarterly* 28: 123-131.

Kemp, J., and Vincent, M. F. 1968. Kemp-Vincent rally test of tennis skill. *Research Quarterly* 39: 1000-1004.

Purcell, K. 1981. A tennis forehand-backhand drive skill test which measures ball control and stroke firmness. *Research Quarterly* 52: 238-245.

Volleyball

Brady, G. F. 1945. Preliminary investigation of volleyball playing ability. *Research Quarterly* 16: 14-17.

Clifton, M. A. 1962. Single hit volley test for women's volleyball. *Research Quarterly* 33: 208-211.

Crogen, C. 1943. A simple volleyball classification test for high school girls. *The Physical Educator* 4: 34-37.

Cunningham, P., and Garrison, J. 1968. High wall volley test for women's volleyball. *Research Quarterly* 39: 486-490.

French, E. L., and Cooper, B. I. 1937. Achievement test in volleyball for high school girls. *Research Quarterly* 8: 150-157.

Kronquist, R. A., and Brumbach, W. B. 1968. A modification of the Brady volleyball test for high school boys. *Research Quarterly* 39: 116-120.

Liba, M. R., and Stauff, M. R. 1963. A test for the volleyball pass. *Research Quarterly* 34: 56-63.

Mohr, D. R., and Haverstick, M. V. 1955. Repeated volleys test for women's volleyball. *Research Quarterly* 26: 179-184.

Russell, N., and Lange, E. 1940. Achievement tests in volleyball for junior high school girls. *Research Quarterly* 11: 33-41.

18

Affective Behavior

Upon completion of this chapter, you should be able to:
1. List components of affective behavior;
2. Describe the uses of affective behavior measurement;
3. Describe the Likert scale, semantic differential, rating scale and questionnaire as they are used in the measurement of social behavior; and
4. Select an instrument to measure social behavior, attitudes, sportsmanship and leadership.

Affective behavior (also called affective domain) involves the interests, appreciations, attitudes, values and emotional biases of an individual. It is reflected through an individual's feelings and emotions. Although many teachers are concerned with the affective behavior of students, not all physical educators agree upon how this concern should be expressed. Many physical education teachers list affective objectives for their classes, but because of discomfort in measuring them, they do not attempt to determine if the objectives have been reached. In addition, there are physical educators who believe that if proper cognitive and psychomotor objectives are attained, the appropriate corresponding affective behavioral objectives will be attained also. Furthermore, for the following reasons some physical educators feel that the affective domain should not be measured at all (Phillips and Hornak 1979; Mood 1982).

1. Behaviors change slowly. Knowledge and skills can change in relatively short periods of time, but an individual's attitude, appreciation and values usually require a longer period of time for change.
2. It is difficult to define and evaluate adjustments, interests, attitudes, appreciations and values. In addition, affective behavior evaluation procedures are unreliable for everyday use.
3. Feelings are not teachable. How do you teach someone to have a positive attitude toward physical fitness, tennis, golf, etc.?
4. Self-reporting inventories or questionnaires depend on the

277

willingness of the students to state their true beliefs. On occasion, students will provide answers that best please the instructors.

5. Physical educators are not adequately trained to evaluate affective behavior.

6. Why should physical education assume responsibility for the development of affective behavior? English and math teachers seldom include the affective objective.

7. There is not adequate time in the physical education class to measure physical skills, knowledge and affective behavior.

In some teaching environments the above are valid arguments against measurement of affective behavior, and all physical educators should be aware of these concerns prior to any attempt to measure in this domain. There are, however, important uses of affective behavior measurement, and if suitable instruments are properly administered, these uses can be of value to the physical educator.

WHY MEASURE AFFECTIVE BEHAVIOR?

McGee (1982) provides the following uses of measurement of affective behavior.

Uses for Groups

Measurement of affective behavior can be used to identify the present status of the group. How do students feel about the physical activity that is to be taught? Concerns about sportsmanship and group cohesiveness may also be addressed. This measurement should not be used to evaluate or judge; rather, it should be used to make the teacher aware of the group's attitude toward a particular activity.

Affective behavior measurement can also be used for program evaluation and planning. The strengths and weaknesses of physical education programs may be identified through attitude measurement. If groups repeatedly have no interest or a bad attitude toward certain activities, it may be wise to make curriculum revisions.

Another important use of affective behavior evaluation is to aid in the establishment of teacher-student rapport. If students and the teachers work together to plan and implement affective objectives, students usually will know that teachers care about them. When students know the teacher cares about their feelings, they are more likely to cooperate with the teacher.

Finally, affective behavior measurement can be useful for motivation. The planning of affective objectives by both teacher and students can serve to motivate the students to work for attainment of the objectives.

Uses for Individuals

The application of affective behavior measurement to individuals must be done with caution. In fulfilling their counseling responsibilities, all teachers should be aware that some students are more sensitive than others. Receiving a low score in group acceptability may negatively influence many students. When measurement of affective behavior is done for individual use, the teacher must apply the results wisely.

Perhaps the most important individual use of affective behavior measurement is to help students know themselves. Students can become more aware of their attitudes, group acceptance, behavior, values and self-esteem. Once aware of these measurement results, the students, with the assistance of the teacher, can plan and work for self-improvement. However, programs for self-improvement will not be the same for everyone. Some individuals may not need self-improvement programs.

Furthermore, students who need to be referred to school counselors can be identified, but the physical educator should not attempt to perform this identification and referral alone. There should be consultation with individuals who are better qualified to make these important decisions.

Finally, affective behavior measurement can be used to help select individuals for important roles in class and varsity athletic teams. Attitude, competitiveness and leadership scores may be used for this purpose.

CATEGORIES OF MEASURES

Many instruments are available for measurement of affective behavior in physical education. They can be classified into the following categories.

Attitude inventories: Through responses to the inventory an individual's feelings about events, people, activities, ideas, policies or institutions are revealed. One's attitude about an activity will influence future participation in the activity. For example, if an individual has a negative attitude about an activity, it is unlikely that he or she will participate in the activity.

Interest inventories: An individual's likes and dislikes for certain activities and programs are expressed in interest inventories which may be used in selecting activities to be taught and establishing new programs.

Leadership: Usually members of a group are asked to identify individuals in the group who would make good leaders. These inventories are sometimes used to identify leaders for athletic teams.

Sportsmanship: An individual's responses, or a group's responses, on this survey determine if an individual will abide by the rules, make sacrifices for the good of the group and be a gracious winner or loser.

Social behavior: Through self-reporting, teacher ratings or peer ratings, the individual's social development is determined. This instrument is often used to determine the student's acceptance by the group or the student's acceptance of the class and school environment.

Personality inventories: Traits such as emotional control, self-confidence, motivation, aggressiveness, determination, poise and mental toughness may be measured with these inventories. Numerous other personality traits also may be measured.

Behavior ratings: After observing a student over a period of time, the teacher rates the affective behavior of the student. The ratings may include many different aspects of behavior, such as sportsmanship, leadership, attitude, self-control, cooperation and peer relations.

TYPES OF ITEMS

The types of items most often used in physical education to measure affective behavior are Likert scales, the semantic differential, rating scales and questionnaires.

Likert Scale

The Likert scale requires individuals to indicate their agreement or disagreement with a series of statements. Typically each statement allows for five degrees of responses. The following are two examples of how the Likert scale may be used for student evaluation of a teacher.

The instructor was enthusiastic about the subject.

1	2	3	4	5
Strongly Disagree	Disagree	Undecided	Agree	Strongly Agree

The instructor was concerned about each student.

1	2	3	4	5
Strongly Disagree	Disagree	Undecided	Agree	Strongly Agree

The responses that best describe the feeling of the respondent are circled. Phrasing the statements so that the high scores reflect the best feeling or attitude provides a basis for statistical analysis of the statements. Thus, a score of 5 is assigned to the most favorable response, 1 to the least favorable, and 2, 3, and 4 to the intervening responses. A group's feeling about a statement is usually reported by averaging the responses.

Fewer or more than five responses can be used. It is not uncommon to find a Likert scale with seven responses, and with younger children, two categories such as yes-no, like-dislike or present-absent are sometimes used.

Semantic Differential

The semantic differential scale requires the individual to respond to bipolar adjectives. The bipolar adjectives represent opposite meanings, such as new-old, good-bad and fair-unfair. The respondent is asked to mark one of seven points that best reflects his or her feelings about a concept. The score for each item ranges from 1 to 7 if the positive adjective of the pair is listed to the right, and from 7 to 1 if the positive adjective is placed to the left.

Three dimensions of a concept can be measured with the semantic differential. Evaluation, the most common dimension, involves the "goodness" of the concept. Typical bipolar adjectives used with this concept are good-bad, beautiful-ugly, pleasant-unpleasant and fair-unfair. A second dimension, potency, involves the strength of the rated concept. Examples of bipolar adjectives used to measure this dimension are heavy-light, full-empty, hard-soft and strong-weak. The third dimension, activity, involves action and is measured by such adjectives as happy-sad, fast-slow, tense-relaxed and active-passive. A semantic differential scale should include at least three items for each dimension.

Bipolar adjectives can measure many different concepts. The following is an example of a semantic differential scale that may be used to evaluate a teacher. With no or only minor adjustments the same scale may be used to rate other concepts or a physical activity.

Student's Feelings About The Teacher

Pleasant	__:__:__:__:__:__:__	Unpleasant	(Evaluation)
Lazy	__:__:__:__:__:__:__	Busy	(Activity)
Weak	__:__:__:__:__:__:__	Strong	(Potency)
Fast	__:__:__:__:__:__:__	Slow	(Activity)
Good	__:__:__:__:__:__:__	Bad	(Evaluation)
Relaxed	__:__:__:__:__:__:__	Tense	(Activity)
Unsuccessful	__:__:__:__:__:__:__	Successful	(Evaluation)
Dominant	__:__:__:__:__:__:__	Submissive	(Potency)
Hard	__:__:__:__:__:__:__	Soft	(Potency)
Fair	__:__:__:__:__:__:__	Unfair	(Evaluation)
Excitable	__:__:__:__:__:__:__	Calm	(Activity)
Deep	__:__:__:__:__:__:__	Shallow	(Potency)

The dimension for each item is identified in the example, but should not be included on the form administered to the group. The adjective pairs should be randomly ordered to prevent the clustering of a single factor, and both negative and positive adjectives should appear in each column.

Rating Scales
Rating scales are similar in form to Likert scales. Rather than using a standard set of response categories for each statement, however, descriptive terms are presented. The use of descriptive terms assures that all respondents will rate specific boundaries of behavior. The following examples illustrate how a rating scale may be used to determine the group's feelings toward the teacher.

Concern for Students

1	2	3	4	5
Indifferent	Self-centered	Somewhat concerned	Generally concerned	Deeply and actively concerned

Enthusiasm of Instructor

1	2	3	4	5
No enthusiasm	Occasional enthusiastic	Usually enthusiastic	Consistently enthusiastic	Effectively enthusiastic

Questionnaire

A questionnaire consists of a series of questions and is useful for obtaining information from a large number of people. Typically, questionnaires are administered to survey interests, ask opinions, determine values or gather factual information. Responses are usually in the form of one word, a brief statement or selection of a response from a set of options. The responses should be made easily and lend themselves to tabulation.

> Are you able to:
> to list the components of affective behavior?
> describe the uses of affective behavior measurement?
> describe the Likert scale, semantic differential, rating scale and questionnaire as they are used in the measurement of social behavior?

INSTRUMENTS FOR MEASUREMENT OF AFFECTIVE BEHAVIOR

Many instruments have been developed to measure affective behavior. Examples of instruments that measure social behavior, attitudes, sportsmanship and leadership are presented. All of the described instruments may be used with males and females.

Social Behavior
COWELL SOCIAL ADJUSTMENT INDEX (Cowell 1958)
Test Objective. To measure the degree of the students' positive and negative social adjustment within their social groups.
Age Level. 12 through 17.
Validity. Using the Pupil Who's Who Ratings as a criterion measure, a coefficient of .63 was obtained.
Reliability. .82.
Norms. The original source reports norms for junior high school boys.
Administration and Directions. The student is rated by the teacher on the 10 positive items in Form A and the 10 negative items in Form B. A mark is placed in the cell that is judged to reflect the degree to which the behavior is displayed. Forms A and B are shown in Figure 18-1.
Scoring. The score is the sum of the points for the items in Form A minus the sum of the points for the items in Form B.

Figure 18-1. *Cowell Social Adjustment Index**
Form A

Instructions: *Think carefully of the student's behavior in group situations; check each behavior trend according to its degree of descriptiveness.*

	Descriptive of the Student			
Behavior Trends	Markedly (+3)	Somewhat (+2)	Only Slightly (+1)	Not at All (+0)
1. Enters heartily and with enjoyment into the spirit of social intercourse				
2. Frank; talkative and sociable, does not stand on ceremony				
3. Self-confident and self-reliant, tends to take success for granted, strong initiative, prefers to lead				
4. Quick and decisive in movement, pronounced or excessive energy output				
5. Prefers group activities, work or play; not easily satisfied with individual projects				
6. Adaptable to new situations, makes adjustments readily, welcomes change				
7. Is self-composed, seldom shows signs of embarrassment				
8. Tends to elation of spirits, seldom gloomy or moody				
9. Seeks a broad range of friendships, not selective or exclusive in games and the like				
10. Hearty and cordial, even to strangers, forms acquaintanceships very easily				

Figure 18-1. *Cowell Social Adjustment Index**
Form B

Instructions: Think carefully of the student's behavior in group situations; check each behavior trend according to its degree of descriptiveness.

Behavior Trends	Descriptive of the Student			
	Markedly (−3)	Somewhat (−2)	Only Slightly (−1)	Not at All (−0)
1. Somewhat prudish, awkward, easily embarrassed in his social contacts				
2. Secretive, seclusive, not inclined to talk unless spoken to				
3. Lacking in self-confidence and initiative, a follower				
4. Slow in movement, deliberative or perhaps indecisive. Energy output moderate or deficient				
5. Prefers to work and play alone, tends to avoid group activities				
6. Shrinks from making new adjustments, prefers the habitual to the stress of reorganization required by the new				
7. Is self-conscious, easily embarrassed, timid or "bashful"				
8. Tends to depression, frequently gloomy or moody				
9. Shows preference for a narrow range of intimate friends and tends to exclude others from his association				
10. Reserved and distant except to intimate friends, does not form acquaintanceships readily				

*From C. C. Cowell, Validating an index of social adjustment for high school use. *Research Quarterly* 29:7-10, 1958.

BLANCHARD BEHAVIOR RATING SCALE (Blanchard 1936)

Test Objective. To measure the character and personality of students.

Age Level. 12 through 17.

Validity. Using the criterion of the average of the correlations of each item with the remainder of the items in its category, a coefficient of .93 was found.

Reliability. A coefficient of .71 was found for the correlation between the scores of the teacher and the student raters.

Norms. No norms reported.

Administration and Directions. The scale includes 24 items to rate nine character and personality traits of the student. The teacher circles the number (1 through 5) that is judged to reflect the degree to which the behavior is displayed. The scale is shown in Figure 18-2.

Scoring. The score is the sum of the numbers that have been circled for the 24 items.

COWELL'S PERSONAL DISTANCE SCALE (Cowell 1958)

Test Objective. To measure a student's degree of acceptance by a social group.

Age Level. 12 through college.

Validity. Using Who's Who in My Group ratings as the criterion, a coefficient of .84 was found.

Reliability. .93.

Norms. No norms reported.

Administration and Directions. Using the scale shown in Figure 18-3, each student is asked to rate all other students.

Scoring. The average score (to the nearest whole number) for each student is determined. The lower the student's score, the greater the degree of acceptance by the group.

Attitudes

ADAMS PHYSICAL EDUCATION ATTITUDE SCALE (Adams 1963)

Test Objective. To measure individual and group attitudes toward physical education.

Age Level. High school through college.

Validity. A coefficient of .77 was found when correlating the set 1 scoring scale against the Likert scoring scale.

Reliability. A coefficient of .71 was reported.

Norms. No norms reported.

Administration and Directions. Two alternate sets of scales were developed. Set 1 is shown in Figure 18-4. The students indicate if they agree or disagree with the statement by placing a check mark on the appropriate blank. Each statement has a designated weight. These weights should not be printed on the scales that are completed by the students.

Scoring. The total score is the sum of the weights of the "agree" items divided by the number of "agree" items (i.e., the average of the scores for the "agree" items).

Figure 18-2. *Blanchard Behavior Frequency Rating Scale**

Personal information	Frequency of observation: No opportunity to observe	Never	Seldom	Fairly often	Frequently	Extremely often	Score
Leadership							
1. He is popular with classmates		1	2	3	4	5	
2. He seeks responsibility in the classroom		1	2	3	4	5	
3. He shows intellectual leadership in the classroom		1	2	3	4	5	
Positive active qualities							
4. He quits on tasks requiring perseverance		5	4	3	2	1	
5. He exhibits aggressiveness in his relationship with others		1	2	3	4	5	
6. He shows initiative in assuming responsibility in unfamiliar situations		1	2	3	4	5	
7. He is alert to new opportunities		1	2	3	4	5	
Positive mental qualities							
8. He shows keenness of mind		1	2	3	4	5	
9. He volunteers ideas		1	2	3	4	5	
Self-control							
10. He grumbles over decisions of classmates		5	4	3	2	1	
11. He takes a justified criticism by teacher or classmate without showing anger or pouting		1	2	3	4	5	
Cooperation							
12. He is loyal to his group		1	2	3	4	5	
13. He discharges his group responsibilities well		1	2	3	4	5	
14. He is cooperative in his attitude toward the teacher		1	2	3	4	5	
Social action standards							
15. He makes loud-mouthed criticisms and comments		5	4	3	2	1	
16. He respects the rights of others		1	2	3	4	5	
Ethical social qualities							
17. He cheats		5	4	3	2	1	
18. He is truthful		1	2	3	4	5	
Qualities of efficiency							
19. He seems satisfied to "get by" with tasks assigned		5	4	3	2	1	
20. He is dependable and trustworthy		1	2	3	4	5	
21. He has good study habits		1	2	3	4	5	
Sociability							
22. He is liked by others		1	2	3	4	5	
23. He makes a friendly approach to others in the group		1	2	3	4	5	
24. He is friendly		1	2	3	4	5	

*From B. E. Blanchard, A behavior frequency rating scale for the measurement of character and personality traits in a physical education classroom situation. *Research Quarterly* 7:56-66, 1936.

Figure 18-3. *Cowell's Personal Distance Scale**

WHAT TO DO:	I WOULD BE WILLING TO ACCEPT HIM:						
If you had full power to treat each student on this list as you feel, just how would you consider him? How near would you like to have him to your family? Check each student in *one* column as to your feeling toward him. Circle your own name.	Into my family as a brother	As a very close "pal" or "chum"	As a member of my "gang" or club	On my street as a "next-door neighbor"	Into my class at school	Into my school	Into my city
	1	2	3	4	5	6	7
1. List should							
2. include							
3. names of all							
4. students in							
5. class							

*From C. C. Cowell, Validating an index of social adjustment for high school use. *Research Quarterly* 29:7-10, 1958.

Figure 18-4. *Adams Physical Education Attitude Scale**

			Weightings (Not for inclusion in questionnaire)
A = Agree D = Disagree			

A	D	Set I	
____	____	1. Physical education gets very monotonous.	3.50
____	____	2. I only feel like doing physical education now and then.	5.95
____	____	3. Physical education should be disposed of.	1.58
____	____	4. Physical education is particularly limited in its value.	4.50
____	____	5. I suppose physical education is all right but I don't much care for it.	5.03
____	____	6. Physical education is the most hateful subject of all.	1.02
____	____	7. I do not want to give up physical education.	8.64
____	____	8. On the whole I think physical education is a good thing.	8.00
____	____	9. People who like physical education are nearly always good to know.	7.71
____	____	10. Anyone who likes physical education is silly.	2.65
____	____	11. Physical education has some usefulness.	6.45
____	____	12. Physical education is the ideal subject.	10.66
____	____	13. Physical education develops good character.	8.92
____	____	14. (School) College would be better without physical education.	2.30
____	____	15. Physical education has little to offer.	9.39
____	____	16. Physical education is my favorite subject.	3.93
____	____	17. Physical education gives lasting satisfaction.	9.60
____	____	18. Physical education's good and bad points balance out each other.	5.99
____	____	19. Physical education is a pleasant break.	7.11
____	____	20. Physical education seems useless to me.	3.08

*From R. S. Adams, Two scales for measuring attitude toward physical education. *Research Quarterly* 34: 91-94, 1963.

WEAR ATTITUDE SCALE (Wear 1955)
Test Objective. To measure attitudes toward physical education.
Age Level. College.
Validity. Face validity.
Reliability. Coefficients of .94 and .96 were reported for Form A and Form B, respectively.
Norms. No norms reported.
Administration and Directions. Two alternate forms of the scale, Form A and Form B, were developed. Form A is shown in Figure 18-5. The students are instructed to respond to each statement as if physical education is an activity course taught during a regular class period and to let their personal experiences determine their answers. They should answer anonymously, or they

should be advised their responses will not affect their physical education grades. The five possible responses are: strongly agree, agree, undecided, disagree, and strongly disagree.

Scoring. Positively worded items are scored 5-4-3-2-1, and negatively worded items are scored 1-2-3-4-5. The total test score is the sum of the scores of the 30 items; a high score indicates a positive attitude toward physical education.

Figure 18-5. *Wear Attitude Scale**

Form A

1. If for any reason a few subjects have to be dropped from the school program, physical education should be one of the subjects dropped.
2. Physical education activities provide no opportunities for learning to control the emotions.
3. Physical education is one of the more important subjects in helping to establish and maintain desirable social standards.
4. Vigorous physical activity works off harmful emotional tensions.
5. I would take physical education only if it were required.
6. Participation in physical education makes no contribution to the development of poise.
7. Because physical skills loom large in importance in youth, it is essential that a person be helped to acquire and improve such skills.
8. Calisthenics taken regularly are good for one's general health.
9. Skill in active games or sports is not necessary for leading the fullest kind of life.
10. Physical education does more harm physically than it does good.
11. Associating with others in some physical education activity is fun.
12. Physical education classes provide situations for the formulation of attitudes, which make one a better citizen.
13. Physical education situations are among the poorest for making friends.
14. There is not enough value coming from physical education to justify the time consumed.
15. Physical education skills make worthwhile contributions to the enrichment of living.
16. People get all the physical exercise they need in just taking care of their daily work.
17. All who are physically able will profit from an hour of physical education each day.
18. Physical education makes a valuable contribution toward building up an adequate reserve of strength and endurance for everyday living.
19. Physical education tears down sociability by encouraging people to attempt to surpass each other in many of the activities.
20. Participation in physical education activities makes for a more wholesome outlook on life.
21. Physical education adds nothing to the improvement of social behavior.
22. Physical education class activities will help to relieve and relax physical tensions.

Wear Attitude Scale (Continued)

23. Participation in physical education activities helps a person to maintain a healthful emotional life.
24. Physical education is one of the more important subjects in the school program.
25. There is little value in physical education as far as physical well-being is concerned.
26. Physical education should be included in the program of every school.
27. Skills learned in physical education class do not benefit a person.
28. Physical education provides situations for developing character qualities.
29. Physical education makes for more enjoyable living.
30. Physical education has no place in modern education.

*From C. L. Wear, Construction of equivalent forms of an attitude scale. *Research Quarterly* 26:113-119, 1955.

KENYON ATTITUDE SCALES (Kenyon 1968a, 1968b)

Test Objective. To measure six attitudes toward physical activity.
Age Level. High school through college.
Validity. Generally, scale scores differed between athletes and nonathletes, and expert opinion confirmed that the six dimensions adequately differentiated between active and passive involvement in physical activity.
Reliability. Coefficients ranged from .72 to .89 for the various scales.
Norms. No norms reported.
Administration and Directions. All six scales are administered.
The six scales are:
(1) Social experience: A high score on this scale indicates the student values physical activities that provide an opportunity for social relationships.
(2) Health and fitness: A high score on this scale indicates the student values activities that contribute to the improvement of physical health and fitness.
(3) Pursuit of vertigo: A high score on this scale indicates the student values physical activities that provide an element of thrill or risk to the participant through speed, acceleration, change of direction or exposure to dangerous situations.
(4) Aesthetic experience: A high score on this scale indicates the student values physical activities that are generally pleasing to the observer.
(5) Catharsis: A high score on this scale indicates the student values physical activities that provide a release from frustration through some vicarious means.
(6) Ascetic experience: A high score on this scale indicates the student values dedication required for championship performance.
Separate scales were developed for males (59 items) and females (54 items). Each item is scored on a 7-point scale, ranging from very strongly disagree to very strongly agree.
Scoring. Each scale is scored separately, so the student will receive six scores. The six scores should not be summed to obtain a single score.
Comments. The Kenyon Attitude Scales may be obtained from ADI Auxiliary Publications Project, Photoduplication Service, Library of Congress, Washington, D.C. 20540. Cite document number 9983. A fee is charged for the photoprints.

CHILDREN'S ATTITUDE TOWARD PHYSICAL ACTIVITY INVENTORY (Simon and Smoll 1974)

Test Objective. To measure children's attitudes toward vigorous physical activity.

Age Level. Elementary through junior high school.

Validity. Since the Kenyon Attitude Scales were used as a model for this inventory, validity was assumed for the Children's Attitude Toward Physical Activity Inventory.

Reliability. Within a day coefficients ranged from .80 to .89 and test-retest coefficients ranged from .44 to .62.

Norms. No norms reported.

Administration and Directions. The authors advise that this inventory be used to assess groups and changes in group attitudes, not to evaluate individuals. A semantic differential is used, and the students are asked to respond to six dimensions and statements.

1. Physical activity as a social experience: Physical activities which give you a chance to meet new people and be with your friends.
2. Physical activity for health and fitness: Taking part in physical activities to make your health better and to get your body in better condition.
3. Physical activities as a thrill but involving some risk: Physical activities are dangerous. They also can be exciting because you move very fast and must change directions quickly.
4. Physical activity as the beauty in human movement: Physical activities which have beautiful movements. Examples are ballet dancing, gymnastics-tumbling and figure skating on ice.
5. Physical activity for the release of tension: Taking part in physical activities to get away from problems you might have. You can also get away from problems by watching other people in physical activities.
6. Physical activity as long and hard training: Physical activities that have long and hard practices. To spend time in practice you need to give up other things you like to do.

Each dimension is rated on the basis of eight pairs of bipolar adjectives, which are separated by a 7-point continuum. Figure 18-6 illustrates one dimension with the bipolar adjectives.

Scoring. Each of the six scales is scored separately. The maximum score for each dimension is 56.

Sportsmanship

LAKIE ATTITUDE TOWARD ATHLETIC COMPETITION SCALE (Lakie 1964)

Test Objective. To measure the student's attitude toward competition.

Age Level. College.

Validity. Face validity.

Reliability. .81.

Norms. No norms reported.

Administration and Directions. Lakie's scale is shown in Figure 18-7. The students are advised to circle the number of the response that best reflects their feelings about each described action.

Scoring. The score is the sum of the item scores. Negative items are scored in a reverse order (5-4-3-2-1). The higher the score, the greater the competitive attitude of the student.

How do you feel about the idea in the box?

Physical Activity for Health and Fitness
Taking part in physical activities to make your health
better and to get your body in better condition

Always think about the idea in the box.

1.	Good	___: 1	___: 2	___: 3	___: 4	___: 5	___: 6	___: 7 : Bad
2.	Of no use	___: 1	___: 2	___: 3	___: 4	___: 5	___: 6	___: 7 : Useful
3.	Not pleasant	___: 1	___: 2	___: 3	___: 4	___: 5	___: 6	___: 7 : Pleasant
4.	Bitter	___: 1	___: 2	___: 3	___: 4	___: 5	___: 6	___: 7 : Sweet
5.	Nice	___: 1	___: 2	___: 3	___: 4	___: 5	___: 6	___: 7 : Awful
6.	Happy	___: 1	___: 2	___: 3	___: 4	___: 5	___: 6	___: 7 : Sad
7.	Dirty	___: 1	___: 2	___: 3	___: 4	___: 5	___: 6	___: 7 : Clean
8.	Steady	___: 1	___: 2	___: 3	___: 4	___: 5	___: 6	___: 7 : Nervous

J. A. Simon and F. L. Smoll, An instrument for assessing children's attitude toward physical activity. *Research Quarterly* 45: 407-415, 1974.

Figure 18-7. *Lake Attitude Toward Athletic Competition Scale**

The following situations describe behavior demonstrated in sports. Circle the category that indicates your feeling toward the behavior described in each of the situations.

1. Strongly approve 2. Approve 3. Undecided 4. Disapprove
5. Strongly disapprove

1 2 3 4 5   1. During a football game team A has the ball on its own 34-yard line, fourth down and 1 yard to go for a first down. The coach of team A signals to the quarterback the play that he wants the team to run.

1 2 3 4 5   2. Team A is the visiting basketball team; and each time a member of the team is given a free shot, the home crowd sets up a continual din of noise until the shot has been taken.

1 2 3 4 5   3. Tennis player A frequently calls out, throws up his arms, or otherwise tries to indicate that his opponent's serve is out of bounds when it is questionable.

1 2 3 4 5   4. In a track meet, team A enters a man in the mile run who is to set a fast pace for the first half of the race and then drop out.

1 2 3 4 5   5. In a football game, team B's quarterback was tackled repeatedly after handing off and after he was out of the play.

1 2 3 4 5   6. Sam, playing golf with his friends, hit a drive into the rough. He accidentally moved the ball with his foot; although not improving his position, he added a penalty stroke to his score.

1 2 3 4 5   7. A basketball player was caught out of position on defense; and rather than allow his opponent to attempt a field goal, he fouled him.

1 2 3 4 5   8. Player A during a golf match made quick noises and movements when player B was getting ready to make a shot.

1 2 3 4 5   9. School A has a powerful but quite slow football team. The night before playing a smaller but faster team, they allowed the field sprinkling system to remain on, causing the field to be heavy and slow.

1 2 3 4 5   10. A basketball team used player A to draw the opponent's high scorer into fouling situations.

1 2 3 4 5   11. The alumni of College A pressured the Board of Trustees to lower the admission and eligibility requirements for athletes.

1 2 3 4 5   12. Team A, by use of fake injuries, was able to stop the clock long enough to get off the play that resulted in the winning touchdown.

1 2 3 4 5   13. A tennis player was given the advantage of a bad call in a close match. He then "evened up" the call by intentionally hitting the ball out of bounds.

1 2 3 4 5   14. The coach of basketball team A removed his team from the floor in protest of an official's decision.

1 2 3 4 5   15. Between seasons a coach moved from College A to College B, and he then persuaded three of College A's athletes to transfer to College B.

1 2 3 4 5   16. After losing a close football game, the coach of the losing team publicly accused the game officials of favoritism when the game movies showed the winning touchdown had been scored by using an illegal maneuver.

1 2 3 4 5   17. College C lowered the admission requirements for boys awarded athletic scholarships.

1 2 3 4 5   18. Team A's safety man returned a punt for a touchdown. Unseen by the officials, he had stepped out of bounds in front of his team's bench. His coach notified the officials of this fact.

1 2 3 4 5   19. A college with very few athletic scholarships to offer gives athletes preference on all types of campus jobs.

1 2 3 4 5   20. Several wealthy alumni of College C make a monthly gift to several athletes who are in need of financial assistance.

1 2 3 4 5   21. College K has a policy of not allowing any member of a varsity squad to associate with the visiting team until the contest or meet is completed.

1 2 3 4 5   22. The Board of Trustees of College C fired the football coach and gave as the reason for his dismissal his failure to win a conference championship during the past five years.

---

*From W. L. Lakie, Expressed attitude of various groups of athletes toward athletic competition. *Research Quarterly* 35: 497-503.

JOHNSON SPORTSMANSHIP ATTITUDE SCALES (Johnson 1969)

Test Objective. To measure the student's attitude toward competition.

Age Level. 12 through 14.

Validity. Empirical validity coefficients ranging from -.01 to .43 were found by correlating test scores and behavior ratings.

Reliability. A coefficient of .86 was found between scores of Form A and Form B.

Norms. No norms reported.

Administration and Directions. Johnson developed alternate forms of the scales. Form A is provided in Figure 18-8. The students are advised to read each statement carefully and to decide if they approve or disapprove of the action taken by the person. They then circle the one response that tells the way they feel.

Scoring. No total test score is recorded. The scale is used to detect attitudes, changes in attitudes, and as material for class discussion.

Figure 18-8. *Johnson Sportsmanship Attitude Scale* *
_____

Directions: Read each statement carefully and decide whether you approve or disapprove of the action taken by the person. Circle the ONE response category that tells the way you feel. PLEASE COMPLETE EVERY ITEM.

Example: A pitcher in a baseball game threw a fast ball at the batter to scare him.

~~Strongly approve~~   Approve   Disapprove   Strongly Disapprove

(If you strongly approve of this action by the pitcher, you circle the first response category as shown.)

The responses can appear after each item or on an answer sheet.

1. After a basketball player was called by the official for traveling, he slammed the basketball onto the floor.

2. A baseball player was called out as he slid into home plate. He jumped up and down on the plate and screamed at the official.

3. After a personal foul was called against a basketball player, he shook his fist in the official's face.

4. A basketball coach talked very loudly in order to annoy an opponent who was attempting to make a very important free throw shot.

5. After a baseball game, the coach of the losing team went up to the umpire and demanded to know how much money had been paid to "throw" the game.

6. A basketball coach led the spectators in jeering at the official who made calls against his team.

7. After two men were put out on a double play attempt, a baseball coach told the players in his dugout to boo the umpire's decision.

8. As the basketball coach left the gymnasium after the game, he shouted at the officials, "You lost me the game; I never saw such lousy officiating in my life."

9. A basketball coach put sand on the gym floor to force the opponents into traveling penalties.

10. A football coach left the bench to change the position of a marker dropped by an official to indicate where the ball went out of bounds.

11. During the first half of a football game a touchdown was called back. At halftime the football coach went into the officials' dressing room and cursed the officials.

12. A football player was taken out of the game for unsportsmanlike conduct. The player changed jerseys and the coach sent him back into the game.

13. Following a closely played basketball game, the coach of the losing team cursed his boys for not winning.

14. After a basketball game the losing team's coach yelled at spectators to "Go get the Ump."

15. A baseball coach permitted players to use profanity loud enough for the entire park to hear when the players did not like a decision.

16. The basketball coach drank alcoholic beverages while supervising his basketball team on a trip.

17. A college football player was disqualified for misconduct. While on the way to the sideline, the player attacked the official.

18. During a time-out in a basketball game, the clock was accidentally left running. The coach whose team was behind ran over to the scoring table and struck the timekeeper.

19. After a basketball player was knocked into a wall, his coach rushed onto the court and hit the player who had fouled.

20. After a baseball player had been removed from the game, the coach met him at the sidelines and hit him.

21. After a runner was called out at first base, the baseball coach went onto the field and wrestled the umpire down to the ground.

---

*From M. L. Johnson, Construction of sportsmanship attitude scales. *Research Quarterly* 40:312-316, 1969.

Leadership

NELSON SPORTS LEADERSHIP QUESTIONNAIRE (1966)

Test Objective. To measure athletic leadership.
Age Level. Junior high through college.
Validity. Face validity.
Reliability. Coefficients of .96 with ninth-grade football players, and .78 with varsity college basketball players were reported in Johnson and Nelson (1986).
Norms. No norms reported.
Administration and Directions. Two questionnaires are designed, one for the coaches and one for the students. The students are advised to list a first and second choice in all cases, excluding his or her own name. An athlete's name can be used any number of times. Students do not sign their name. The questionnaire for the students is provided in Figure 18-9.
Scoring. Five points are awarded for a name appearing in response number 1 and three points are awarded for a name appearing in response number 2.

Figure 18-9. *Nelson Sport Leadership Questionnaire**

Do not sign your name to the questionnaire. Fill in the name or names of the squad member that, in your opinion, best fit the question. Give your first and second choice in all cases. *Do not use your own name* on any of the answers. The names of the same players can be used any number of times, and your answers will be kept confidential.

1. If you were on a trip and had a choice of the players you would share the hotel room with, who would they be?
   1. _____ 2. _____
2. Who are the most popular men on the squad?
   1. _____ 2. _____
3. Who are the best scholars on the squad?
   1. _____ 2. _____
4. Which players on the team know the most basketball, in terms of strategy, team play, etc.?
   1. _____ 2. _____
5. If the coach were not present for a workout, which players would be the most likely to take charge of the practice?
   1. _____ 2. _____
6. Which players would you listen to first if the team appeared to be disorganized during a crucial game?
   1. _____ 2. _____
7. Your team is behind 1 point with 10 seconds remaining in the game and you could pass to anyone on the squad. Who would it be?
   1. _____ 2. _____
8. Of all the players on your team, who exhibits the most poise on the floor during the crucial parts of the game?
   1. _____ 2. _____
9. Who are the "take charge" men on your team?
   1. _____ 2. _____
10. Who are the most consistent ball handlers on your squad?
    1. _____ 2. _____
11. Who are the most consistent shooters on your squad?
    1. _____ 2. _____
12. Who are the most valuable players on your squad?
    1. _____ 2. _____
13. Who are the most unselfish players who are interested most in the team as a whole and who play most "for the team"?
    1. _____ 2. _____
14. Which players have the most overall ability of the squad?
    1. _____ 2. _____
15. Who are the most likable players on the squad?
    1. _____ 2. _____
16. Which players on your team have influenced you the most?
    1. _____ 2. _____
17. Which players have actually helped you the most?
    1. _____ 2. _____
18. Which players do you think would make the best coaches?
    1. _____ 2. _____
19. Which players do you most often look to for leadership?
    1. _____ 2. _____
20. Who are the hardest workers on the squad?
    1. _____ 2. _____

*From D. O. Nelson, Nelson Sports Leadership Questionnaire. *Research Quarterly* 37:268-275, 1966.

1. Select one of the tests described in this chapter and administer it to a group of students. Score the scale and interpret the results for the group.
2. Review at least one test from each of the areas listed at the conclusion of this chapter.

SOURCES OF ADDITIONAL INSTRUMENTS FOR MEASUREMENT OF AFFECTIVE BEHAVIOR

Attitudes

McCue, B. F. 1953. Constructing an instrument for evaluating attitudes toward intensive competition in team games. *Research Quarterly* 24: 205-210.

McPherson, B. D., and Yuhasz, M. S. 1968. An inventory for assessing men's attitudes toward exercise and physical activity. *Research Quarterly* 39: 218-219.

Richardson, C. E. 1960. Thurston scale for measuring attitudes of college students toward physical fitness and exercise. *Research Quarterly* 31: 638-643.

Scott, P. M. 1953. Attitudes toward athletic competition in elementary school. *Research Quarterly* 24: 352-361.

Seaman, J. A. Attitudes of physically handicapped children toward physical education. *Research Quarterly* 41: 439-445.

Body Image

Secord, P. F., and Jourard, S. M. 1953. The appraisal of body cathexis: body cathexis and the self. *Journal of Consulting Psychology* 17: 343-347.

Competition Anxiety

Martens, R. 1977. *Sport competition anxiety test.* Champaign, Ill.: Human Kinetics Publishers.

Perceived Exertion

Borg, G. A. V. 1973. Perceived exertion: a note on "history" and methods. *Medicine and Science in Sports* 5: 90-93.

Self-Esteem

Sonstroem, R. J. 1978. Physical estimation and attraction scales: rationale and research. *Medicine and Science in Sports* 10: 97-102.

Self-Motivation

Dishman, R. K., Ickes, W., and Morgan, W. P. 1981. Self-motivation and adherence to therapeutic exercise. *Journal of Behavior Medicine* 4: 421-436.

Sportsmanship

Boyer, G. 1963. Children's concepts of sportsmanship in the fourth, fifth, and sixth grades. *Research Quarterly* 34: 282-287.

McAfee, R. A. 1955. Sportsmanship attitudes of sixth, seventh, and eighth grade boys. *Research Quarterly* 26: 120.

References

AAHPERD health related physical fitness test manual. 1980. Reston, Va.: American Alliance for Health, Physical Education, Recreation and Dance.

AAHPERD youth fitness test manual. 1976. Reston, Va.: American Alliance for Health, Physical Education, Recreation and Dance.

AAU physical fitness program. 1986. Bloomington, Indiana: American Athletic Union.

Adams, R. S. 1963. Two scales for measuring attitude toward physical education. *Research Quarterly* 34: 91-94.

Ahmann, J. S., and Glock, M. D. 1958. *Evaluating pupil growth.* Boston: Allyn and Bacon.

American Association for Health, Physical Education and Recreation. 1967. *Archery for boys and girls: skills test manual.* Washington, D. C.: AAHPER.

American Association for Health, Physical Education and Recreation. 1965. *Football: skills test manual.* Washington, D. C.: AAHPER.

Arnheim, D. D., and Sinclair, W. A. 1985. *Physical education for special populations: a developmental, adapted, and remedial approach.* Englewood Cliffs, N. J.: Prentice-Hall.

Arnheim, D. D., and Sinclair, W. A. 1979. *The clumsy child: a program of motor therapy.* 2d ed. St. Louis: C. V. Mosby.

Barrow, H. M. 1954. Tests of motor ability for college men. *Research Quarterly* 25: 253-260.

Barrow, H. M., and McGee, R. 1979. *A practical approach to measurement in physical education.* 3d ed. Philadelphia: Lea & Febiger.

Bass, R. I. 1939. An analysis of the components of tests of semi-circular canal function and of static and dynamic balance. *Research Quarterly* 10 (May): 33-52.

Baumgartner, T. A., and Jackson, A. S. 1982. *Measurement for evaluation in physical education.* 2d ed. Dubuque, Iowa: Wm. C. Brown.

Baumgartner, T. A. et al. 1984. Equipment improvements and additional norms for the modified pull-up test. *Research Quarterly for Exercise and Sport* 55: 64-68.

Baumgartner, T. A., and Wood, S. S. 1984. Development of shoulder-girdle strength endurance in elementary children. *Research Quarterly for Exercise and Sport* 55: 169-171.

Bennett, C. L. 1956. Relative contributions of modern dance, folk dance, basketball, and swimming to motor abilities of college women. *Research Quarterly* 27: 253-257.

Blanchard, B. E. 1936. A behavior frequency rating scale for the measurement of character and personality traits in a physical education classroom situation. *Research Quarterly* 7 (May): 56-66.

Bloom, S. B., Madaus, G. F., and Hastings, J. T. 1981. *Evaluation to improve learning.* New York: McGraw-Hill.

Body composition (a round table). 1986. *The Physician and Sportsmedicine* 14(3): 144-152, 157, 161-162.

Bonci, C. M., Hensel, F. J., and Torg, J. S. 1986. A preliminary study on the measurement of static and dynamic motion at the glenohumeral joint. *The American Journal of Sports Medicine* 14: 12-17.

Bosco, J. S., and Gustafson, W. F. 1983. *Measurement and evaluation in physical education, fitness, and sports.* Englewood Cliffs, N.J.: Prentice-Hall.

Bowerman, W. J., and Harris, W. D. 1967. *Jogging.* New York: Grosset and Dunlap.

Brady, G. F. 1945. Preliminary investigations of volleyball playing ability. *Research Quarterly* 16: 14-17.

Broer, M. R. 1973. *Efficiency of human movement.* 3d ed. Philadelphia: W. B. Saunders.

Brouha, L. 1943. The step test: a simple method of measuring physical fitness for muscular work in young men. *Research Quarterly* 14: 31-36.

Brouha, L. and Ball, M. V. 1952. *Canadian Red Cross Society's School Meal Study.* Toronto: University of Toronto Press.

Brown, F. G. 1983. *Principles of educational and psychological testing.* 3d ed. New York: Holt, Rinehart and Winston.

Brumbach, W. B. 1967. *Beginning volleyball, a syllabus for teachers.* Revised ed. Eugene, Oregon: W. B. Brumbach. In Collins, D. R.,and Hodges, P. B. 1978. *A comprehensive guide to sports skills tests and measurement.* Springfield, Illinois: Charles C. Thomas.

Bucher, C. A., and Prentice, W. E. 1985. *Fitness for college and life.* St. Louis: Times Mirror/Mosby.

Buell, C. E. 1982. *Physical education and recreation for the visually handicapped.* Reston, Virginia: American Alliance for Health, Physical Education, Recreation and Dance.

Bunn, J. W. 1955. *Scientific principles of coaching.* Englewood Cliffs, N. J.: Prentice-Hall.

Chapman, N. L. 1982. Chapman ball control test - field hockey. *Research Quarterly for Exercise and Sport* 53: 239-242.

Chase, C. I. 1978. *Measurement for educational evaluation.* 2d ed. Reading, Mass.: Addison-Wesley Publishing.

Cirn, J. T. 1986. True/false versus short answer questions. *College Teaching* 34(4): 34-37.

Clark, H. H., ed. 1975. Exercise and fat reduction. *Physical fitness research digest.* Washington, D. C.: President's Council on Physical Fitness, Series 5, April.

Clark, H. H., ed. 1979. Posture. *Physical fitness research digest.* Washington, D. C.: President's Council on Physical Fitness and Sports, Series 9, January.

Clark, H. H., and Clark, D. H. 1987. *Application of measurement to physical education.* 6th ed. Englewood Cliffs, N. J.: Prentice-Hall.

Clevett, M. A. 1931. An experiment in teaching methods of golf. *Research Quarterly* 2: 104-112.

Collins, D. R., and Hodges, P. B. 1978. *A comprehensive guide to sports skills tests and measurement.* Springfield, Illinois: Charles C. Thomas.

Cooper, K. H. 1982. *The aerobics program for total well-being.* New York: M. Evans and Company, Inc.

Corbin, C. H., and Lindsey, R. 1985. *Concepts of physical fitness.* 5th ed. Dubuque, Iowa: Wm. C. Brown.

Corbin, C. B., and Noble, L. 1980. Flexibility: a major component of physical fitness. *Journal of Physical Education and Recreation* 51(6): 23-24,57-60.

Cornelius, W. L., and Hinon, M. M. 1980. The relationship between isometric contractions of hip extensors and subsequent flexibility in males. *The Journal of Sports Medicine and Physical Fitness* 20: 75-80.

Cowell, C. C. 1958. Validating an index of social adjustment for high school use. *Research Quarterly* 29: 7-10.

Cratty, B. J. 1975. *Remedial motor activity for children.* Philadelphia: Lea and Febiger.

Custer, S. J., and Chaloupka, V. A. 1977. Relationship between predicted maximal oxygen consumption and running performance of college females. *Research Quarterly* 48: 47-50.

Doolittle, T. L., and Bigbee, R. 1968. The twelve-minute run-walk: a test of cardiorespiratory fitness of adolescent boys. *Research Quarterly* 39: 491-495.

Dotson, C. O., and Kirkendall, D. R. 1974. *Statistics for physical education, health, and recreation.* New York: Harper & Row.

Downie, N. M., and Heath, R. W. 1974. *Basic statistical methods.* 4th ed. New York: Harper & Row.

Dunn, J. M., Morehouse, J. W., and Fredericks, H. D. 1986. *Physical education for the severely handicapped: a systematic approach to a data based gymnasium.* Austin, Texas: Pro-Ed.

Ebel, R. L. 1979. *Essentials of educational measurement.* 3d ed. Englewood Cliffs, N.J.: Prentice-Hall.

Edgren, H. 1932. An experiment in the testing of ability and progress in basketball. *Research Quarterly* 3: 159-171.

Fait, H. F., and Dunn, J. M. 1984. *Special physical education: adapted, individualized, and developmental.* 5th ed. Philadelphia: Saunders College Publishing.

Franks, B. D., and Deutsch, H. 1973. *Evaluating performance in physical education.* New York: Academic Press.

French, R. W., and Jansma, P. 1982. *Special physical education.* Columbus: Charles E. Merrill.

Fringer, M. N. 1961. A battery of softball skill tests for senior high school girls. Master's thesis, Eugene, Oregon. In Collins, D. R., and Hodges, P. B. 1978. *A comprehensive guide to sports skills tests and measurement.* Springfield, Illinois: Charles C. Thomas.

Fry, P. F. 1983. Measurement of psychosocial aspects of physical education. *Journal of Physical Education, Recreation and Dance* 54(8): 26-27.

Gabbard, C. et al. 1983. Effects of grip and forearm position on flexed-arm hang performance. *Research Quarterly for Exercise and Sport* 54: 198-199.

Gallagher, J. R., and Brouha, L. 1943. A simple method for testing the physical fitness of boys. *Research Quarterly* 14, no. 1: 24-30.

Gates, D. P., and Sheffield, R. P. 1940. Tests of change of direction as measurement of different kinds of motor ability in boys of 7th, 8th, and 9th grades. *Research Quarterly* 11: 136-147.

Golding, L. A., Meyers, C. R., and Sinning, W. E. 1982. *The Y's way to physical fitness.* 2d ed. Chicago, Ill.: National Board of YMCA.

Green, J. A. 1975. *Teacher-made tests.* 2d ed. New York: Harper & Row.

Griffin, P. S. 1982. Second thoughts on affective evaluation. In Wiese, C. E. (Ed.). Doing well and feeling good. *Journal of Physical Education, Recreation and Dance* 53(2): 15-25, 86.

Harris, M. L. 1969. A factor analytic study of flexibility. *Research Quarterly* 40: 62-70.

Hensley, L. D., East, W. B., and Stillwell, J. L. 1979. A racquetball skills test. *Research Quarterly* 50: 114-118.

Hewitt, J. E. 1966. Hewitt's tennis achievement test. *Research Quarterly* 37: 231-237.

Hewitt, J. E. 1965. Revision of the Dyer Backboard Tennis Test. *Research Quarterly* 36: 153-157.

Hodgkins, J., and Skubic, V. 1963. Cardiovascular efficiency scores for college women in the United States. *Research Quarterly* 34: 454-461.

Holt, L. E., Travis, T. M., and Okita, T. 1970. A comparative study of three stretching techniques. *Perceptual and Motor Skills* 31: 611-616.

Hopkins, D. R., Shick, J., and Plack, J. J. 1984. *Basketball for boys and girls: skills test manual.* Reston, Va.: American Alliance for Health, Physical Education, Recreation and Dance.

Humphrey, L. D. 1981. Flexibility. *Journal of Physical Education, Recreation and Dance* 52(7): 41-43.

Jackson, A. et al. 1982. Baumgartner's modified pull-up test for male and female elementary school aged children. *Research Quarterly for Exercise and Sport* 53: 163-164.

Jackson, A. S., and Coleman, E. 1976. Validation of distance run tests for elementary school children. *Research Quarterly* 47: 86-94.

Jackson, A. S., and Pollock, M. L. 1985. Practical assessment of body composition. *The Physician and Sportsmedicine* 13(5): 76-90.

Jensen, C. R., Schultz, G. W., and Bangerter, B. L. 1983. *Applied kinesiology and biomechanics.* 3d ed. New York: McGraw-Hill.

Jensen, C. R., and Hirst, C. C. 1980. *Measurement in physical education and athletics.* New York: Macmillan.

Johnson, B. L., and Nelson, J. K. 1986. *Practical measurements for evaluation in physical education.* 4th ed. Edina, Minn.: Burgess.

Johnson, L., and Londeree, B. 1976. *Motor fitness testing manual for the moderately mentally retarded.* Reston, Virginia: American Alliance for Health, Physical Education, Recreation and Dance.

Johnson, M. L. 1969. Construction of sportsmanship attitude scales. *Research Quarterly* 40: 312-316.

Johnson, P. B. et al. 1975. *Sport, exercise and you.* New York: Holt, Rinehart and Winston.

Johnson, R., and Christian, V. 1982. *Laboratory experiences in measurement and evaluation: theory to application.* Boone, N. C.: Appalachian State University.

Kalakian, L. H., and Eichstaedt, C. B. 1982. *Developmental/adapted physical education: making ability count.* Minneapolis: Burgess Publishing.

Katch, F. I., and McArdle, W. D. 1977. *Nutrition, weight control, and exercise.* Boston: Houghton Mifflin.

Kenyon, G. S. 1968a. A conceptual model for characterizing physical activity. *Research Quarterly* 39: 96-105.

Kenyon, G. S. 1968b. Six scales for assessing attitude toward physical activity. *Research Quarterly* 39: 566-574.

Kirby, R. F. 1971. A simple test of agility. *Coach and Athlete*: June: 30-31.

Kirkendall, D. R., Gruber, J. J., and Johnson, R. E. 1980. *Measurement and evaluation for physical educators.* Dubuque, Iowa: Wm. C. Brown.

Kryspin, W. J, and Feldusen, J. F. 1974. *Developing classroom tests: a guide for writing and evaluating test items.* Edina, Minn.: Burgess.

Lafuze, M. 1951. A study of the learning of fundamental skills by college freshman women of low motor ability. *Research Quarterly* 22: 149-157.

Lakie, W. L. 1964. Expressed attitudes of various groups of athletes toward athletic competition. *Research Quarterly* 35: 497-503.

Logan, G. A., and McKinney, W. C. 1982. *Anatomic kinesiology.* 3d ed. Dubuque, Iowa: Wm. C. Brown.

Lohman, T. G. 1982. Body composition methodology in sports medicine. *The Physician and Sports Medicine.* 10(12): 46-58.

Lohman, G. A. 1982. Measurement of body composition in children. *Journal of Physical Education, Recreation and Dance* 53(7): 67-70.

Lohman, G. A., and Pollack, M. L. 1981. Which caliper? how much training? *Journal of Physical Education, Recreation and Dance* 52(1): 27-29.

Luttgens, K., and Wells, K. F. 1982. *Kinesiology: scientific basis of human motion.* 7th ed. Philadelphia: Saunders College.

Lyman, H. B. 1963. *Test scores and what they mean.* Englewood Cliffs, N.J.: Prentice-Hall.

Manitoba physical fitness performance test manual and fitness objectives. 1977. Manitoba, Canada: Manitoba Department of Education.

Marsh, J. J. 1984. Measuring affective objectives in physical education. *Physical Educator* 41(2): 77-81.

Masley, J. W., Hairabedian, A., and Donaldson, D. N. 1953. Weight training in relation to strength, speed, and coordination. *Research Quarterly* 24: 308-315.

Masters, L. F., Mori, A. A., and Lange, E. K. 1983. *Adapted physical education: a practitioner's guide.* Rockville, Maryland: Aspen Publication.

Mattson, D. E. 1981. *Statistics: difficult concepts, understandable explanations.* St. Louis: C. V. Mosby.

McArdle, W. D. et al. 1972. Reliability and interrelationships between maximal oxygen intake, physical work capacity, and step test scores in college women. *Medicine and Science in Sports* 4: 182-186.

McClenaghan, B. A., and Gallahue, D. L. 1978. *Fundamental movement: a developmental and remedial approach.* Philadelphia: W. B. Saunders.

McCloy, C. H., and Young, N. D. 1954. *Tests and measurements in health and physical education.* 3d ed. New York: Appleton-Century-Crofts.

McDonald, L. G. 1951. The construction of a kicking test as an index of general soccer ability. Master's thesis, Springfield, Mass., Springfield College. In Collins, D. R., and Hodges, P. B. 1978. *A comprehensive guide to sports skills tests and measurement.* Springfield, Illinois: Charles C. Thomas.

McGee, R. 1982. Uses and abuses of affective measurement. In Wiese, C. E. (Ed.). Doing well and feeling good. *Journal of Physical Education, Recreation and Dance* 53(2): 15-25, 86.

McKeachie, W. J. 1969. *Teaching tips: a guidebook for the beginning college teacher.* Lexington, Mass.: D. C. Heath.

Metheny, E. 1952. *Body mechanics.* New York: McGraw-Hill.

Metropolitan Life Insurance Company. 1983. *1983 height and weight tables announced.* New York: Metropolitan Life Insurance Company.

Miller, A. G., and Sullivan, J. V. 1982. *Teaching physical activities to impaired youth: an approach to mainstreaming.* New York: John Wiley & Sons.

Miller, D. K. 1970. A comparison of the effects of individual and team sports programs on the motor ability of male college freshmen. Unpublished doctoral dissertation, Florida State University.

Miller, D. K. 1983. *The well being-good health handbook.* New York: Leisure Press.

Miller, D. K., and Allen, T. E. 1986. *Fitness: a lifetime commitment.* 3d ed. Edina, Minn.: Burgess.

Mitchell, J. R. 1963. The modification of the McDonald soccer skill test for upper elementary school boys. Master's thesis, Eugene, Oregon, University of Oregon. In Collins, D. R., and Hodges, P. B. 1978. *A comprehensive guide to sports skills tests and measurement.* Springfield, Illinois: Charles C. Thomas.

Mood, D. P. 1982. Evaluation in the affective domain? No! In Wiese, C. E. (Ed.). Doing well and feeling good. *Journal of Physical Education, Recreation and Dance* 53(2): 15-25, 86.

Mood, D. P. 1980. *Numbers in motion: a balanced approach to measurement and evaluation in physical education.* Palo Alto, Calif.: Mayfield.

Moore, M. 1983. New height-weight tables gain pounds, lose status. *The Physician and Sportsmedicine* 11(5): 25.

Morehouse, C. A., and Stull, G. A. 1975. *Statistical principles and procedures with applications for physical education.* Philadelphia: Lea & Febiger.

Nelson, D. O. 1966. Leadership in sports. *Research Quarterly* 37: 268-275.

Nichols, D. B., Arsenault, D. R., and Giuffre, D. L. 1980. *Motor activities for the underachiever.* Springfield, Ill.: Charles C. Thomas.

Pate, R. R. 1985. *Norms for college students: health related physical fitness test.* Reston, Va.: American Alliance for Health, Physical Education, Recreation and Dance.

Pate, R. R., ed. 1978. *South Carolina physical fitness test manual.* Columbia, S. C.: Governor's Council on Physical Fitness.

Phillips, D. A., and Hornak, J. E. 1979. *Measurement and evaluation in physical education.* New York: John Wiley and Sons.

Physical Fitness - Motor Ability Test. 1973. Austin, Texas: Texas Governor's Commission on Physical Fitness.

Piscopo, J., and Baley, J. A. 1981. *Kinesiology: the science of movement.* New York: John Wiley & Sons.

Pollock, M. L., Wilmore, J. H., and Fox, S. M. 1978. *Health and fitness through physical activity.* New York: John Wiley and Sons.

Poole, J., and Nelson, J. K. 1970. Construction of a badminton skills test battery. Unpublished study. In Johnson, B. L., and Nelson, J. K. 1986. *Practical measurements for evaluation in physical education.* 4th ed. Edina, Minn.: Burgess Publishing.

Presidential physical fitness award program. 1986. Washington, D. C.: The President's Council on Physical Fitness and Sports.

Rarick, G. L., Widdop, J. H., and Broadhead, G. D. 1970. The physical fitness and motor performance of educable mentally retarded children. *Exceptional Children* 36: 509-519.

Roach, E. G., and Kephart, N. C. 1966. *The Purdue perceptual-motor survey.* Columbus, Ohio: Charles E. Merrill.

Rothstein, A. L. 1985. *Research design and statistics for physical education.* Englewood Cliffs, N.J.: Prentice-Hall.

Russell, N., and Lange, E. 1940. Achievement tests in volleyball for junior high school girls. *Research Quarterly* 11: 33-41.

Safrit, M. J. 1981. *Evaluation in physical education.* 2d ed. Englewood Cliffs, N.J.: Prentice-Hall.

Safrit, M. J. 1986. *Introduction to measurement in physical education and exercise science.* St. Louis: Times Mirror/Mosby College.

Sargent, D. A. 1921. The physical test of a man. *American Physical Education Review* 26(4): 188-194.

Scott, M. G., Carpenter, A., French, E., and Kuhl, L. 1941. Achievement examination in badminton. *Research Quarterly* 12: 242-253.

Scott, M. G., and French, E. 1959. *Measurement and evaluation in physical education.* Dubuque, Iowa: Wm. C. Brown.

Seashore, H. G. 1947. The development of a beam-walking test and its use in measuring development of balance in children. *Research Quarterly* 18: 246-258.

Seils, L. G. 1951. The relationship between measures of physical growth and gross motor performance of primary-grade school children. *Research Quarterly* 22: 244-260.

Sheehan, T. J. 1971. *An introduction to the evaluation of measurement data in physical education.* Reading, Mass.: Addison-Wesley.

Sheldon, W., Stevens, S. S., and Tucker, W. B. 1970. *The varieties of human physique.* Darien, Conn.: Hafner.

Sherrill, C. 1976. *Adapted physical education and recreation.* Dubuque, Iowa: Wm. C. Brown.

Shick, J. 1970. Battery of defensive softball skills tests for college women. *Research Quarterly* 41: 82-87.

Shick, J., and Berg, N. G. 1983. Indoor golf skill test for junior high school boys. *Research Quarterly for Exercise and Sport* 54: 75-78.

Simon, J. A., and Smoll, F. L. 1974. An instrument for assessing children's attitude toward physical activity. *Research Quarterly* 45: 407-415.

Skubic, V., and Hodgkins, J. 1963. Cardiovascular efficiency test for girls and women. *Research Quarterly* 34: 191-198.

Skubic, V., and Hodgkins, J. 1964. Cardiovascular efficiency test scores for junior and senior high school girls in the United States. *Research Quarterly* 35: 184-192.

Smith, J. A. 1956. Relation of certain physical traits and abilities to motor learning in elementary school children. *Research Quarterly* 27: 220-228.

Special fitness test manual for mildly mentally retarded persons. 1976. Reston, Virginia: American Alliance for Health, Physical Education, Recreation and Dance.

Spence, J. T. et al. 1968. *Elementary statistics.* 2d ed. New York: Appleton-Century-Crofts.

Sterner, T. G., and Burke, E. J. 1986. Body fat assessment: a comparison of visual estimation and skinfold techniques. *The Physician and Sportsmedicine* 14(4): 101-107.

Stamford, B. 1986. Somatotypes and sports selection. *The Physician and Sportsmedicine* 14(7): 176.

Stodola, Q., and Stordahl, K. 1967. *Basic educational tests and measurements.* Chicago: Science Research Associates.

Stoner, L. J. 1982. Evaluation in the affective domain? Yes! In Wiese, C. E. (Ed.). Doing well and feeling good. *Journal of Physical Education, Recreation and Dance* 53(2): 15-25, 86.

Technical manual for health related physical fitness. 1984. Reston, Va.: American Alliance for Health, Physical Education, Recreation and Dance.

Testing for impaired, disabled and handicapped individuals. 1980. Reston, Virginia: American Alliance for Health, Physical Education, Recreation and Dance.

Thomas, J. R., Pierce, C., and Ridsale, S. 1977. Age differences in children's ability to model motor behavior. *Research Quarterly* 48: 592-597.

Torshen, K. P. 1977. *The mastery approach to competency-based education.* New York: Academic Press.

Tyson, K. W. 1970. A handball skill test for college men. Master's thesis, Austin, University of Texas. In Collins, D. R., and Hodges, P. B. 1978. *A comprehensive guide to sports skills tests and measurement.* Springfield, Illinois: Charles C. Thomas.

Vars, G. F. 1983. Missiles, marks, and the middle level student. *NASS Principal's Bulletin* 67(5): 72-77.

Vicent, W. J. 1976. *Elementary statistics in physical education.* Springfield, Ill.: Charles C. Thomas.

Verducci, F. M. 1980. *Measurement concepts in physical education.* St. Louis: C. V. Mosby.

Wallin, D. et al. 1985. Improvement in muscle flexibility; a comparison between two techniques. *The American Journal of Sports Medicine.* 13:263-268.

Wear. C. L. 1955. Construction of equivalent forms of an attitude scale. *Research Quarterly* 26: 113-119.

Weber, J. C., and Lamb, D. R. 1970. *Statistics and research in physical education.* St. Louis: C. V. Mosby.

Wessel, J. 1961. *Movement fundamentals.* 2d ed. Englewood Cliffs, N. J.: Prentice-Hall.

Wiese, C. E. 1982. Is affective evaluation possible? In Wiese, C. E. (Ed.). Doing well and feeling good. *Journal of Physical Education, Recreation and Dance* 53(2): 15-25, 86.

Williford, N. H. 1986. Evaluation of warm-up for improvement in flexibility. *The American Journal of Sports Medicine* 14: 316-319.

Williford, N. H., and Smith, J. F. 1985. A comparison of proprioceptive neuromuscular facilitation and static stretching techniques. *American Corrective Therapy Journal* 39: 30-33.

Appendix A
Square Root Example

Find the square root of 595.8

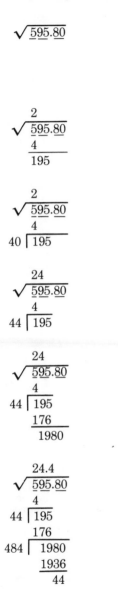

1. Begin at the decimal point and mark off two places at a time to the right and to the left. If there is an odd number to the left, mark the one digit. If there is an odd number to the right, add a zero.

2. Estimate the square root of the first number (or first two numbers). Square the number (2) and place it under the 5. Subtract 4 from 5 and bring down the next pair of numbers (95).

3. Multiply the first root by 2 and add a zero (2 × 2 = 4, add a zero = 40). This number is the new divisor.

4. Divide 40 into 195 (195 ÷ 40 = 4). Place 4 as the next digit of the square root. Replace the zero of 40 with 4.

5. Multiply 44 by 4 (4 × 44 = 176) and place the answer under 195. Subtract 176 from 195 (195 − 176 = 19). Bring down the next two digits (80).

6. Multiply 24 by 2 (2 × 24 = 48) and add a zero. Divide 480 into 1980 (1980 ÷ 480 = 4). Place 4 as the next digit of the square root. Replace the zero of 480 with 4. Multiple 484 by 4 (484 × 4 = 1936) and place the answer under 1980.

7. If you want to determine another decimal place in the answer, add two zeros and repeat the procedure.

Appendix B
Critical Values of t (two-tailed test)

df	.05	.01
1	12.706	63.657
2	4.303	9.925
3	3.182	5.841
4	2.776	4.604
5	2.571	4.032
6	2.447	3.707
7	2.365	3.499
8	2.306	3.355
9	2.262	3.250
10	2.228	3.169
11	2.201	3.106
12	2.179	3.055
13	2.160	3.012
14	2.145	2.977
15	2.131	2.947
16	2.120	2.921
17	2.110	2.898
18	2.101	2.878
19	2.093	2.861
20	2.086	2.845
21	2.080	2.831
22	2.074	2.819
23	2.069	2.807
24	2.064	2.797
25	2.060	2.787
26	2.056	2.779
27	2.052	2.771
28	2.048	2.763
29	2.045	2.756
30	2.042	2.750
40	2.021	2.704
60	2.000	2.660
120	1.980	2.617
∞	1.960	2.576

Adapted from Table 12 of E. S. Pearson and H. O. Hartley (Eds.), *Biometrika Tables for Statisticians*, Vol. 1, Cambridge University Press for the Biometrika Trustees, 1966. Used with the permission of the editor of *Biometrika*.

Appendix C
F Distribution

F Distribution

p = .05 values

Degrees of freedom for the numerator, v_1

Degrees of freedom for denominator v_2	1	2	3	4	5	6	7	8	9	10	12	15	20	30	40	60	120	∞
1	161.4	199.5	215.7	224.6	230.2	234.0	236.8	238.9	240.5	241.9	243.9	245.9	248.0	250.1	251.1	252.2	253.3	254.3
2	18.51	19.00	19.16	19.25	19.30	19.33	19.35	19.37	19.38	19.40	19.41	19.43	19.45	19.46	19.47	19.48	19.49	19.50
3	10.13	9.55	9.28	9.12	9.01	8.94	8.89	8.85	8.81	8.79	8.74	8.70	8.66	8.62	8.59	8.57	8.55	8.53
4	7.71	6.94	6.59	6.39	6.26	6.16	6.09	6.04	6.00	5.96	5.91	5.86	5.80	5.75	5.72	5.69	5.66	5.63
5	6.61	5.79	5.41	5.19	5.05	4.95	4.88	4.82	4.77	4.74	4.68	4.62	4.56	4.50	4.46	4.43	4.40	4.36
6	5.99	5.14	4.76	4.53	4.39	4.28	4.21	4.15	4.10	4.06	4.00	3.94	3.87	3.81	3.77	3.74	3.70	3.67
7	5.59	4.74	4.35	4.12	3.97	3.87	3.79	3.73	3.68	3.64	3.57	3.51	3.44	3.38	3.34	3.30	3.27	3.23
8	5.32	4.46	4.07	3.84	3.69	3.58	3.50	3.44	3.39	3.35	3.28	3.22	3.15	3.08	3.04	3.01	2.97	2.93
9	5.12	4.26	3.86	3.63	3.48	3.37	3.29	3.23	3.18	3.14	3.07	3.01	2.94	2.86	2.83	2.79	2.75	2.71
10	4.96	4.10	3.71	3.48	3.33	3.22	3.14	3.07	3.02	2.98	2.91	2.85	2.77	2.70	2.66	2.62	2.58	2.54
11	4.84	3.98	3.59	3.36	3.20	3.09	3.01	2.95	2.90	2.85	2.79	2.72	2.65	2.57	2.53	2.49	2.45	2.40
12	4.75	3.89	3.49	3.26	3.11	3.00	2.91	2.85	2.80	2.75	2.69	2.62	2.54	2.47	2.43	2.38	2.34	2.30
13	4.67	3.81	3.41	3.18	3.03	2.92	2.83	2.77	2.71	2.67	2.60	2.53	2.46	2.38	2.34	2.30	2.25	2.21
14	4.60	3.74	3.34	3.11	2.96	2.85	2.76	2.70	2.65	2.60	2.53	2.46	2.39	2.31	2.27	2.22	2.18	2.13
15	4.54	3.68	3.29	3.06	2.90	2.79	2.71	2.64	2.59	2.54	2.48	2.40	2.33	2.25	2.20	2.16	2.11	2.07
16	4.49	3.63	3.24	3.01	2.85	2.74	2.66	2.59	2.54	2.49	2.42	2.35	2.28	2.19	2.15	2.11	2.06	2.01
17	4.45	3.59	3.20	2.96	2.81	2.70	2.61	2.55	2.49	2.45	2.38	2.31	2.23	2.15	2.10	2.06	2.01	1.96
18	4.41	3.55	3.16	2.93	2.77	2.66	2.58	2.51	2.46	2.41	2.34	2.27	2.19	2.11	2.06	2.02	1.97	1.92
19	4.38	3.52	3.13	2.90	2.74	2.63	2.54	2.48	2.42	2.38	2.31	2.23	2.16	2.07	2.03	1.98	1.93	1.88
20	4.35	3.49	3.10	2.87	2.71	2.60	2.51	2.45	2.39	2.35	2.28	2.20	2.12	2.04	1.99	1.95	1.90	1.84
21	4.32	3.47	3.07	2.84	2.68	2.57	2.49	2.42	2.37	2.32	2.25	2.18	2.10	2.01	1.96	1.92	1.87	1.81
22	4.30	3.44	3.05	2.82	2.66	2.55	2.46	2.40	2.34	2.30	2.23	2.15	2.07	1.98	1.94	1.89	1.84	1.78
23	4.28	3.42	3.03	2.80	2.64	2.53	2.44	2.37	2.32	2.27	2.20	2.13	2.05	1.96	1.91	1.86	1.81	1.76
24	4.26	3.40	3.01	2.78	2.62	2.51	2.42	2.36	2.30	2.25	2.18	2.11	2.03	1.94	1.89	1.84	1.79	1.73
30	4.17	3.32	2.92	2.69	2.53	2.42	2.33	2.27	2.21	2.16	2.09	2.01	1.93	1.84	1.79	1.74	1.68	1.62
40	4.08	3.23	2.84	2.61	2.45	2.34	2.25	2.18	2.12	2.08	2.00	1.92	1.84	1.74	1.69	1.64	1.58	1.51
60	4.00	3.15	2.76	2.53	2.37	2.25	2.17	2.10	2.04	1.99	1.92	1.84	1.75	1.65	1.59	1.53	1.47	1.39
120	3.92	3.07	2.68	2.45	2.29	2.17	2.09	2.02	1.96	1.91	1.83	1.75	1.66	1.55	1.50	1.43	1.35	1.25
∞	3.84	3.00	2.60	2.37	2.21	2.10	2.01	1.94	1.88	1.83	1.75	1.67	1.57	1.46	1.39	1.32	1.22	1.00

Adapted from Table 18 of E. S. Pearson and H. O. Hartley (Eds.), *Biometrika Tables for Statisticians*, Vol. 1, Cambridge University Press for the Biometrika Trustees, 1966. Used with the permission of the editor of *Biometrika*.

Appendix C
F Distribution (continued)

F Distribution

p = .01 values

Degrees of freedom for denominator	Degrees of freedom for the numerator, v_1																	
	1	2	3	4	5	6	7	8	9	10	12	15	20	30	40	60	120	∞
1	4052	4999.5	5403	5625	5764	5859	5928	5981	6022	6056	6106	6157	6209	6261	6287	6313	6339	6366
2	98.50	99.00	99.17	99.25	99.30	99.33	99.36	99.37	99.39	99.40	99.42	99.43	99.45	99.47	99.47	99.48	99.49	99.50
3	34.12	30.82	29.46	28.71	28.24	27.91	27.67	27.49	27.35	27.23	27.05	26.87	26.69	26.50	26.41	26.32	26.22	26.13
4	21.20	18.00	16.69	15.98	15.52	15.21	14.98	14.80	14.66	14.55	14.37	14.20	14.02	13.84	13.75	13.65	13.56	13.46
5	16.26	13.27	12.06	11.39	10.97	10.67	10.46	10.29	10.16	10.05	9.89	9.72	9.55	9.38	9.29	9.20	9.11	9.02
6	13.75	10.92	9.78	9.15	8.75	8.47	8.26	8.10	7.98	7.87	7.72	7.56	7.40	7.23	7.14	7.06	6.97	6.88
7	12.25	9.55	8.45	7.85	7.46	7.19	6.99	6.84	6.72	6.62	6.47	6.31	6.16	5.99	5.91	5.82	5.74	5.65
8	11.26	8.65	7.59	7.01	6.63	6.37	6.18	6.03	5.91	5.81	5.67	5.52	5.36	5.20	5.12	5.03	4.95	4.86
9	10.56	8.02	6.99	6.42	6.06	5.80	5.61	5.47	5.35	5.26	5.11	4.96	4.81	4.65	4.57	4.48	4.40	4.31
10	10.04	7.56	6.55	5.99	5.64	5.39	5.20	5.06	4.94	4.85	4.71	4.56	4.41	4.25	4.17	4.08	4.00	3.91
11	9.65	7.21	6.22	5.67	5.32	5.07	4.89	4.74	4.63	4.54	4.40	4.25	4.10	3.94	3.86	3.78	3.69	3.60
12	9.33	6.93	5.95	5.41	5.06	4.82	4.64	4.50	4.39	4.30	4.16	4.01	3.86	3.70	3.62	3.54	3.45	3.36
13	9.07	6.70	5.74	5.21	4.86	4.62	4.44	4.30	4.19	4.10	3.96	3.82	3.66	3.51	3.43	3.34	3.25	3.17
14	8.86	6.51	5.56	5.04	4.69	4.46	4.28	4.14	4.03	3.94	3.80	3.66	3.51	3.35	3.27	3.18	3.09	3.00
15	8.68	6.36	5.42	4.89	4.56	4.32	4.14	4.00	3.89	3.80	3.67	3.52	3.37	3.21	3.13	3.05	2.96	2.87
16	8.53	6.23	5.29	4.77	4.44	4.20	4.03	3.89	3.78	3.69	3.55	3.41	3.26	3.10	3.02	2.93	2.84	2.75
17	8.40	6.11	5.18	4.67	4.34	4.10	3.93	3.79	3.68	3.59	3.46	3.31	3.16	3.00	2.92	2.83	2.75	2.65
18	8.29	6.01	5.09	4.58	4.25	4.01	3.84	3.71	3.60	3.51	3.37	3.23	3.08	2.92	2.84	2.75	2.66	2.57
19	8.18	5.93	5.01	4.50	4.17	3.94	3.77	3.63	3.52	3.43	3.30	3.15	3.00	2.84	2.76	2.67	2.58	2.49
20	8.10	5.85	4.94	4.43	4.10	3.87	3.70	3.56	3.46	3.37	3.23	3.09	2.94	2.78	2.69	2.61	2.52	2.42
21	8.02	5.78	4.87	4.37	4.04	3.81	3.64	3.51	3.40	3.31	3.17	3.03	2.88	2.72	2.64	2.55	2.46	2.36
22	7.95	5.72	4.82	4.31	3.99	3.76	3.59	3.45	3.35	3.26	3.12	2.98	2.83	2.67	2.58	2.50	2.40	2.31
23	7.88	5.66	4.76	4.26	3.94	3.71	3.54	3.41	3.30	3.21	3.07	2.93	2.78	2.62	2.54	2.45	2.35	2.26
24	7.82	5.61	4.72	4.22	3.90	3.67	3.50	3.36	3.26	3.17	3.03	2.89	2.74	2.58	2.49	2.40	2.31	2.21
30	7.56	5.39	4.51	4.02	3.70	3.47	3.30	3.17	3.07	2.98	2.84	2.70	2.55	2.39	2.30	2.21	2.11	2.01
40	7.31	5.18	4.31	3.83	3.51	3.29	3.12	2.99	2.89	2.80	2.66	2.52	2.37	2.20	2.11	2.02	1.92	1.80
60	7.08	4.98	4.13	3.65	3.34	3.12	2.95	2.82	2.72	2.63	2.50	2.35	2.20	2.03	1.94	1.84	1.73	1.60
120	6.85	4.79	3.95	3.48	3.17	2.96	2.79	2.66	2.56	2.47	2.34	2.19	2.03	1.86	1.76	1.66	1.53	1.38
∞	6.63	4.61	3.78	3.32	3.02	2.80	2.64	2.51	2.41	2.32	2.18	2.04	1.88	1.70	1.59	1.47	1.32	1.00

Adapted from Table 18 of E. S. Pearson and H. O. Hartley (Eds.), Biometrika Tables for Statisticians, Vol. 1, Cambridge University Press for the Biometrika Trustees, 1966. Used with the permission of the editor of Biometrika.

Appendix D
Statistical Software

The packages listed below are examples of microcomputer statistics programs. Other programs may be purchased.

PROGRAM TITLE	PUBLISHER
CISP (IBM PC and compatibles)	Crunch Software Corporation 2547-22nd Avenue San Francisco, CA 94116
PC STATISTICIAN (IBM PC and compatibles)	Human Systems Dynamics 9010 Reseda Boulevard, Suite 222 Northridge, CA 91324
PROSTAT (IBM PC and compatibles)	COMPress P. O. Box 102 Wentworth, NH 03282
SPSS/PC+ (IBM PC and compatibles)	SPSS Inc. 444 N. Michigan Avenue Chicago, IL 60611
STATA (IBM PC and compatibles)	Computing Resource Center 10801 National Boulevard Los Angeles, CA 90064
STATGRAPHICS (IBM PC and compatibles)	STSC, Inc. Software Publishing Group 2115 East Jefferson Street Rockville, MD 20852
STATPAK (IBM PC and compatibles)	Northwest Analytical, Inc. 520 NW Davis Portland, OR 97209
Statpro (IBM PC and compatibles)	Wadsworth Professional Software, Inc. Statler Office Building 20 Park Plaza Boston, MA 02116
STATS PLUS (Apple II, II+, IIe, IIc)	Human Systems Dynamics 9010 Reseda Boulevard, Suite 222 Northridge, CA 91324
Systat (IBM PC and compatibles)	Systat Inc. 2902 Central Street Evanston, IL 60201

Index